Color Atlas of

Clinical Application of Fiberoptic Bronchoscopy

Color Atlas of

Clinical Application of Fiberoptic Bronchoscopy

Mosby
Year Book

St. Louis Baltimore Boston Chicago London Philadelphia Sydney Toronto

Mosby Year Book

Dedicated to Publishing Excellence

Mosby–Year Book, Inc.
11830 Westline Industrial Drive
St. Louis, MO 63146

Published with rights in the USA, Canada and Puerto Rico by Mosby–Year Book, Inc.
A Year Book Medical Publishers imprint of Mosby–Year Book, Inc.

From the Japanese edition of 'Clinical application of fiberoptic bronchoscopy', © 1987, Published by: Nankodo Co. Ltd., Tokyo, Japan. Printed in Japan.

English translation first published by Wolfe Publishing Ltd, 2–16 Torrington Place, London WC1E 7LT, UK.

Library of Congress Cataloging–in–Publication Data

Kitamura, Satoshi, 1939–
Color atlas of fiberoptic bronchoscopy/Satoshi Kitamura.
p. cm.
Includes bibliographies and index.
ISBN 0-8151-5141-1
1. Bronchoscopy—Atlases. I. Title.
[DNLM: 1. Bronchoscopy—methods—atlases. 2. Fiber Optics—atlases. WF 17 K62c]
RC734.B7K57 1990
GIG.2'307545 –dc20
DNLM/DLC
for Library of Congress 89-14827
CIP

Contents

Acknowledgements

With any project there are usually many individuals who contribute to its successful conclusion.

Some have made such important contributions that I take special pleasure in acknowledging my deep indebtedness to them: Yukihiko Sygiyama, MD, Tomoaki Iwanaga, MD, Yasuo Sugama, MD, Jun Kobayashi, MD and Tatsuya Saitoh, MD in my department.

Although publishing is a publisher's duty, this should not be taken for granted and it is with pleasure that I record the patience, meticulous attention to detail and courtesy of the senior staff of Nankodo Co., Mr Hideaki Saito.

1 History of bronchoscopy

Bronchoscopy procedures began about 80 years ago. Professor Gustav Killian[1] was the first to use this technique. However, from 1905, Professor Chevalier Jackson[2] improved on the rigid bronchoscope and established bronchoscopy as a standard diagnostic tool. In Japan Professor Inokichi Kubo of Kyushu University, who studied at Professor Killian's laboratory in 1907, was the first to practise bronchoscopy. Previously bronchoscopy was used mainly for extracting foreign bodies from the trachea or bronchus, and also for extracting small tumours.

In spite of many improvements, the rigid bronchoscope, the early Jackson type, had a low level of illumination and a limited visual field. However, with the progress of thoracic surgery, the need for bronchoscopy increased. This led to an improved bronchoscope and the development of new fields of diagnosis. Professor Yuzuru Ono, of Keio University, who studied under Professor Jackson, established the Japanese Bronchoesophagology Society; as a result tracheo-oesophagology made rapid progress in Japan. The widespread use of the improved Jackson-type bronchoscope furthered the development of thoracic surgery in Japan and also accelerated the improvement of the bronchoscope. Kozuki and Horie[3] developed and improved the high-powered illumination system using a xenon discharge as a source of light. They also developed the rigid bronchoscope using glass fibres as a light guide. As a result of these improvements, which significantly increased the visual field, the operators could get more precise results.

In 1966, Ikeda developed the first flexible fibreoptic bronchoscope. This new instrument made it possible to see easily the upper segmental bronchi of the left upper lobe and the subsegmental bronchi of B^6; these bronchi were not clearly viewed with the old type of bronchoscope. According to users of this new fibreoptic bronchoscope, the value and usefulness of this instrument as a diagnostic tool increased markedly. With the technical progress of producing glass fibre, the flexible fibreoptic bronchoscope, which has a diameter ranging from 2.4 mm to 3.2 mm, was developed and used widely. It is 15 years since the bronchofibrescope was first developed, and it has been greatly improved during the intervening period.

Currently four Japanese companies and one American company have produced bronchoscopes; over 95 per cent of these are made in Japan.

The flexible fibreoptic bronchoscope, which has an outer diameter of 4–6 mm, is soft; its tip can be widely moved through an angle of 150–180°. This fibrescope is capable of an angle of viewing ranging from 55–120° at the tip; in addition, its visual image is strikingly clear in spite of using glass fibres. Therefore the old bronchoscope, which showed the proximal bronchus only, has been largely superseded; the new instrument alters the conception of bronchoscopy itself. It shows the area from the lobar bronchus to the fourth order subsegmental bronchi; it also helps the collection of specimens by using biopsy forceps or brushes and these specimens can be examined in a variety of ways.

Now the rigid bronchoscope, which normally needs general anaesthesia, and the flexible fibreoptic bronchoscope are widely used for investigating various pulmonary diseases. The use of the flexible fibreoptic bronchoscope has spread widely and the procedure using this instrument is now becoming routine for the physician, surgeon and radiologist.

References

[1] Killian, G., Direct endoscopy of the upper air-passages and esophagus: Its diagnostic and therapeutic value in the search for and removal of foreign bodies. *J. Laryng.* **18:** 461, 1902.

[2] Jackson, C., Foreign bodies in the trachea, bronchi and esophagus. *Laryngoscope,* **15:** 527, 1905.

[3] Kozuki, H., *et al.,* Analysis of transbronchial examinations in the diagnosis of lung cancer. *Thoracic Disease,* **5:** 436, 1961.

[4] Ikeda, M., Flexible fibreoptic bronchoscope. *J. Jpn. Bronchoesophagol. Soc.,* **19:** 54, 1968.

2 Usefulness of flexible fibreoptic bronchoscopy

Since the mid-seventies we have performed brush cytology of the bronchus, using fluoroscopic television as a diagnostic tool for lung cancer. We used lignocaine as a local anaesthetic on the pharynx and a rubber cannula with a characteristic curve for each bronchus. Through the cannula, we inserted sharp forceps (Tsuboi type) into the affected bronchus and obtained tissue specimens or cells for pathological examination. This method was very useful. However, we could not see directly into the orifices of each bronchus, especially the orifices of the subsegmental bronchi, and sometimes we could not reach peripheral coin lesions. In some instances where squamous cell carcinoma or bronchial adenoma is present, such abnormalities may not show up on radiography at all; it is extremely difficult to diagnose such abnormalities by this method. In addition, the blind operation of a cannula and forceps under TV fluoroscopy prolonged the period of examination and caused considerable pain to the patients.

Our department introduced the flexible fibreoptic bronchoscope in 1975 and we have used it since for various examinations. Up to 1979, patients had a vinyl tracheal tube inserted. This tube had been previously curved into a suitable shape and was attached to the patient's face with adhesive tape; the examiner then inserted the bronchoscope through this tube (**2.1**). As a result we needed more time for preparation and therefore could not perform as many examinations as we would have liked.

Since 1979 we have tried to insert the fibreoptic bronchoscope directly without such a tube; this has helped to shorten examination time significantly. At first, an assistant would pull out the patient's tongue with gauze, while the examiner inserted the fibreoptic bronchoscope. In later procedures the examiner inserted the bronchoscope through a mouthpiece. This is our standard technique. In the USA the bronchoscope was mainly introduced through a nostril. This method is also used by us where nervous patients are involved and for those who have a prominent pharyngeal reflex or difficulty of insertion per os. This is a good method because it causes less pharyngeal reflex and no problems at transbronchial lung biopsy. The disadvantage is that insertion is very difficult in patients who suffer from hypertrophic rhinitis or a nasal polyp.

We carry out between 10 and 20 cases of bronchoscopy every week, approximately 800–900 per annum. The time taken for these examinations has shortened significantly. For example, if we need to get information about the larger bronchi using the fibreoptic bronchoscope in patients who are complaining of a haemoptysis or cough, we need 5 minutes for local anaesthesia with the Jackson-type spray, and 3 minutes for inserting the bronchoscope and taking 28 photographs of the vocal cords, trachea, carina, and the orifices of the segmental bronchi in both lungs. All procedures take about 8 minutes. If we carry out bronchography on one side, we only need

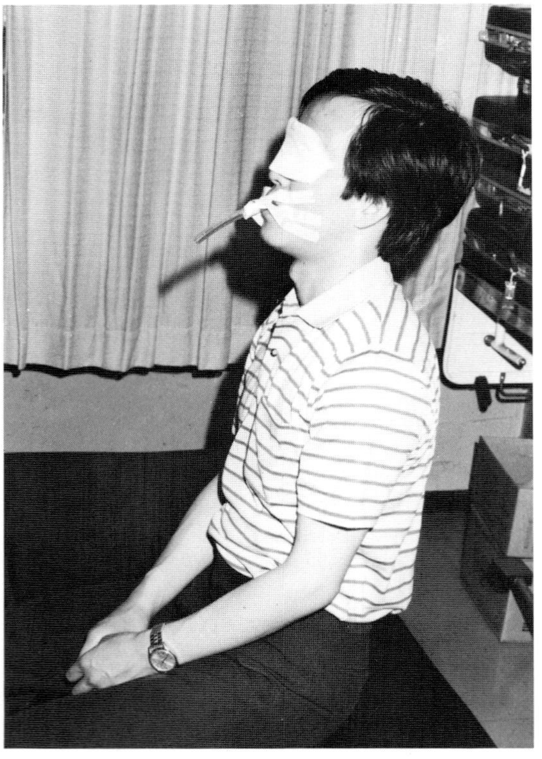

2.1 Tracheal tube inserted and attached to patient's face with adhesive tape.

7–8 minutes more for taking about 8 radiographs; during the observation period with the aid of fluoroscopy, the contrast medium is sucked out. The significantly shorter time taken for these procedures made things easier for the patients. These procedures, including transbronchial lung biopsy, have become routine examinations at the outpatients' clinic.

In the area of otorhinolaryngology, many doctors prefer to use the rigid bronchoscope for removing a foreign body from the bronchus[1]. Fibreoptic bronchoscopy is useful in almost all cases where a foreign body has lodged in the bronchus.

Many doctors say that the use of a rigid bronchoscope is indicated where massive haemoptysis or profuse bleeding occurs during examination[2]. In the past we experienced massive haemoptysis because of the presence of bronchiectasis or lung cancer, and profuse bleeding as a result of biopsy of bronchial tumours. In each case we succeeded in controlling the haemorrhage by using the fibreoptic bronchoscope, which was inserted per os directly without a tracheal tube.

In case of massive haemorrhage, if enough information is available about the haemorrhagic site, the most important step is to make the patient lie on the affected side. To prevent blood entering the healthy lung, the examiner inserts the tip of the bronchoscope (BF-1 T10 with a big hole for suction is suitable) into the orifice of the main bronchus of the bleeding side and extracts the blood continuously. When the bleeding ceases, the tip is slowly advanced, extracting coagula from the bleeding site as one proceeds, searching for the exact place or bronchus that is bleeding. Then epinephrine (Bosmin), diluted 10-20 times, is infused through the bronchoscope. The local injection method of thrombin, our new device, is more effective. This method is that 5–10 ml (1000 u/ml) of thrombin solution is injected directly to the bleeding site or bronchus. When the tip of the bronchoscope is covered with coagula, the instrument is pulled out, the coagula removed and the scope re-inserted. Usually re-insertion takes only a few seconds in the hands of an expert and should cause no problems.

The rigid bronchoscope may be thought to be useful in the case of resection of bronchial tumours or granulomatous tissues. However, in routine work doctors may feel that fibreoptic bronchoscopy is enough as both diagnostic and therapeutic tools. The flexible bronchoscope has various clinical uses. We feel that the advantages and the superiority of the flexible bronchoscope over the rigid one are clear and definitive.

References

[1] Holinger, P.H., Holinger, L.D., Use of open tube bronchoscope in the extraction of foreign bodies. *Chest,* **73:** 721, 1978.

[2] Landa, J.F., Indication of bronchoscopy. *Chest,* **73:** 686, 1978.

[3] Kinoshita, M., Shiraki, R., Wagai, F., Watanabe, H., Kitamura, S., Thrombin instillation therapy through the fibreoptic bronchoscope in cases of haemoptysis. *Jpn. J. Thorac. Dis.,* **20:** 251, 1982.

3 Machine and instrumentation

1 Flexible fibreoptic bronchoscopes

Four Japanese companies, Olympus, Machida, Asahi Kogaku, and Fuji Shashin produce flexible fibreoptic bronchoscopes. Fifteen types of flexible fibreoptic bronchoscope are now available. Each type has its advantages and disadvantages. One has to make a selection according to its purpose.

a) Scopes made by the Olympus Company

Seven types are now available. Figure **3.1** shows the standard and widely applicable type, BF-10, with the biopsy forceps (BF-19C). This is the improved type of BF-B3R previously distributed. The inner diameter of the channel for biopsy is 2 mm and many commercially available accessories like a biopsy forceps, brushes and injection needles can be used. It has a viewing angle of 100 degrees and has an abundant number of fibres which provide an excellent image. It can be used for procedures such as observation of bronchi, bronchography, transbronchial lung biopsy, bronchial tumour biopsy, transbronchial brushing, bronchoalveolar lavage, bronchial toilet and intra-tumour injection of various drugs. This 'scope's tip bends 160 degrees upwards and 130 degrees downwards, so that we can easily observe the left apical and posterior and right apical upper lobe bronchi and both apical lower bronchi. Every year the fibreoptic bronchoscope is improved by manufacturers, paying special attention to the bending angle of tips, the visual angle and the material of optic fibres. Recent developments have made it possible to obtain clear photographs from flexible bronchoscopes which match those taken by rigid bronchoscopes.

Figure **3.2** shows the tips of various bronchoscopes. The right column shows the scheme of shapes of tips and the left column gives the maximum bending angles. The bending angles for BF-10(**A**) are 160 degrees upwards and 130 degrees downwards with a channel (2 mm) for forceps. In addition, because its objective lens is located between the light guides of both sides, lighting of BF-10 is uniform. A BF-10 can take a good photograph because of the high quality of the fibres used. BF-6C10(**F**) has a big objective lens and a wide visual angle, so that we can get a wide-angled photograph. We can also get brushing cytology specimens by using the special cytology brush. But the small diameter (1.5 mm) of its channel hinders suction and yields unclear photographs. Sometimes its one-sided light guide cause darkness of the visual field on the opposite side.

BF-P10(**B**) has a small outer diameter (4.8 mm) and a wide channel diameter (2 mm). Its tip can be turned 180 degrees upwards. It is the most useful 'scope for biopsy of the right apical or left apicoposterior bronchi. BF-3C10(**E**) is easy to insert and is very useful for the observation of narrowed or deep sites because of its small outer diameter (3.6 mm) of insertion area; it is also useful for removal of foreign bodies in infants. Using a cytology brush, we can perform brushing cytology with this scope. BF-1T10 (**C**) has the biggest diameter of the channel (2.6 mm) and various accessories; biopsy forceps with big cups can be used with this 'scope. Therefore, the quantity of tissue

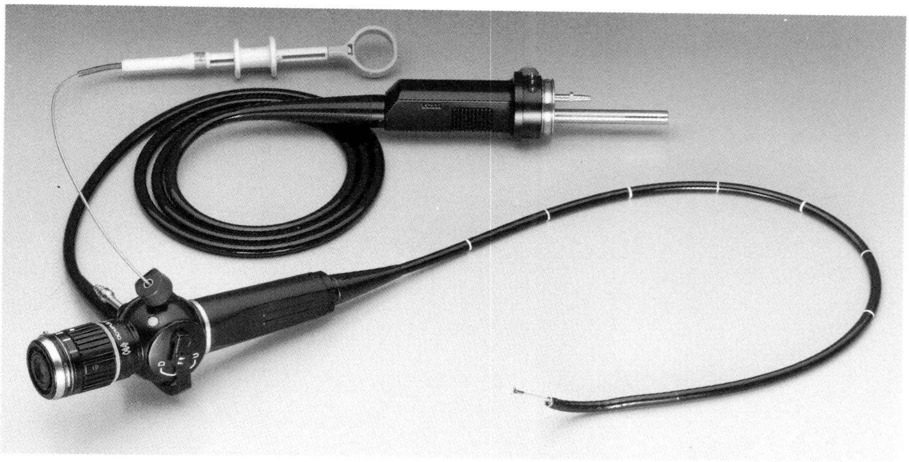

3.1 The biopsy forceps (BF-19C) inserted into an Olympus BF-10.

Table 3.1 Comparison with methods and abilities of Olympus fibreoptic bronchoscopes

	BF type B10	BF type 6C10	BF type P10	BF type 3C10	BF type 1T10	BF type 2T10
Angle of visual fields	100°	120°	90°	75°	90°	90°
Direct vision	3~50 mm	4~50 mm	3~50 mm	3~50 mm	3~50 mm	3~50 mm
Depth of observation	5.3 mm∅	6.0 mm∅	4.8 mm∅	3.5 mm∅	5.9 mm∅	5.9 mm∅
(Fixed focus)	up 160° down 130°	up 160° down 100°	up 180° down 100°	up 160° down 100°	up 160° down 100°	up 160° down 100°
Bending angle	6.0 mm∅	6.0 mm∅	5.0 mm∅	3.6 mm∅	6.0 mm∅	6.0 mm∅
Diameter of the soft part	2.0 mm∅	1.5 mm∅	2.0 mm∅	1.2 mm∅	2.6 mm∅	Diameter of the L-channel 2.0 mm∅
Diameter of the channel						Diameter of the S-channel 1.5 mm∅
Length of the effective portion	550 mm	550 mm	550 mm	550 mm	550 mm	550 mm
Total length	760 mm	760 mm	760 mm	760 mm	760 mm	760 mm

Photograph taking system MODEL SC16-10 and others

specimens is increased. Good aspiration capacity makes it useful in cases of bronchial toilet and for dealing with massive haemorrhage. Two light guides, one on each side of the objective lens, which is similar to BF-10, provide even illumination and relatively good photographs. BF-2T10(**D**) has two channels and has the capacity for carrying out various types of treatment, biopsy and suction.

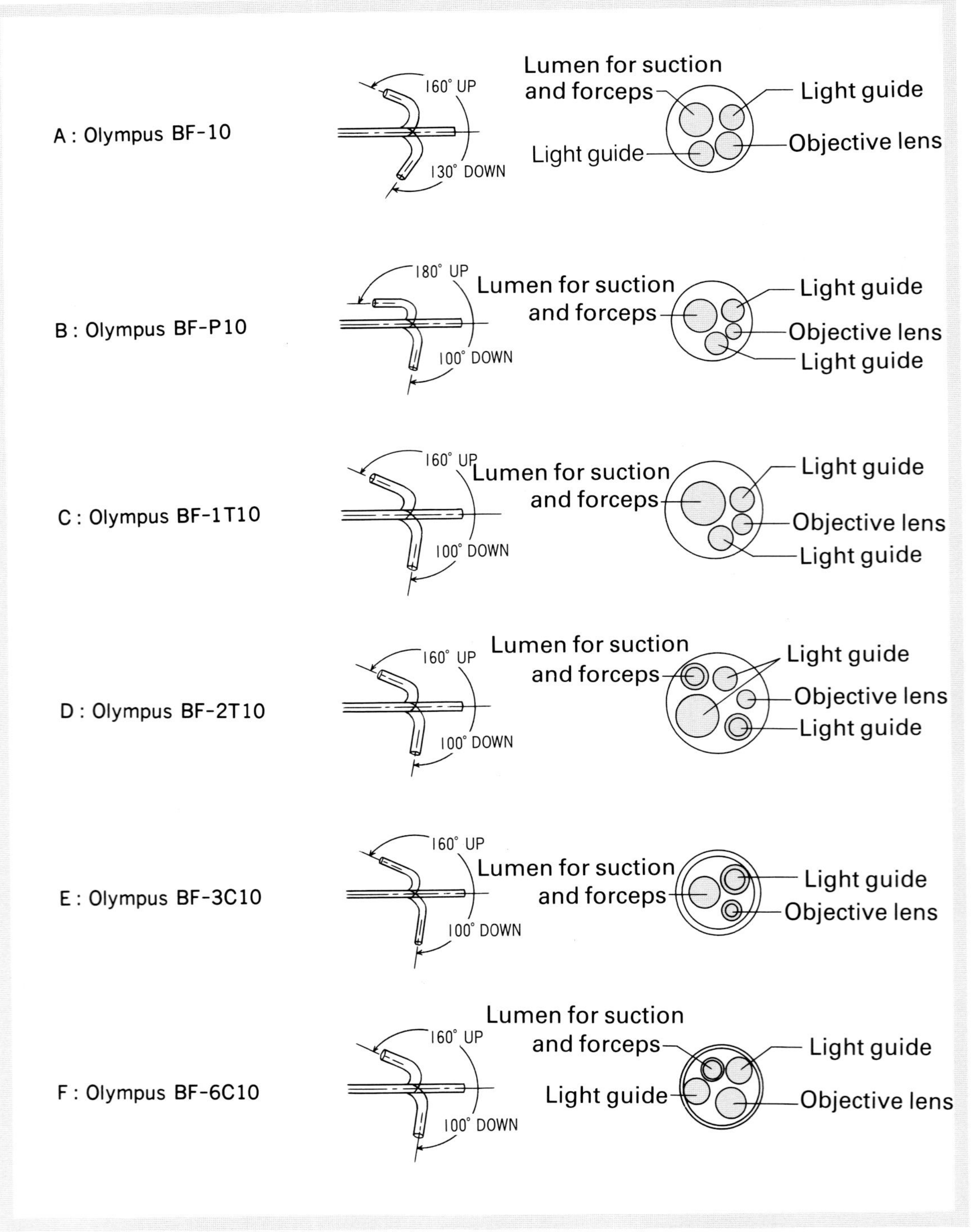

3.2 Tips of various fibreoptic bronchoscopes (Olympus): light guide, objective lens, hole for suction and forceps.

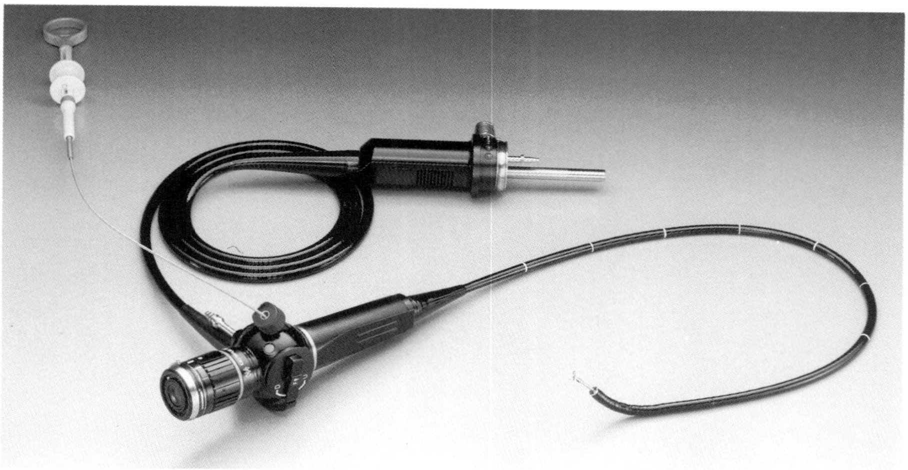

A : BF-1T10

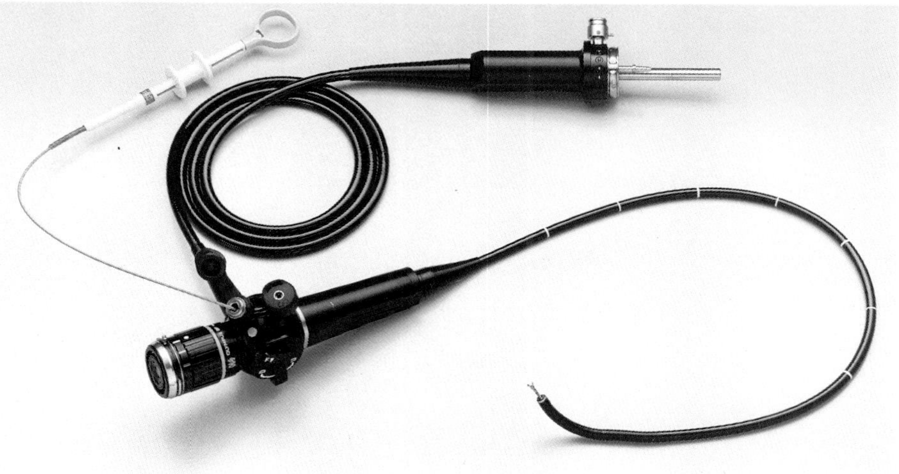

B : BF-2T10

3.3 Fibreoptic bronchoscopes made by Olympus.

Figure **3.3** shows BF-1T10 and BF-2T10: BF-2T10 has two channels—one is large and the other is small. This increases the capacity of suction in case one has to use various accessories such as forceps or inject drugs. The introduction of the automatic suction adapter makes it possible to suck sputum easily. While using the accessory through the big channel, we can suck through the small channel. Therefore, it is very easy to remove opacities from the visual field. When the injection and ventilation holes of the small channel are closed at the same time and the big channel is capped, suction through both channels simultaneously is possible and the suction capacity is markedly increased. Figure **3.4** shows the biopsy procedure using the old type BF-2TR. In this type, there is only one light guide, which is is located to one side, which provides uneven illumination and as a result bad photographs. Table 3.1 compares the various instruments and their capacities.

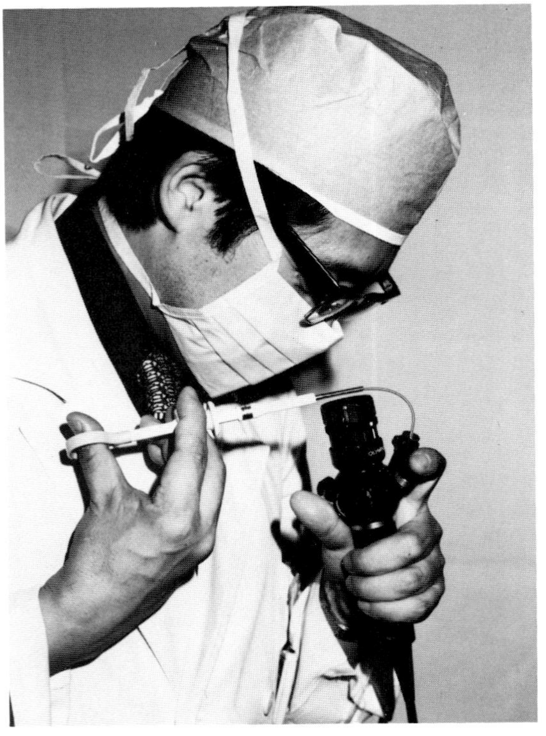

3.4 Performing transbronchial biopsy using a fibreoptic bronchoscope (BF-2TR) and the biopsy forceps.

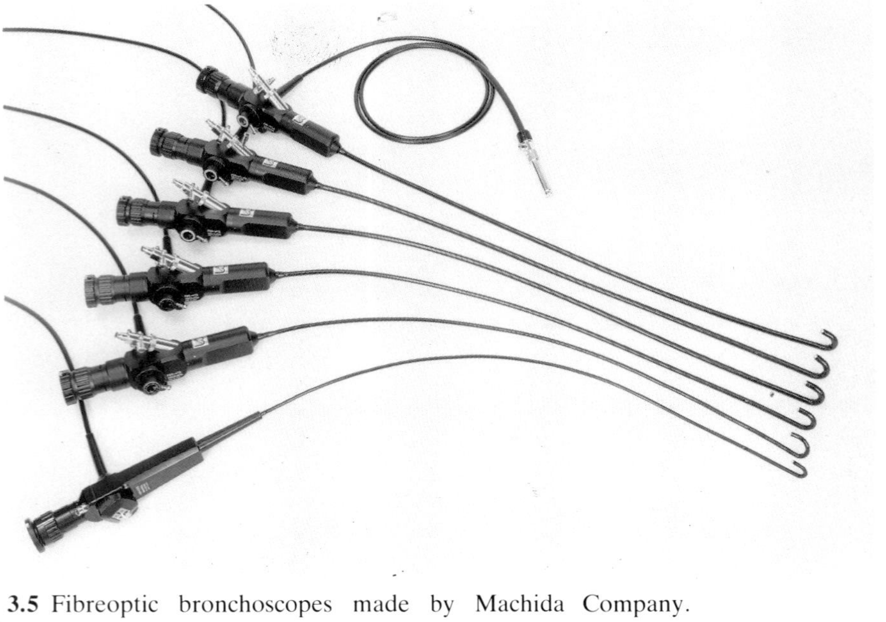

3.5 Fibreoptic bronchoscopes made by Machida Company.

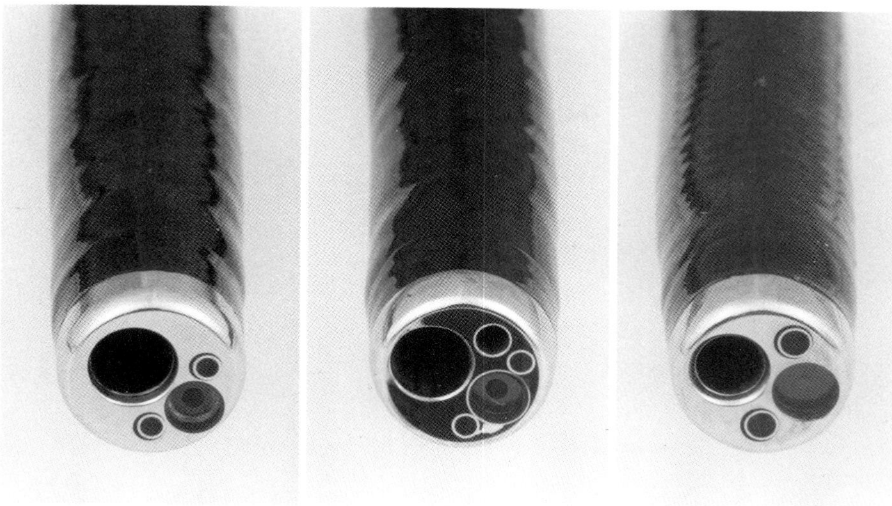

3.6 The tips of bronchoscopes made by Machida Company.

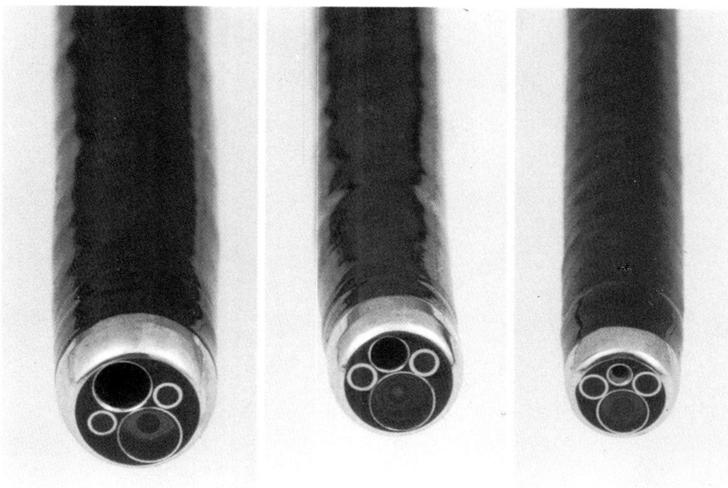

3.7 The tips of bronchoscopes made by Machida Company.

b) Scopes made by the Machida Company

Six types of 'scope are available. Figure **3.5** shows the 'scopes — FBS-6TLII, FBS-6TLWII, FBS-6TII, FBS-5TII, FBS-4TII, and FBS-3.5TII. These 'scopes have the panning system, which means the tips can be moved to both right and left. This system makes selective insertion into a particular bronchus very easy. However, this system weakens the bending portion of tips; many problems have arisen, especially in the USA, when using these 'scopes. Therefore, FBS-T types (FBS-6TII, FBS-5TII) which do not have this rotation system are mainly produced. Figures **3.6** and **3.7** show the tips of these 'scopes. The body of the FBS-T type is soft and the movement of tips can easily follow that of control units. Currently, the FBS-6TII and FBS-6TLII are available. The channels for forceps in these 'scopes differ in diameter. The internal diameter of the latter is large (2.5 mm) and this type is similar to the Olympus BF-1T10.

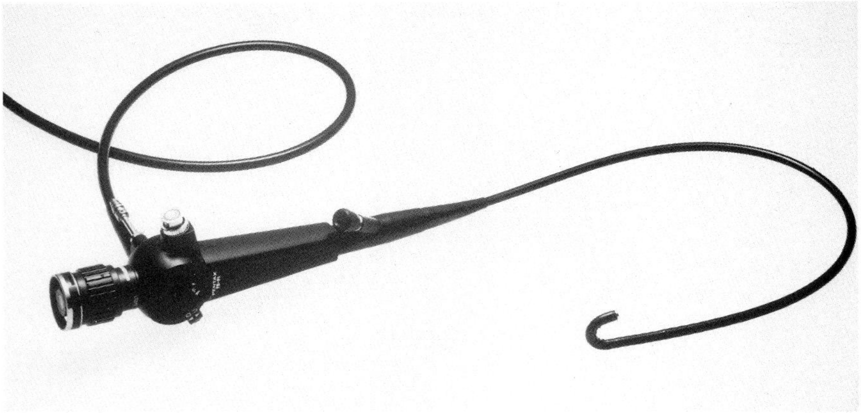

3.8 A fibreoptic bronchoscope made by Asahi Kogaku Company.

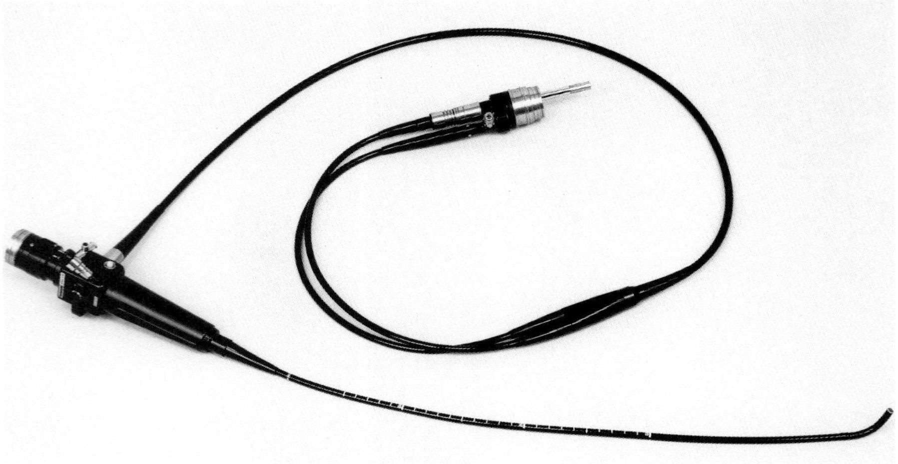

3.9 Fibreoptic bronchoscope made by Fuji Shashin Company.

c) Scopes made by the Asahi Kogaku Company

Bronchoscopes were developed by this company in 1977; currently the FB-19H and FB-15H are available. Figure **3.8** shows the fibreoptic bronchoscope made by Asahi Kogaku (FB-19H). The quality of optic fibres is good and the resolution of the image is excellent.

d) Scopes made by the Fuji Shashin Company

This company's 'scopes were developed in 1978 and three types are available. The wide visual angle (105 degrees) is characteristic. Figure **3.9** shows the fibreoptic bronchoscope made by Fuji Shashin (BRO-Y3S). In addition, BRO-YP2 has a small diameter and BRO-YL2 is the 'scope used for treatment. Figure **3.10** shows the control unit of GRO-YP2.

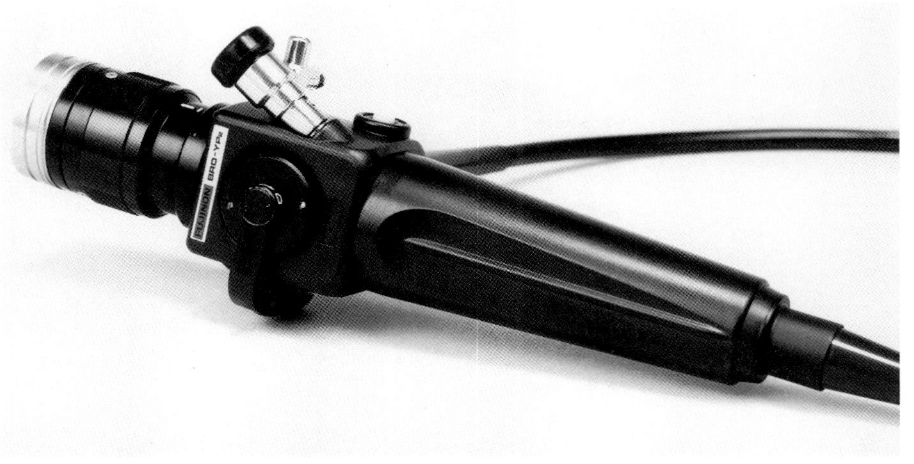

3.10 Control unit of a GRO-YP2.

2 Fibreoptic bronchoscope accessories

Where fibreoptic bronchoscopes are used for examination and treatment, it is desirable to use the most suitable accessories. Figure **3.11** shows tips of various forceps of the fibreoptic bronchoscope. They are roughly divided into biopsy forceps, cytology brushes, grasping forceps, curettes, surgical scissors, washing tubes and injection needles. Among biopsy forceps, the fenestrated alligator jaws (FB-15C(5)) was designed by the author and it makes it possible to obtain a large sample with relatively less tissue crushing.

Figure **3.12** shows the handles of various instruments. For daily clinical use we tend to rely mainly on the fenestrated biopsy forceps (FB-19), oblong biopsy forceps (FB-14C) and biopsy forceps with a needle (FB-18C) for intrabronchial tumour biopsy, and on the fenestrated biopsy forceps (FB-19C) and the fenestrated alligator jaws (FB-15C) for transbronchial lung biopsy. For brush cytology of peripheral foci, the cytology brush (BC-10C), the cytology brush with cover (BC-5C), the double-jointed cytology brush (BC-8C), and the double-jointed curette (CC-3C) are used. In cases of tumour biopsy and lung biopsy, it is better to use the fenestrated biopsy forceps, because the tissue specimens are less likely to be crushed. For a biopsy of a tumour protruding into the bronchial lumen and having a solid and slippery surface, the biopsy forceps with a needle at the joint is very useful. Forceps are seldom used to extricate foreign bodies, but the magnetic extractor (IE-2P) for clips, the grasping forceps with a big mouth (FG-12L) and the W-shaped grasping forceps (FG-4L) may be useful for this purpose. To inject anticancer drugs, the injection catheter is used.

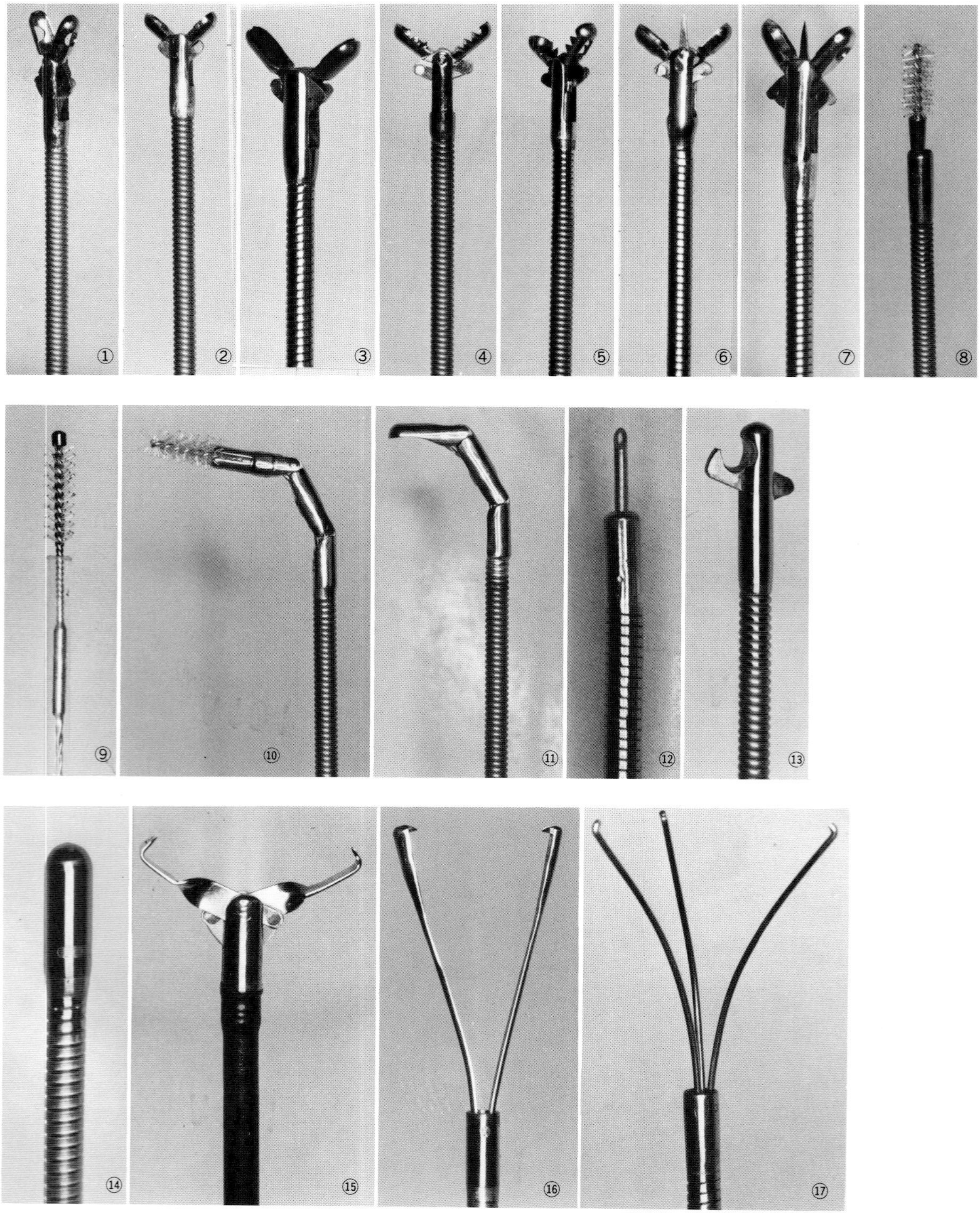

3.11 The various tips and accessories of a fibreoptic bronchoscope:
1 Fenestrated biopsy forceps (standard channel size)
2 Oblong biopsy forceps
3 Biopsy forceps (wide channel size; 2.6 mm)
4 Biopsy forceps with alligator jaws (standard channel size)
5 Fenestrated biopsy forceps with alligator jaws
6 Biopsy forceps with a needle at the joint (wide channel size)
7 Fenestrated biopsy forceps with a needle
8 Cytology brush (standard channel size)
9 Cytology brush with sheath (standard channel size)

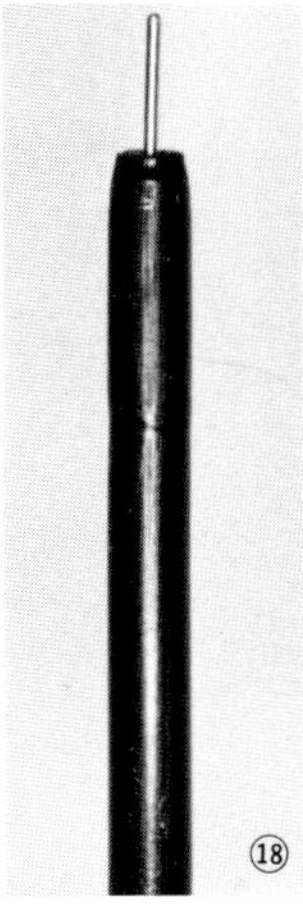

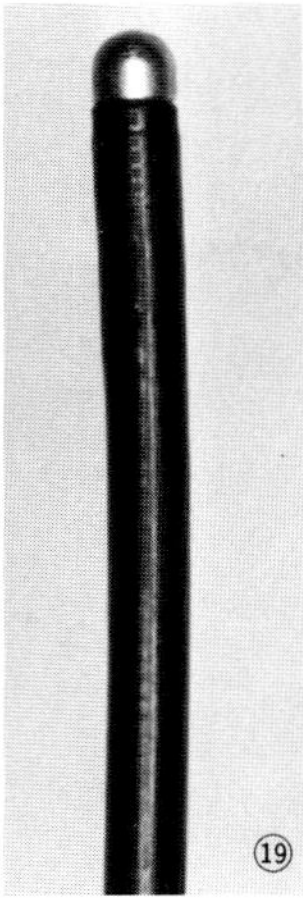

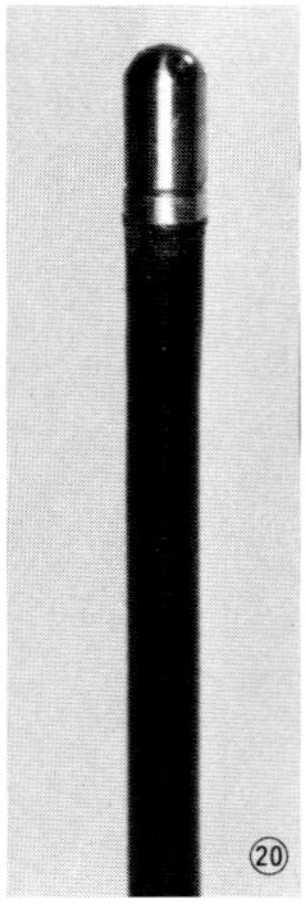

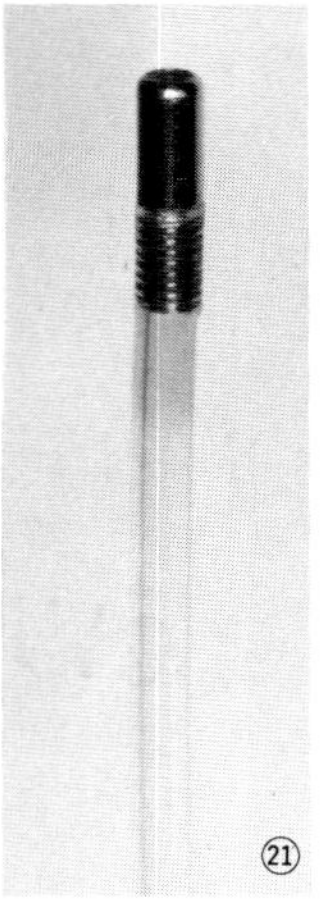

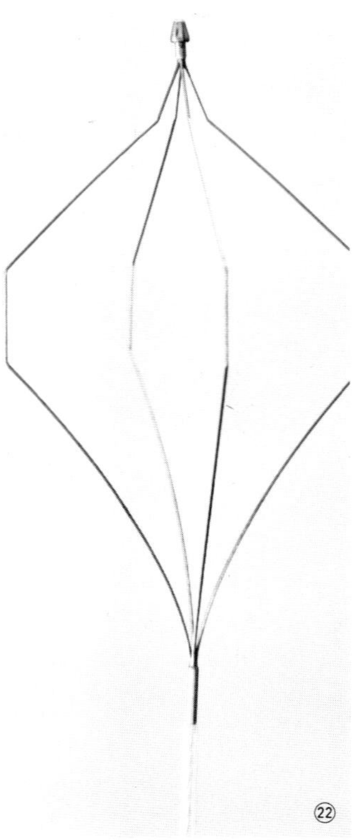

10 Double-jointed cytology brush (standard channel size)
11 Double-jointed curette (standard channel size)
12 Injection catheter (standard channel size)
13 Surgical scissors forceps
14 Magnetic extractor (standard channel size)
15 Grasping forceps with a wide mouth (wide channel size)
16 W-shaped grasping forceps (standard channel size)
17 Grasping forceps, trident type (wide channel size)
18 Diathermic cutter (wide channel size)
19 Diathermic coagulation tip — round type (wide channel size)
20 Diathermic coagulation tip — absorption type (wide channel type)
21 Scattering and washing catheter (wide channel size)
22 Grasping forceps, basket type (wide channel size)

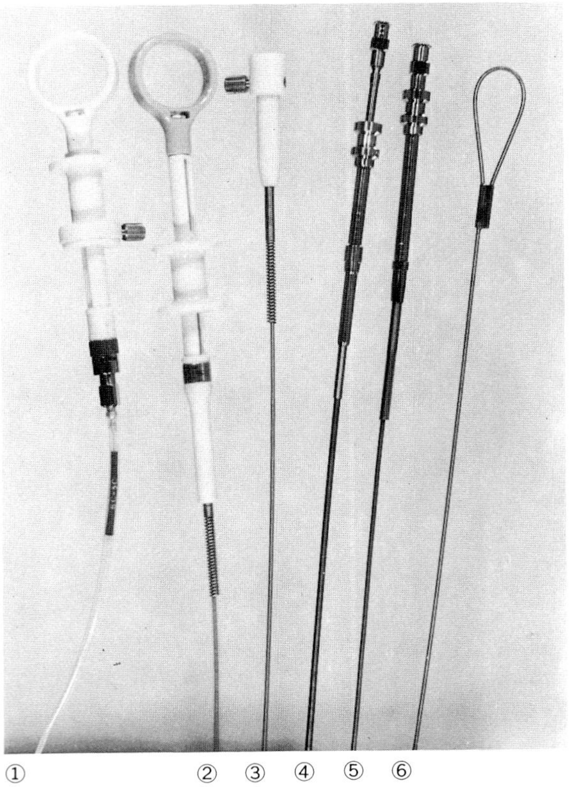

3.12 Control units of a bronchoscope's accessories:
1 Cytology brush with sheath
2 Fenestrated biopsy forceps
3 Cytology brush
4 and 5 Biopsy needles
6 Cleaning brush for biopsy channel

3 Light sources

Several light sources are available from some companies. To obtain good photographs one needs a flash system and use of a high shutter speed (1/150–1/500). Many machines use a xenon lamp and some of them can be used for another company's bronchoscope with a supplementary socket. CLE-F10, CLE-10, FIL-FS, LX-500A and RH-150TL are relatively light and are ideal for bedside or mass survey use. The CLV-F10 and RS-500 are suitable for use in a fixed position. Figures **3.13** and **3.14** show various light sources.

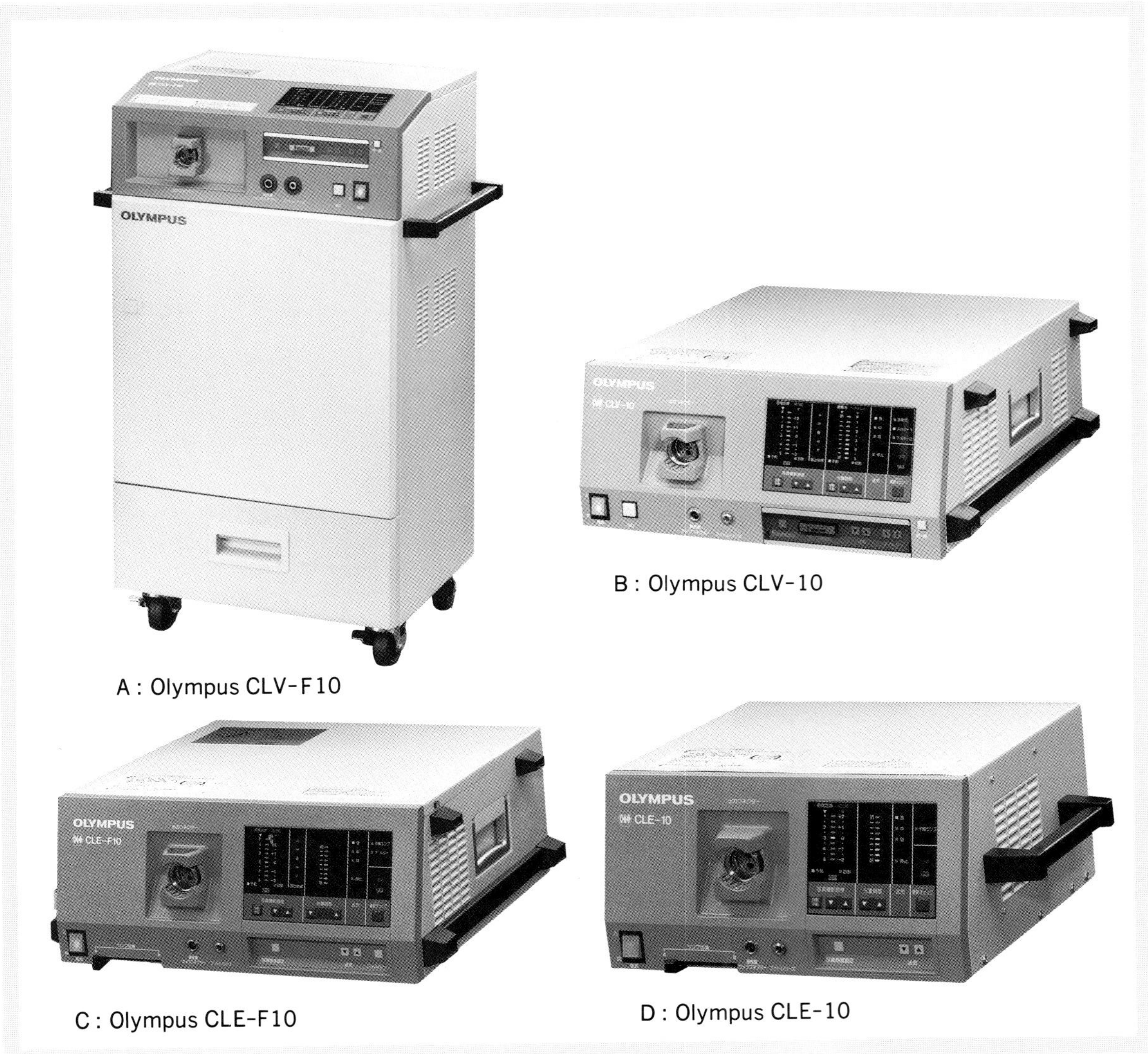

A : Olympus CLV-F10

B : Olympus CLV-10

C : Olympus CLE-F10

D : Olympus CLE-10

3.13 Different light sources

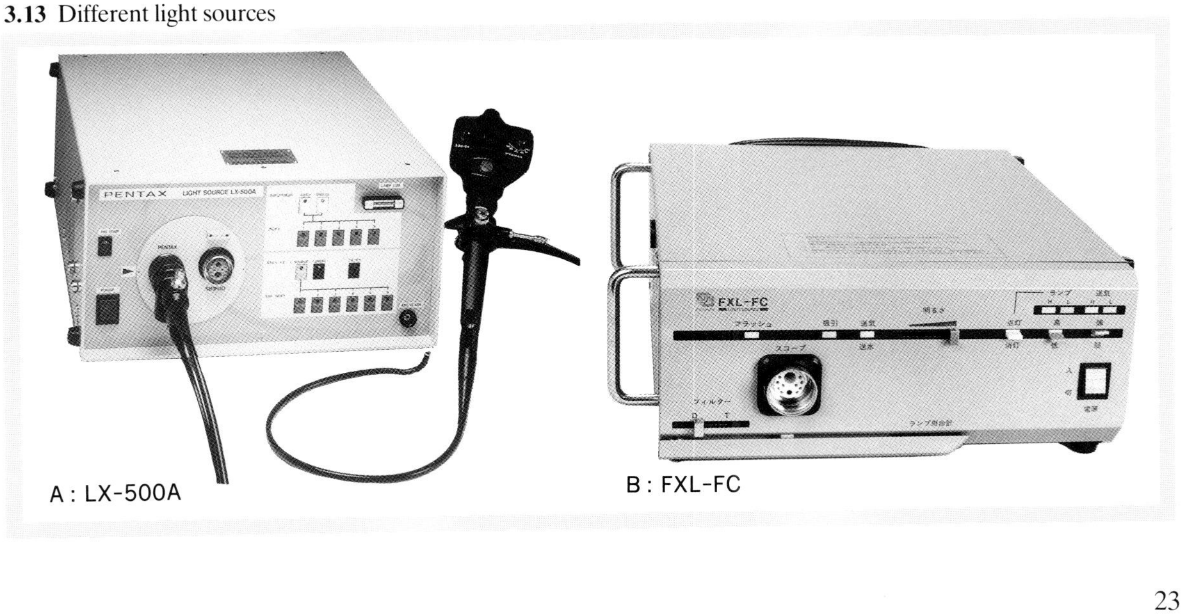

A : LX-500A

B : FXL-FC

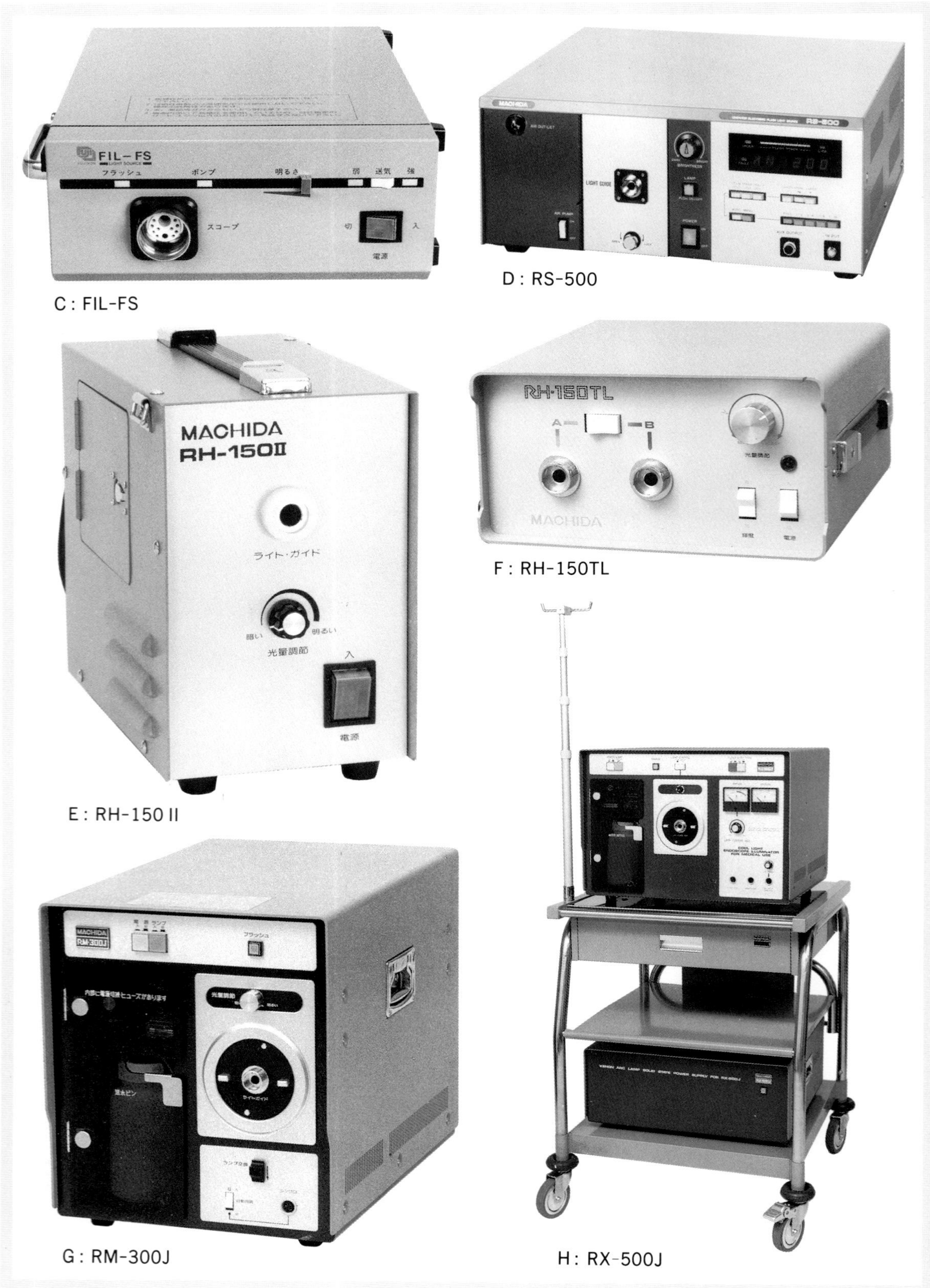

C: FIL-FS

D: RS-500

E: RH-150 II

F: RH-150TL

G: RM-300J

H: RX-500J

3.14 Six different light sources

A: LX-500A
B: FXL-FC } previous page

E: RH-150 11 with a data inprinting system
F: For Machida use, RH-150TL with the adapter

4 Photographing instruments — cameras and adapters

Bronchoscopic findings are routinely sketched on the special recording files. It is very important to record the findings precisely and objectively. For educational purposes, 16 mm cine and videotapes are used frequently. For daily clinical use, where a detailed record of findings of the bronchial mucosa and a tumour protruding in the bronchial lumen is required, the still photograph is the best.

Figure **3.15** shows various cameras which are currently available. **A** is the 35 mm camera, Olympus OM-1N with the enlargement adapter (A10-E). B is a Polaroid camera. This is a useful implement because it has the advantage of providing an instant colour photograph of the findings. However, its images are not so sharp. **C** is the special Olympus camera used for bronchoscopy. This camera is small, light and easy to set up and operate. It has the precise EE system and the automatic system for rolling up the film. Olympus special film (20 frames), 16 mm cassette is used. **D** is a special 35 mm camera (FG110-H2) made by Fuji Shashin Company and it uses a cartridge system. **E** is made by Fuji and this can input data (see below). **F** made by Fuji can be used with a 'scope of the Machida Company using a special adapter. **G** is a 35 mm camera made by Asahi Kogaku Company. **H** (PS-PEII) which is made by Asahi operates on the cartridge system and automatically winds up film and selects exposure time. Figure **3.16** shows an Olympus BF-6C10 being used with SC16-10. It is small, light and easy to handle.

Magnification of findings depends on the type of camera and 'scope used. Magnification can be changed by using adapters. Figures **3.17** and **3.18** show various Olympus adapters. In the middle line of the figure, A10-M1 (0.8x), A10-M2 (1.0x), A10-M3 (1.4x) and A10-M4 (2.0x) are shown; this order shows the progression of enlargement. The author normally uses M4 (2.0x). Figure **3.19** shows the data inprinting system made by Olympus Company. If the patient's name, age, sex or Karte number is registered via the keyboard beforehand, it is recorded on the film. The data of 30 patients can be recorded at the same time.

Figure **3.20** shows the Olympus medical TV system. This system can be used for immediate recording, displaying, transforming and observing by several individuals.

Figure **3.21** shows an Olympus BF-6C10, a 35 mm single lens reflex camera, attached to an OM-1N.

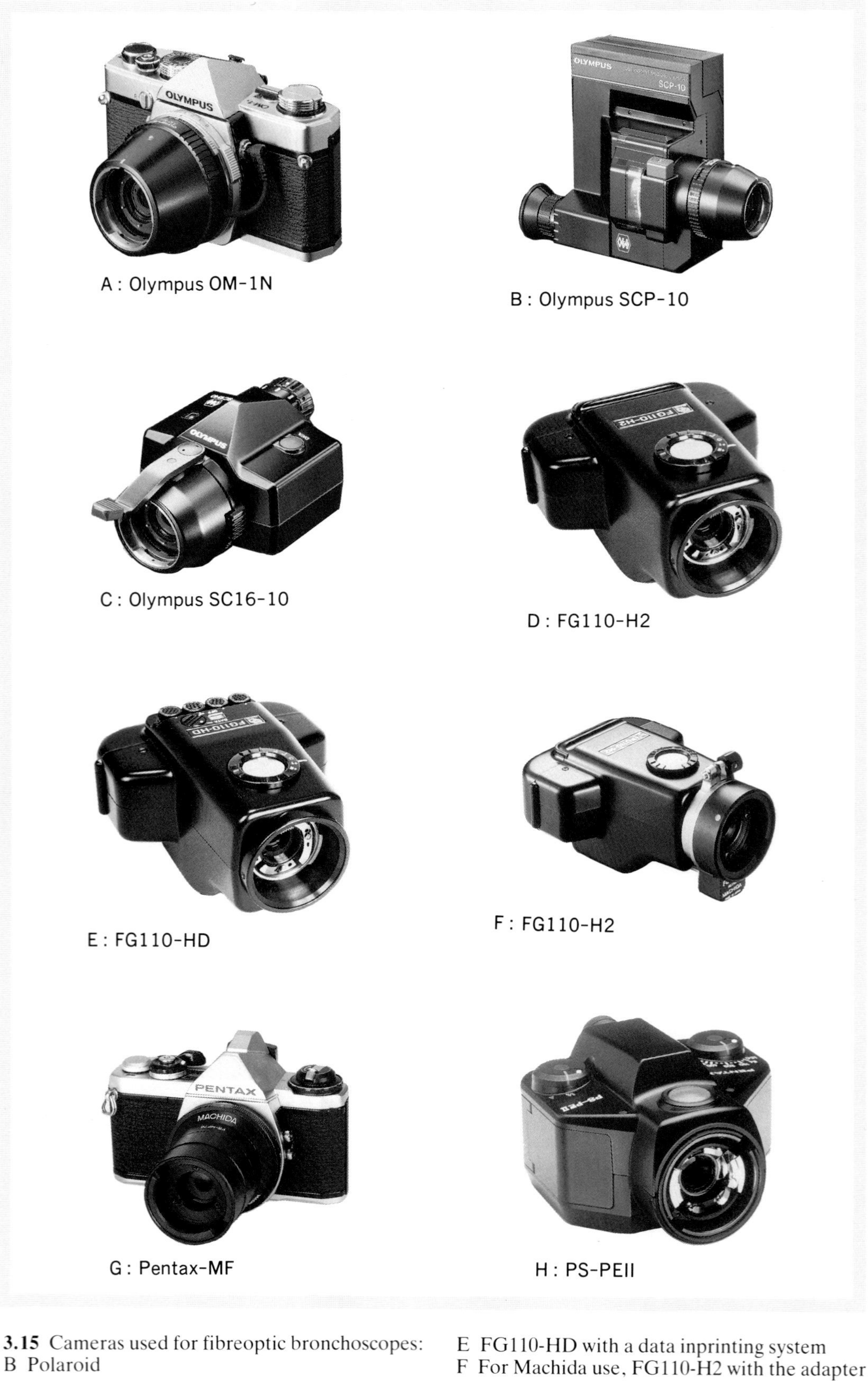
A : Olympus OM-1N
B : Olympus SCP-10
C : Olympus SC16-10
D : FG110-H2
E : FG110-HD
F : FG110-H2
G : Pentax-MF
H : PS-PEII

3.15 Cameras used for fibreoptic bronchoscopes:
B Polaroid
E FG110-HD with a data inprinting system
F For Machida use, FG110-H2 with the adapter

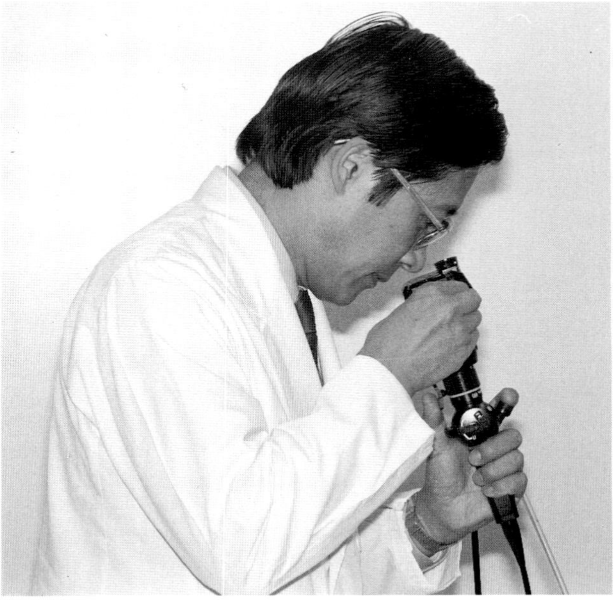

3.16 Taking photographs using the fibreoptic bronchoscope (Olympus BF-6C10) with the camera for endoscopy (SC16-10).

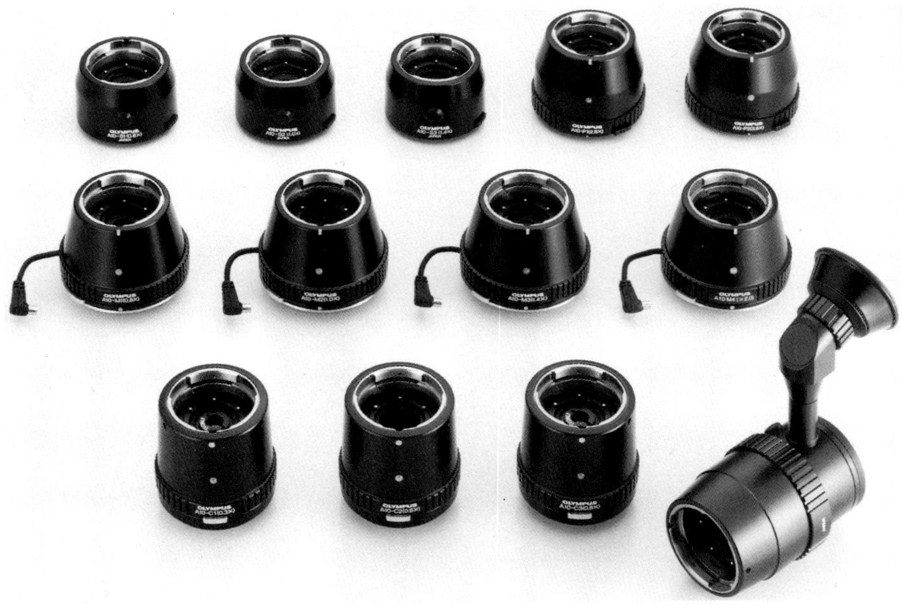

3.17 Various adapters for changing magnification, made by Olympus.

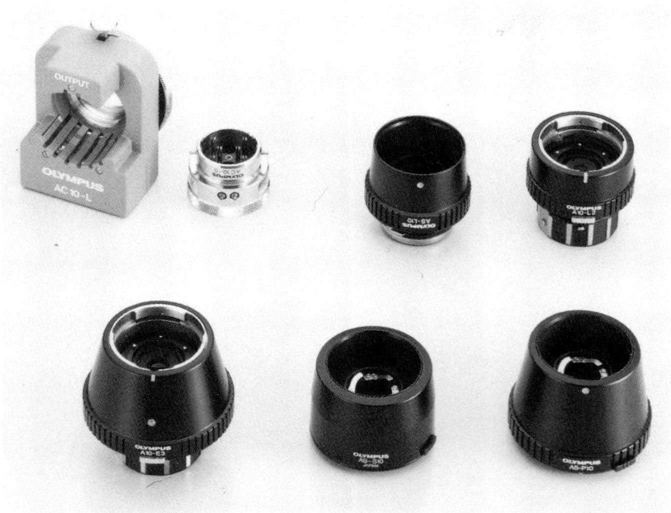

3.18 Exchanging adapters, which can be connected to ordinary cameras and light sources.

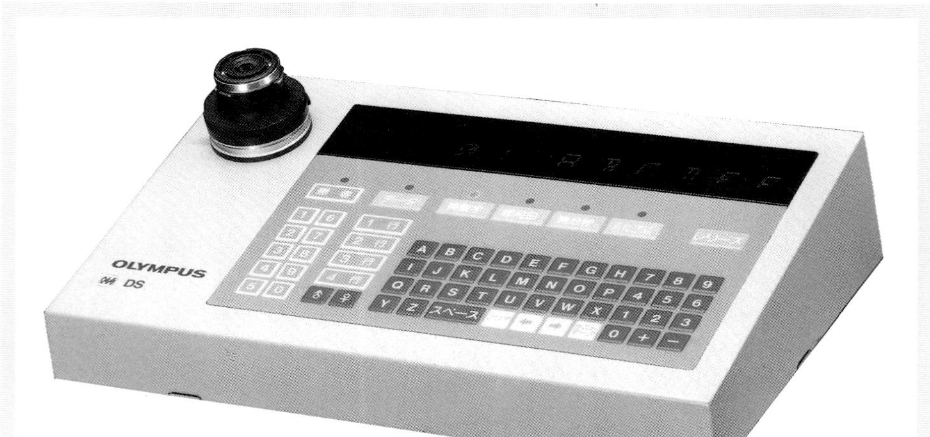

3.19 Data inprinting system.

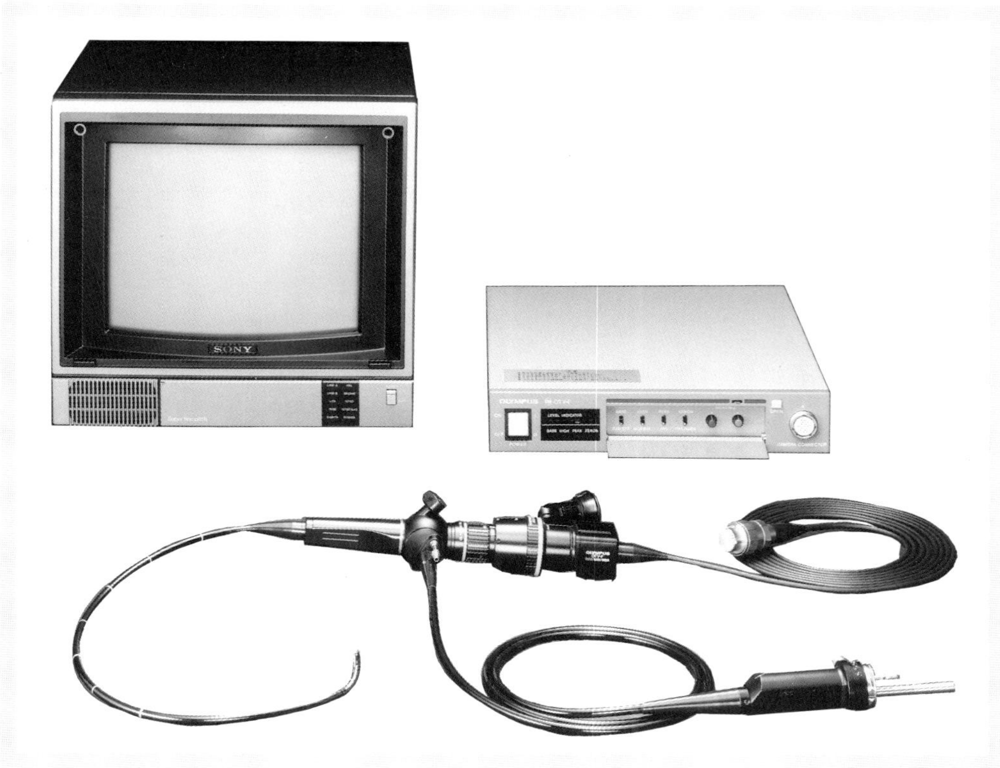

3.20 Medical TV system.

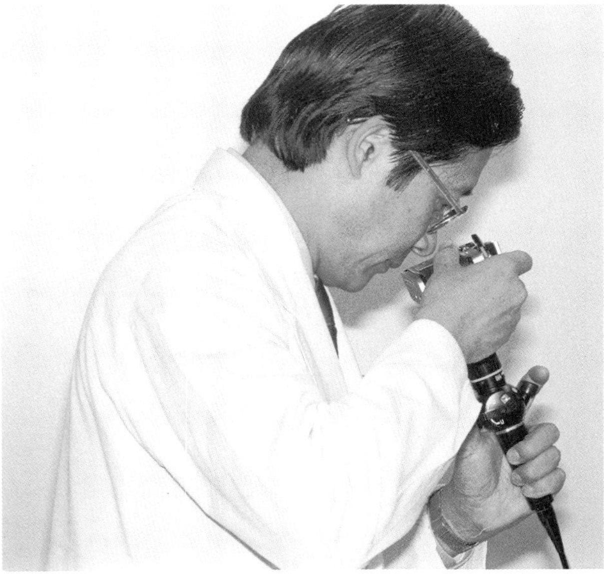

3.21 Taking photographs using a camera (35 mm single lens reflex camera, OM-1N) attached to the fibreoptic bronchoscope (Olympus BF-6C10).

5 Cleaning, sterilisation and storage of fibreoptic bronchoscopes and other accessories

a) Cleaning and sterilisation of fibreoptic bronchoscopes

After a 'scope is used, a solution of invert soap is prepared in a washbowl. For example, 10 per cent Osban is dissolved in 200 times its volume and 10 per cent Hyamine in 100 times its volume. The body of the 'scope is scrubbed with gauze soaked in this solution. The tip that bends must not be wiped too hard (**3.22A**). When washing the channel of the forceps, connect the suction tube to the forceps lumen and suck out the cleaning solution from the tip of the 'scope. Next, all parts of the channel are brushed (**3.22B**). The suction tube is then connected and distilled water and cleaning solution are sucked through alternately. Finally, distilled water is sucked out, followed by air to dry the channel. The part that is inserted into the patient is washed with distilled water and gauze, followed by gauze with 30 per cent alcohol. Next the cap and adapter are removed from the open end of the 'scope's channel and the channel is cleaned with a cotton bud containing 70 per cent alcohol (**3.22C**). The cap and adapter are washed thoroughly with a brush in cleaning solution, rinsed in water, and then reattached to the 'scope. Finally, the control unit is cleaned with gauze dipped in 70 per cent alcohol. Generally, in fibreoptic bronchoscopy, the same scope is used on several patients one after the other, with washing and sterilisation between each patient.

To prevent infection or contamination by tuberculosis, syphilis, HIV, and hepatitis-B, patients with these diseases or suspected of suffering from these diseases, should be scheduled to be examined at the end of the day. An automatic washing machine (EW-D), which can wash the outside and inside of a fibreoptic bronchoscope at the same time, has been developed recently. Figure **3.23** shows an EW-D cleaning machine washing a 'scope. With this machine it is possible to sterilise and dry a bronchoscope in about 7 minutes. The surface of the objective lens is cleaned with gauze dipped in 70 per cent alcohol and the eye lens by using a cotton bud dipped in 70 per cent alcohol (**3.24**). Overnight sterilisation is carried out by using formaldehyde gas, ultraviolet light or anprolene gas (ethylene oxide) (**3.25**).

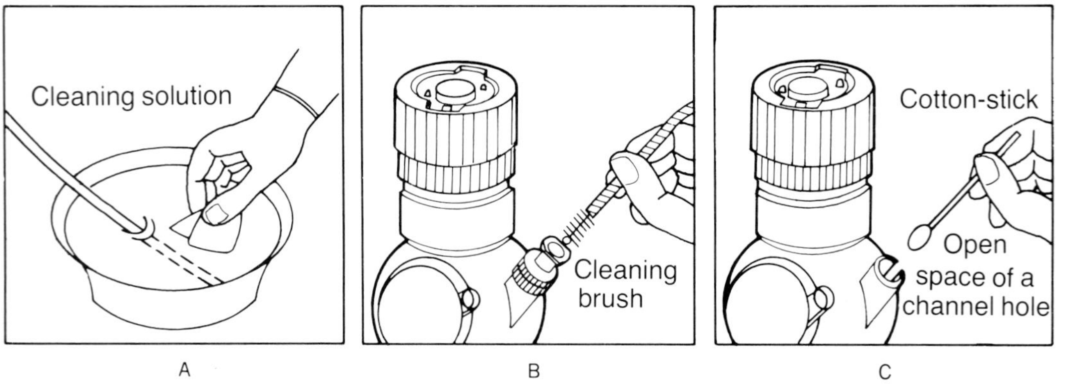

3.22 The stages of cleaning and sterilisation of the body of a bronchoscope: A The instrument being scrubbed in cleaning solution; B A cleaning brush being inserted into the channel; C A cotton bud being inserted into the open space of a channel hole.

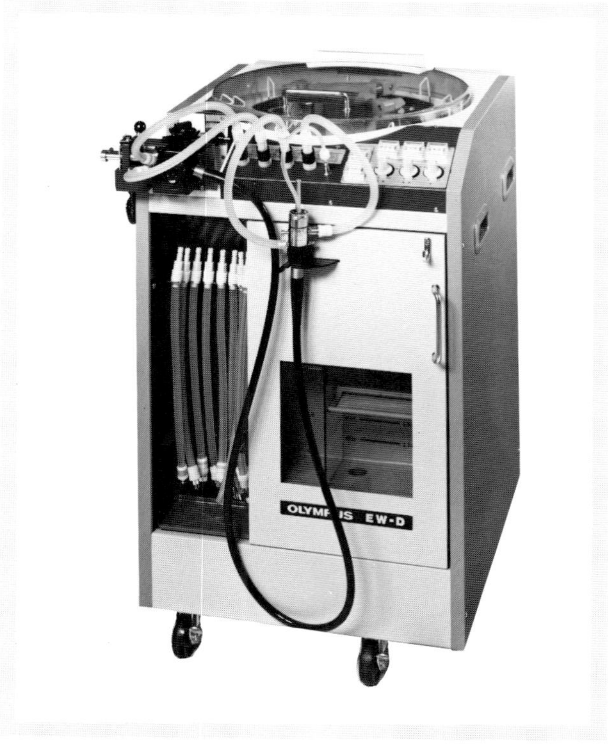

3.23 Cleaning machine for endoscopes.

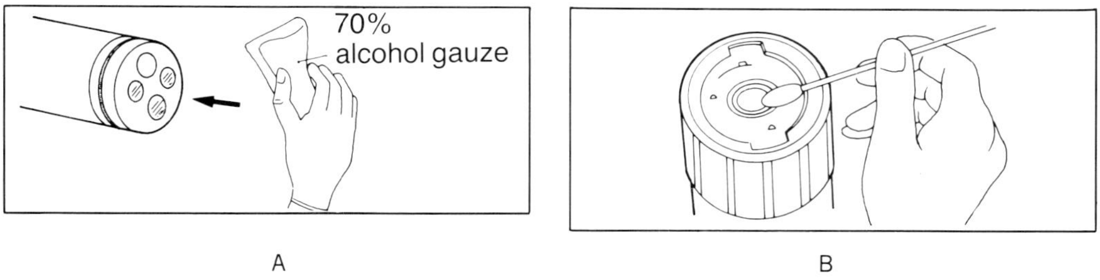

3.24 Cleaning of the surface of the objective lens (A) and the eye lens (B): in A 70 per cent alcohol gauze is being used; in B a cotton bud is being used on the eye lens.

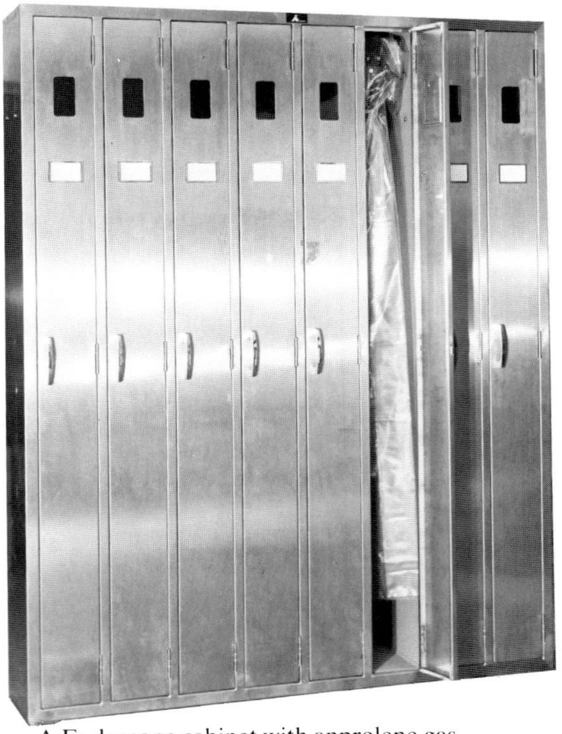

A Endoscope cabinet with anprolene gas sterilisation system

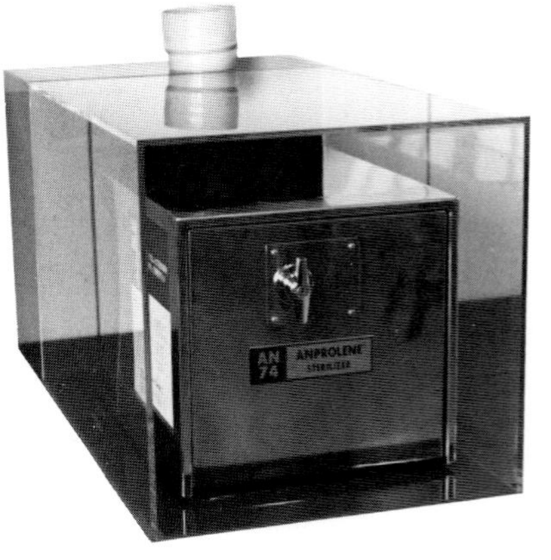

B Anprolene gas sterilisation system

3.25 Sterilisation system with anprolene gas (ethylene oxide) (space for 8 'scopes).

b) Cleaning of biopsy forceps, cytology brushes and injection catheters

After use biopsy forceps should be washed thoroughly by scrubbing in cleaning solution. Carefully rinse away the blood attached to the tips of the cups. Routinely these items are rinsed in water and cleaned with gauze dipped in 70 per cent alcohol. Then one or two drops of silicon oil are poured onto the tips of the forceps and wiped off, the cup is placed in position and the forceps hung in a storage cabinet. We have to use either iodine solution, formaldehyde gas, or ethylene oxide gas for sterilising 'scopes. If heat sterilisation is chosen, the 'scope can be boiled, but not autoclaved.

After use, the knob which holds the cytology brushes is loosened and a brush wire is pulled through it. A sheath of brushes should be washed thoroughly in cleaning solution with gauze. Then the inside of a brush tube should be washed by injecting distilled water and cleaning solution, after which air is sucked through it to dry the inside. A control unit is cleaned with gauze dipped in 70 per cent alcohol. Used brushes must be discarded.

A used injection catheter, its top, needle and control unit should be washed thoroughly with gauze soaked in cleaning solution. Any attached foreign body or blood should be removed by brushing in cleaning solution. Later, cleaning solution is sucked through an injection tube to clean the inside of the catheter (**3.26**). Finally, the inside and outside are washed with distilled water and air is sucked through to dry up the inside. The outside is cleaned with 70 per cent alcohol and a few drops of silicon oil is applied to its top. Sterilisation should be carried out by using iodine, formaldehyde, or ethylene oxide gas. Sterilisation by boiling is suitable but autoclaving must be avoided.

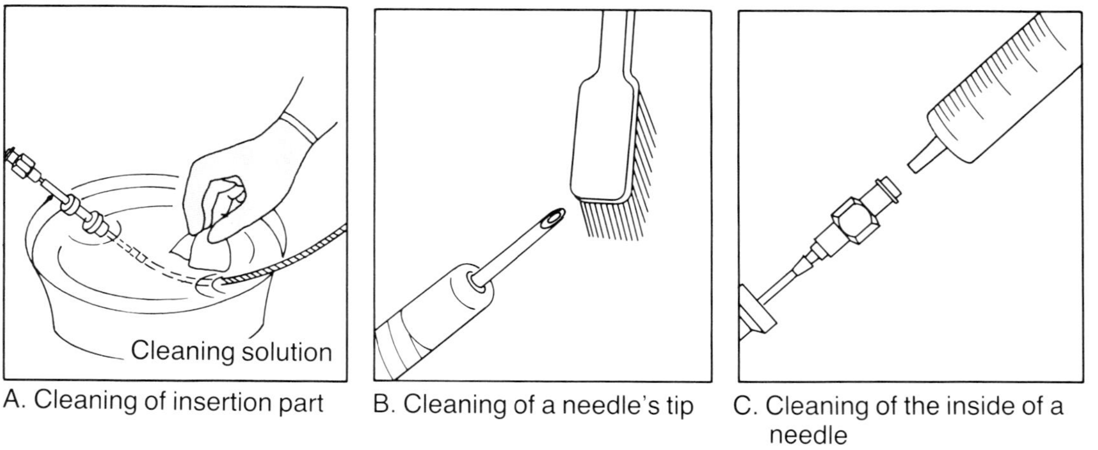

3.26 Cleaning of a needle catheter: A Cleaning of insertion part; B Cleaning of a needle's tip; C Cleaning of the inside of a needle.

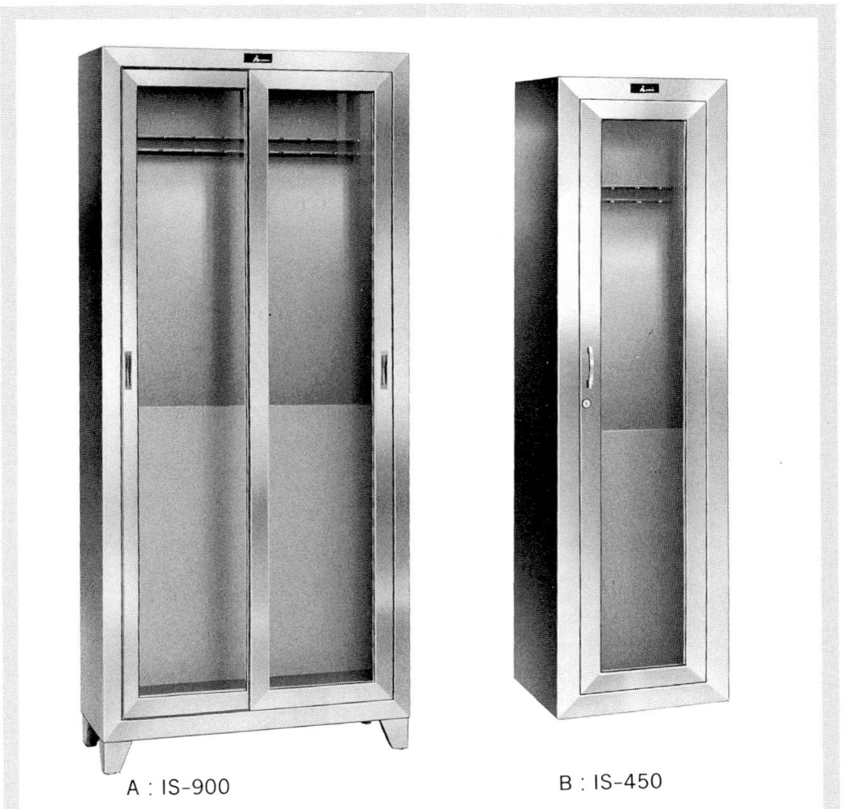

3.27 Cabinets for endoscopes: A Type IS-900; B Type IS-450.

c) Storage and housing of fibreoptic bronchoscopes

When bronchoscopy is completed, the body of 'scopes should be cleaned thoroughly and the water at the tips wiped off. Fully dried 'scopes are then housed in a cabinet for endoscopes and sterilised using either ultraviolet light or ethylene oxide gas. Before this the angulation lever at the control unit should be removed and special caps should be attached to 'scopes, cameras and forceps. Where possible, bronchoscopes should be hung upright. It is ideal to place them in a cabinet for endoscopes (see **3.27**). If you have to store scopes in a curved position, select a curve of greater diameter than those in the carrying case. Scopes, light sources and camera systems should be housed in a room with even temperature and moisture. Avoid areas where there is direct sunlight or Xray equipment. If the carrying case is used for storage, the shaft of the 'scope should be placed in such a way that the curve is retained.

4 Indications and contraindications

1 Indications

All patients with respiratory diseases may be suitable for fibreoptic bronchoscopy. In particular, patients whose chest radiographs reveal abnormal shadows and those with symptoms such as cough, sputum production, haemoptysis and dyspnoea should undergo this procedure.

Recently, we have begun to perform fibreoptic bronchoscopy on men and women over 40 years of age who suffer from cough and sputum production. This procedure is carried out every 6 months to locate any intrabronchial lesions at an early stage. Most patients will readily submit to this procedure.

Drainage of sputa using a fibreoptic bronchoscope is necessary for cases of lung cancer, lung abscess, pneumonia, bronchiectasis and diffuse pan-bronchiolitis, who cannot expectorate. Similarly, those who have undergone thoracic and abdominal surgery may be suitable for this procedure.

When a foreign body is lodged in the bronchus and aspiration pneumonia is present, fibreoptic bronchoscopy may be necessary.

2 Contraindications

Generally there are few contraindications to fibreoptic bronchoscopy. However, patients who are very weak, or suffer from severe cardiac conditions such as acute myocardial infarction and angina pectoris, might worsen their general condition or precipitate an ischaemic attack by submitting to this procedure. It is also worth remembering that those with hypoxaemia of less than 60 Torr, poor pulmonary function, severe laryngeal and tracheal stenosis should not undergo this procedure where possible.

Those who suffer from bronchial asthma and have a history of asthma should not undergo bronchoscopy, because the pharyngolaryngeal anaesthesia and the insertion of the fibrescope may cause severe bronchoconstriction. However, the author and his co-worker carry out this procedure on almost all asthma patients under drip-infusion of steroids and aminophylline.

Although massive haemoptysis is considered to be a contraindication, fibreoptic bronchoscopy is carried out to observe any haemorrhagic condition and to identify the site and drain the blood and coagula in the bronchial lumen. The bleeding is stopped by administering epinephrine and thrombin solution. In such an instance, the skilful operator performs fibreoptic bronchoscopy with great care, because the visual field of the fibrescope is frequently blurred by blood and coagula. New bleeding can easily occur if the tip of the fibrescope disturbs the bronchial mucosa.

Where thrombocytopenia and bleeding are present, transbronchial lung biopsy and transbronchial tumour biopsy should not be performed.

5 Fibreoptic bronchoscopy procedure

1 Premedication and local anaesthesia

While fibreoptic bronchoscopy can be performed under either general or local anaesthesia, only the latter is used in adult cases at present. This procedure can be performed easily and safely by a well-trained operator even on patients in an extremely poor condition, unconscious patients, elderly patients over 80 years of age and patients with severe hypoxaemia. If a general anaesthetic is necessary, because of the patient's extreme anxiety, a suitable endotracheal tube can be inserted.

Patients must not take any food or drink for at least 4 hours before this procedure. This rule must be observed to prevent reflex vomiting during local anaesthesia and fibreoptic bronchoscopy. Occasionally, patients get very nervous, cannot sleep well and become fatigued, which makes the procedure more difficult. The patient should be given a simple but clear explanation of the procedure beforehand to alleviate any anxiety and facilitate co-operation, because the patient is conscious throughout the procedure, although often in a drowsy state. It is important that the patient is told about the safety level of this procedure. If necessary, a mild tranquillizer (5 mg of diazepam) is given the evening before.

From 15–30 minutes before the procedure 0.5 mg atropine sulphate is injected subcutaneously to reduce hypersecretion. If there is an abnormally strong reaction to the instrument, 35–70 mg of meperidine (pethidine hydrochloride) and/or 25–50 mg of hydroxyzine hydrochloride are also injected subcutaneously. If these premedications are not sufficient, 5–10 mg of diazepam is injected intravenously.

The most common local anaesthetic agents are lignocaine, cocaine and tertracaine. The effects of cocaine last longer than those of lignocaine. Cocaine may also be the most effective local anaesthetic, but dosage should be restricted to approximately 200 mg. We use 4 per cent of Xylocaine (lignocaine). Xylocaine is probably the most popular and easiest drug to use of the three above-mentioned drugs, because it has lower toxicity than the other two. Thus, in cases where the effect of lignocaine diminishes, further administration of a small dose of cocaine may be recommended.

Usually, we start the local anaesthesia procedure with the patient seated, with 3 ml of lignocaine given via an electronic nebuliser (**5.1**). Then the oral lumen and pharynx are sprayed using the Jackson-type spray (**5.2**). After this either the operator or the patient himself pulls out the tongue (**5.3**), the elongated nozzle of the spray is gradually inserted and puffs of anaesthetic are sprayed over the vocal cords and trachea at the beginning of each inspiration. Great care must be exercised to avoid unnecessary touching or friction with the spray nozzle. By ensuring that spraying is done at the beginning of each inspiration, once the vicinity of the vocal cords has been reached one can obtain satisfactory anaesthesia with a minimum dose of anaesthetic. It is very important to tell the patient not to swallow anaesthetic mixed with sputum; he should be provided with a paper cup to spit into.

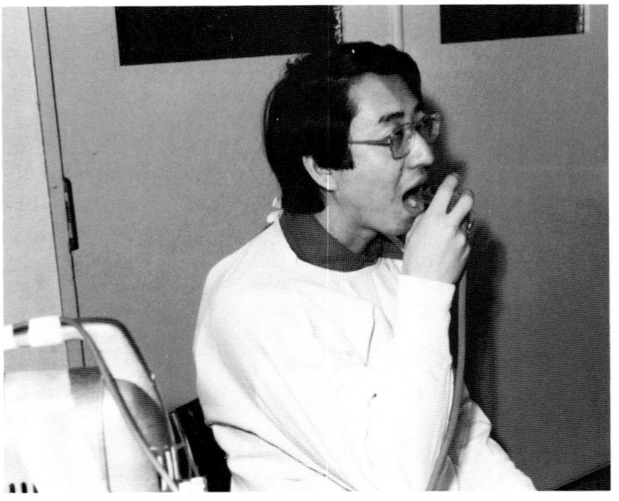

5.1 Aspiration anaesthesia by using an electric nebuliser. A patient inserts a glass apparatus into the mouth and aspirates anaesthetic while he is inhaling.

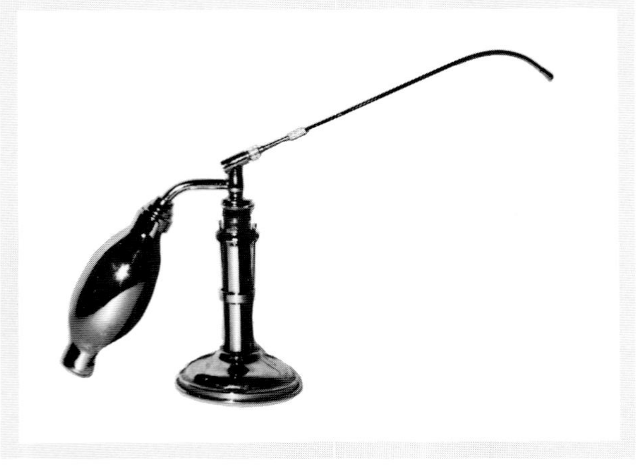

5.2 Jackson-type hand nebuliser being used for local anaesthesia. Four per cent lignocaine is sprayed to anaesthetise the oral cavity, pharynx, larynx, trachea and upper parts of the main bronchi.

Typically, the dose of lignocaine used in this procedure is 5-7.5 ml. Actually one can avoid anaesthesia using an electronic nebuliser. It is thought that the maximum dose of lignocaine should be 400 mg (10 ml of 4 per cent lignocaine solution). Small amounts of lignocaine (1.0-2.0 ml) may be infused via the instrument channel of the bronchoscope, should the patient show any signs of a reflex cough during the procedure. Be extremely aware of lignocaine intoxication; make sure that the total amount used does not exceed 1,000 mg.

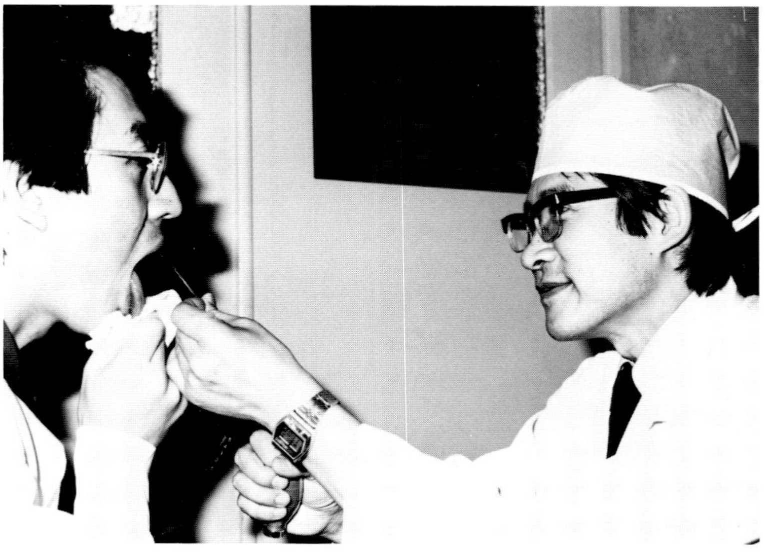

5.3 Local anaesthesia using a Jackson-type spray. The operator advances the tip of the nebuliser into the oral cavity, pharynx and larynx while a patient holds his tongue with his right hand.

2 Insertion of fibreoptic bronchoscope

a) Preparation immediately before insertion

Before starting one should choose the most suitable fibreoptic bronchoscope; this depends on the condition of the patient and the purpose of this procedure. If the patient has a relatively small amount of intrabronchial secretion and the procedure is only for observation, a BF-6C10 (Olympus) is recommended, and in cases with a large amount of intrabronchial secretion where both observation and biopsy are necessary, a BF-10 is recommended. In the patient undergoing bronchial toilet or transbronchial lung biopsy (TBLB) of the middle or lower lobe except the apinal lower, BF-10 is recommended, and for TBLB in the right or left upper lobe segmental bronchi, BF-P10 is recommended. Before the actual insertion of the instrument, check the fibrescope to ensure that it is in good working order and that the locking lever is in the 'off' position. Connect the fibrescope to the light source apparatus. Then disinfect the channel of the fibrescope to the light source apparatus. After this step disinfect the channel of the fibrescope by aspirating the disinfectant solution three or four times followed by distilled water; then dry the channel by aspirating air.

Having completed these steps, wipe the part of the fibrescope and lens that is to be inserted with gauze dipped in 70 per cent ethanol. Polish the lens with lens cleaner (**5.4**) for a good view and adjust the focus. Usually, if the operator is righthanded, the control unit with the ocular lens is held in the left hand to leave the right hand free for inserting forceps, brush and retractable needle or infusing saline to collect broncho-alveolar lavage fluid. The angulation lever which controls the angle of the fibrescope tip is operated by the thumb (**5.5**). The patient is told to lie in a straight supine position on the examination table. Both eyes are covered with gauze fixed with tape.

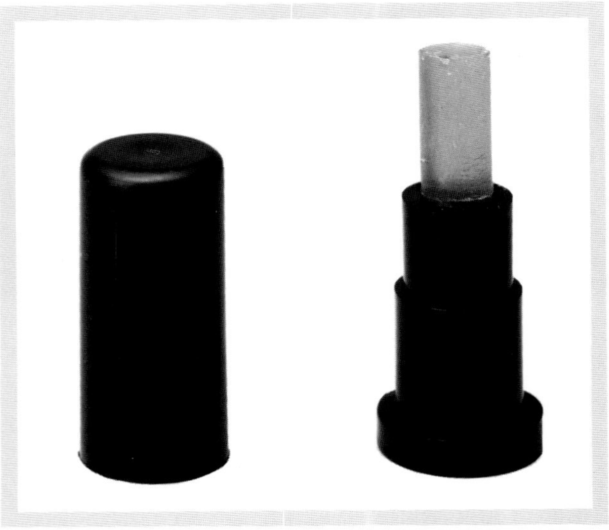

5.4 Lens cleaner. Replace the cap quickly after use because this is a volatile item.

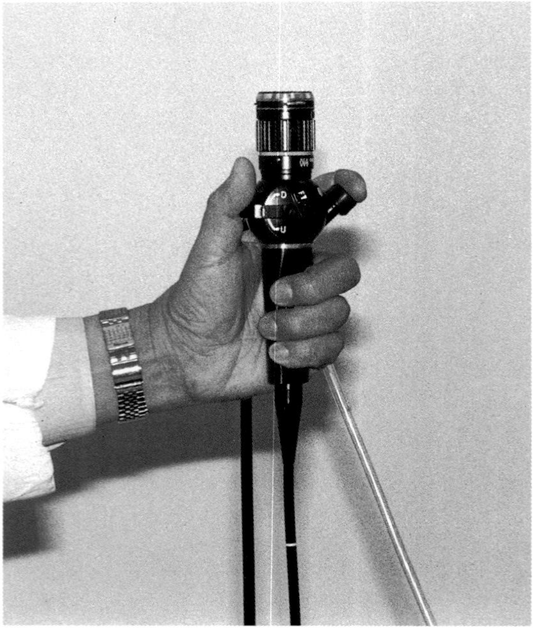

5.5 The correct method of holding the fibreoptic bronchoscope (BF-6C10).

b) Fibreoptic bronchoscopy via direct transoral insertion without a tracheal tube

After instructing the patient to relax and let his shoulders sag, he is told to stick out his chin and put out his tongue. These steps are sufficient for expansion of the laryngeal lumen. A plastic mouthpiece (**5.6**), to protect the instrument from an inadvertent bite, is inserted. Figure **5.7** shows the operator inserting the fibrescope attached with the lecture scope. Figure **5.8** shows the lecture scope. The tip of the instrument is inserted through the mouthpiece and passes over the tongue along the midline of the body with the angle of the tip maintained slightly upwards as far as the epiglottis (**5.9**). Upon reaching the epiglottis, the tip is straightened and advanced, when the vocal cords come into view (**5.10**). Here a small dose of lignocaine (0.5-1.0 ml) may be administered. The bronchoscope is advanced and the tip of the instrument reaches the orifice of the glottis (**5.11**). The bronchoscope is then advanced, keeping the vocal cords in the centre of the field of vision, and passed through the vocal cords. The upper portion of the trachea comes into view (**5.12**). The bronchoscope is further advanced, and the whole trachea and carina come into view (**5.13**), and then the tip is advanced and the orifices of the right and left bronchi come into view (**5.14**). To prevent a severe reflex cough, administer 0.5-1 ml of lignocaine on the upper part of trachea, carina, orifice of the right upper bronchus, right middle lobe bronchus, right lower lobe bronchus, left main bronchus, left upper lobe bronchus and left lower lobe bronchus.

In this procedure nearly all of the instilled lignocaine is aspirated within 2-3 seconds. In spite of following these steps, a severe reflex cough may still occur; therefore the shaft of the bronchoscope (5-10 cm from the tip) is liberally coated with lignocaine gel. This is our routine for fibreoptic bronchoscopy via direct transoral insertion without a tracheal tube. With this procedure one can observe the pharynx, epiglottis, vocal cords and the upper part of the trachea. Additionally, the procedure time is very short.

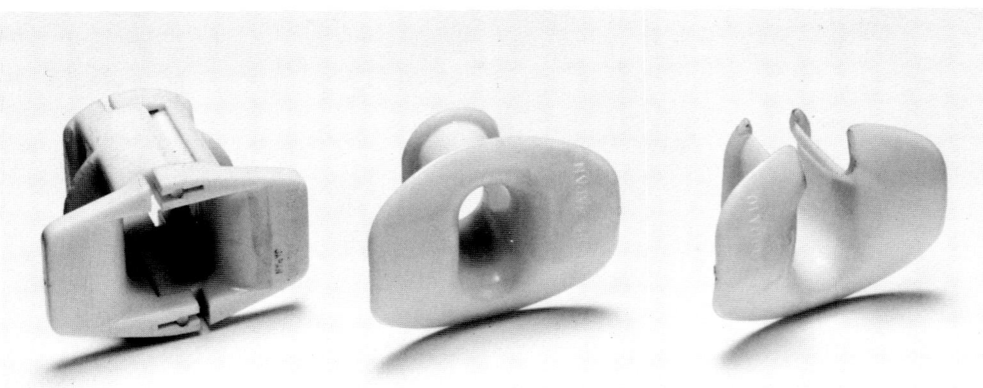

5.6 Three mouthpieces.

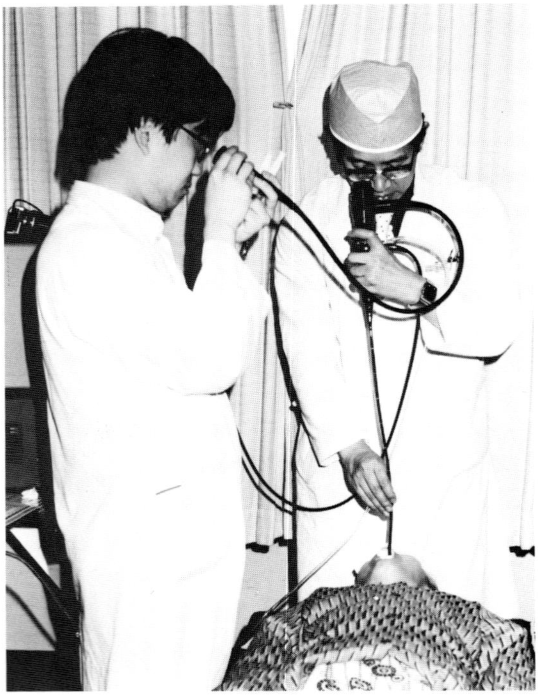

5.7 An operator is inserting a fibreoptic bronchoscope directly into a patient's trachea, while he teaches a student via the attached lecturescope.

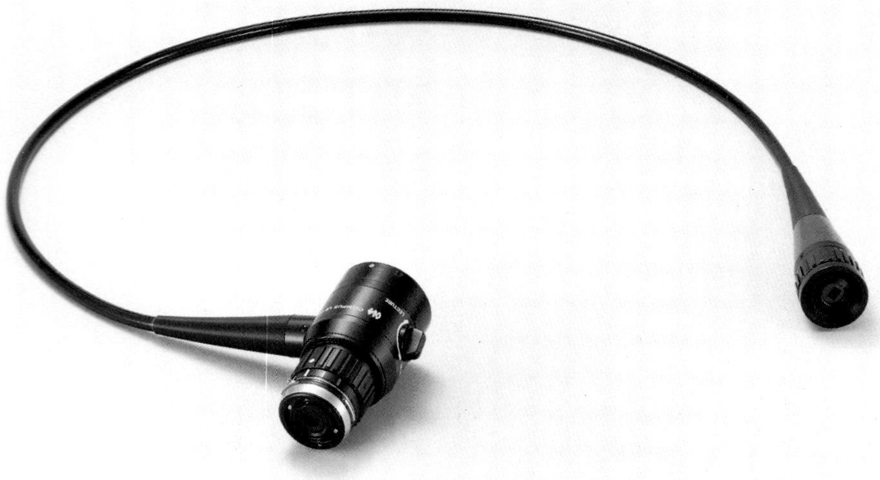

5.8 A lecturescope made by Olympus Co. It is possible for a viewer to observe what an operator is viewing simultaneously.

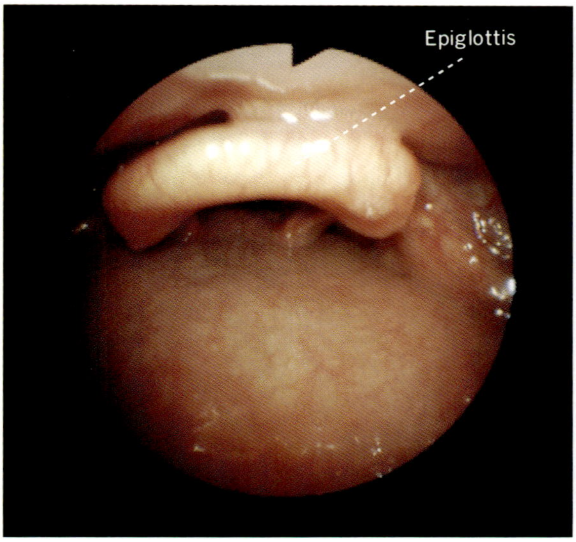

5.9 The tip of the fibrescope at the epiglottis.

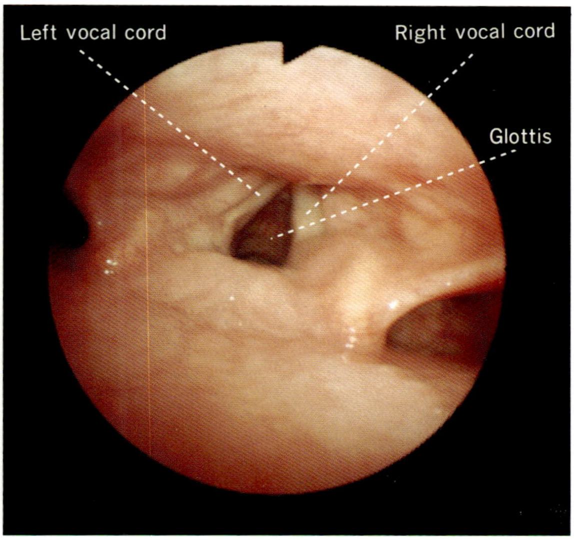

5.10 The vocal cords viewed.

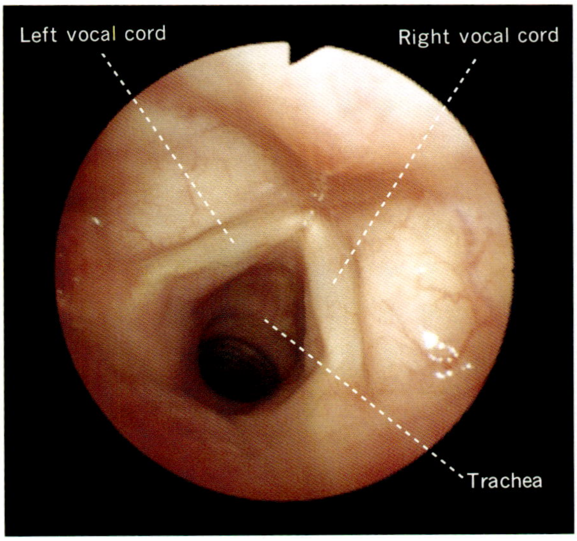

5.11 The vocal cords and glottis viewed together.

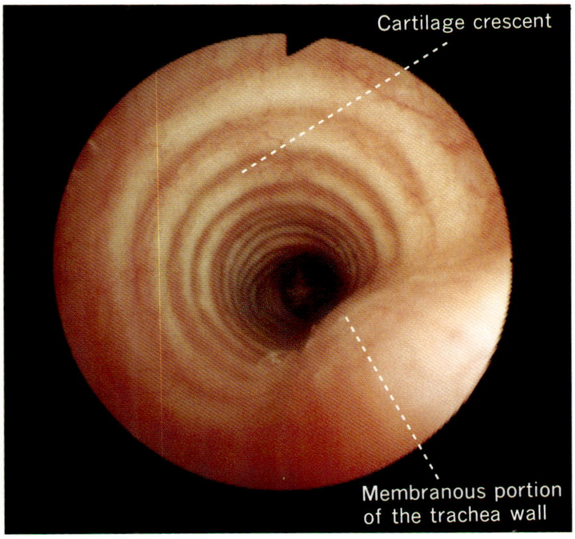

5.12 Passing through the glottis.

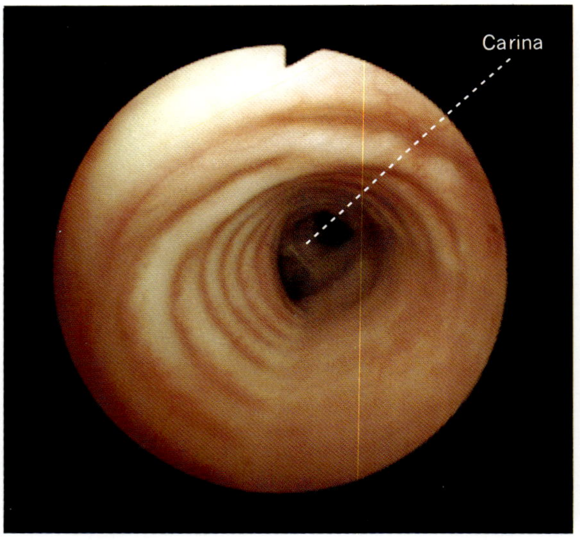

5.13 The whole of the trachea and the carina are visible.

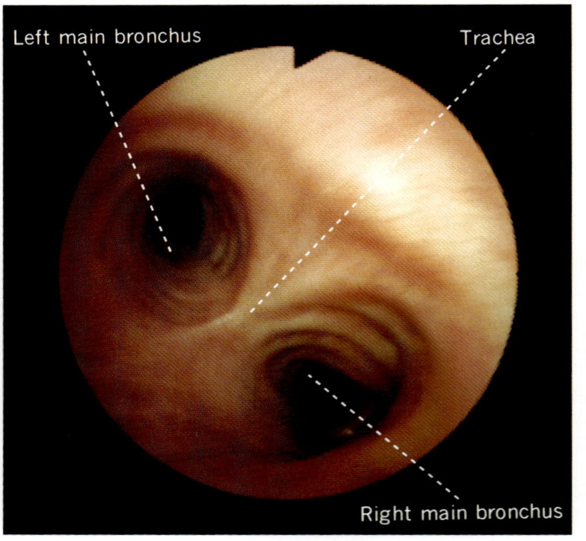

5.14 The carina viewed.

d) Fibreoptic bronchoscopy via transnasal insertion

This method is very useful if the patient has a strong pharyngeal reflex or the patient is comatose and it is difficult to keep the mouth open, or if postoperative bronchial toilet is necessary. The patient should lie or sit comfortably. The widest nostril is anaesthetised with lignocaine spray, then lignocaine gel is applied inside the nostril. After these procedures, the fibreoptic bronchoscope is inserted (**5-17A**). Be extremely careful because nasal bleeding can occur if there is damage to the nasal mucosa.

c) Fibreoptic bronchoscopy via transoral insertion with a tracheal tube

Figure **5.15** shows a tracheal tube and a stylet. First, the stylet is inserted into the tracheal tube and a suitable curve is made. Then, while observing with a laryngoscope, the tracheal tube is inserted into the trachea and the stylet is pulled out. The tracheal tube is fixed to the patient's face with adhesive tape and the bronchoscope is inserted (**5.16**).

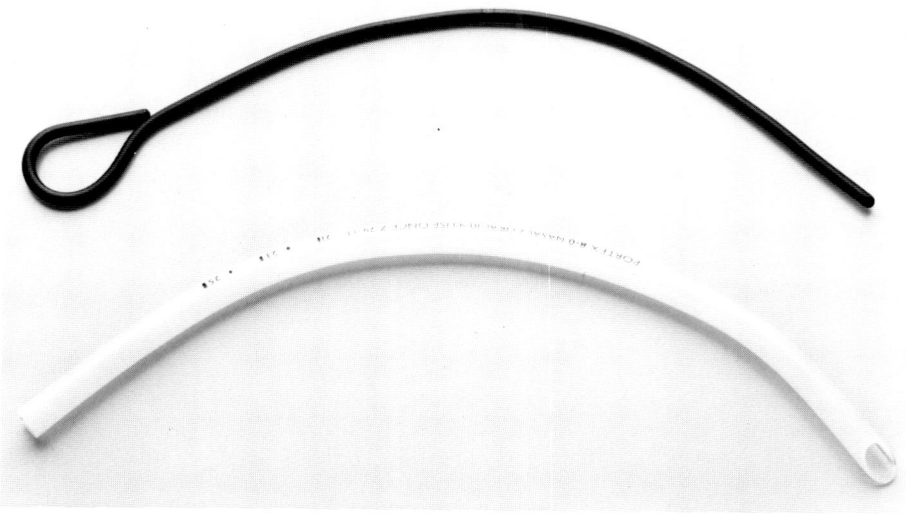

5.15 Tracheal tube and stylet.

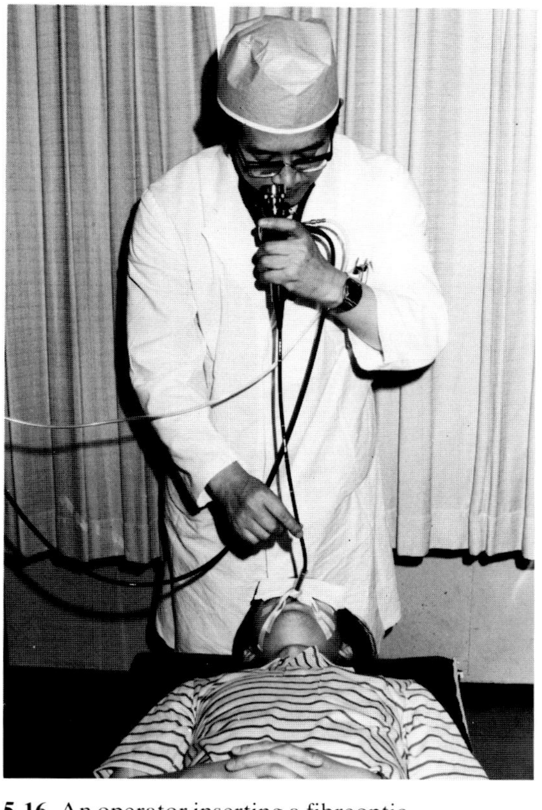

5.16 An operator inserting a fibreoptic bronchoscope through a tracheal tube.

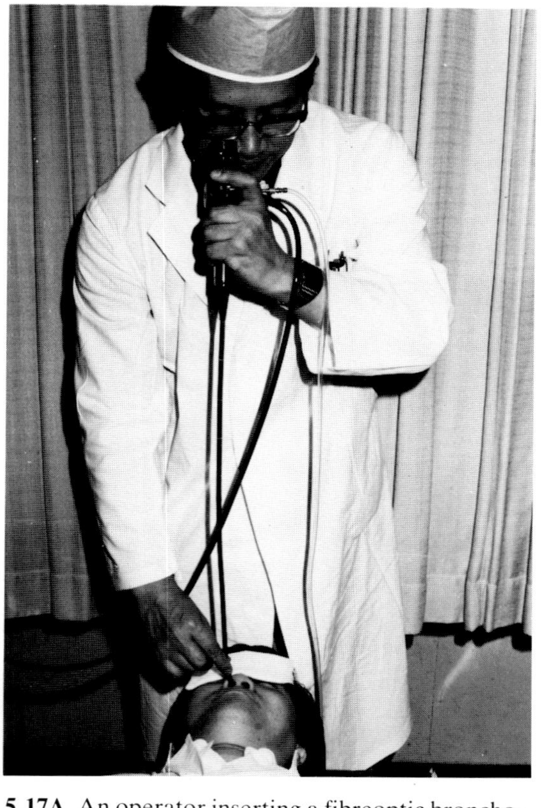

5.17A An operator inserting a fibreoptic bronchoscope transnasally.

3 Taking the photograph

Fibreoptic bronchoscopy is very useful for clinical diagnosis and for therapeutic methods such as transbronchial lung biopsy, transbronchial tumour biopsy, bronchial toilet, brushing or curetting in peripheral pulmonary lesions, bronchography, injection of therapeutic agents directly into endobronchial tumours, aspiration biopsy beyond the tracheal or bronchial wall, electrosurgery and cryosurgery and removal of foreign bodies. Before undertaking such procedures, take a photograph to evaluate the pathological conditions precisely. A good quick photograph is essential. If there is sputum on the bronchial mucosa, aspirate the right upper lobe bronchi. The picture on the left (**5.17B**(a)) shows the orifices covered with sputum, and on the right (**5.17B**(b)) the sputum has been rinsed and aspirated.

Figure **5.18** shows the positions and angles of photography for 25 photographs. First, take a photograph of the vocal cords and glottis (**5.19**), followed by photographs of the carina (**5.20**) from point 1, the right upper lobe bronchus and truncus intermedius (**5.21**) from point 2, the orifices of right B^1, B^2 and B^3 (**5.22**) from point 3, the orifice of right B^1 (**5.23**) from point 4, the orifice of right B^2 (**5.24**) from point 5 and orifice of right B^3 (**5.25**) from point 6.

Thereafter, advance the tip of the bronchoscope to the truncus intermedius and photograph the orifices of the right middle and lower lobe bronchi (**5.26**) from point 7, the orifice of right B^4 and B^5 (**5.27**) from point 8, the orifice of right B^7 and basal lobe bronchi (**5.28**) from point 9, the orifice of B^8, B^9 and B^{10} (**5.29**) from point 10, the orifice of B^8 (**5.30**) from point 11, the orifice of B^9 (**5.31**) from point 12, the orifice of right B^{10} (**5.32**) from point 13 and the orifice of right B^6 (**5.33**) from point 14. Then ease out the tip of the bronchoscope and advance it to the left side.

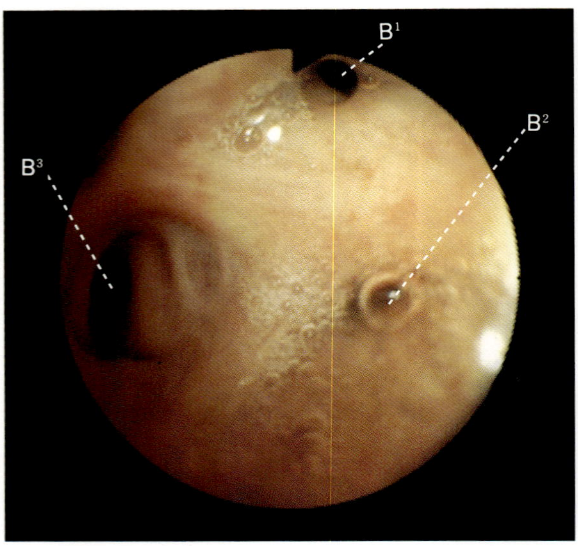

5.17B^a This is an example of bad procedure conditions. Note that the orifices of the right upper lobe bronchi are covered with whitish sputum.

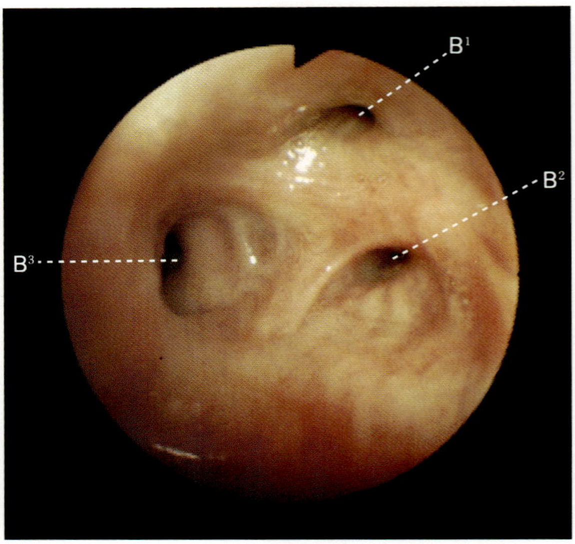

5.17B^b Here the sputum has been aspirated giving the operator a clear view of the orifices.

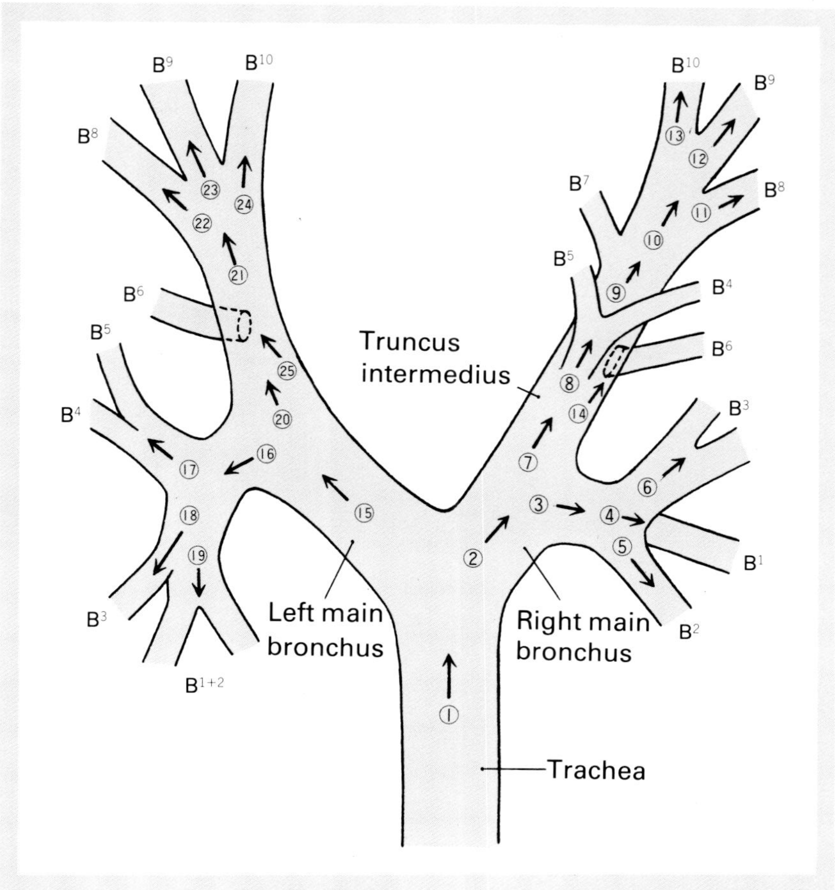

5.18 The various points and angles of photographing while carrying out a fibreoptic bronchoscopy procedure.

First photograph the bifurcation of the left upper and lower bronchi (**5.34**) from point 15, the orifice of left upper bronchus (**5.35**) from point 16, the orifices of left B^4 and B^5 (**5.36**) from point 17, the orifice of left B^3 (**5.37**) from point 18, and the orifices of B^{1+2} (**5.38**) from point 19. Then ease out the tip of the bronchoscope and advance it to the left lower lobe bronchus. First photograph the orifice of the left lower bronchus (**5.39**) from point 20, the orifices of B^8, B^9 and B^{10} (**5.40**) from point 21, the orifice of left B^8 (**5.41**) from point 22, the orifice of left B^9 (**5.42**) from point 23, the orifice of left B^{10} (**5.43**) from point 24, and the orifice of B^6 (**5.44**) from point 25. Usually, the author takes a total of 25 photographs for each case. However, the whole procedure takes only 3-4 minutes.

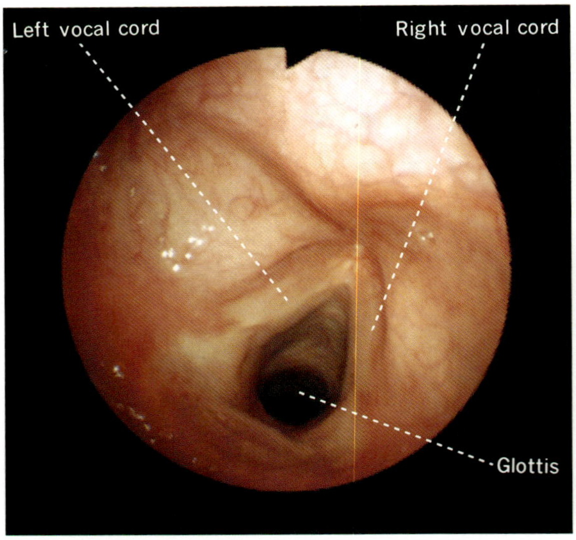

5.19 Vocal cord and glottis.

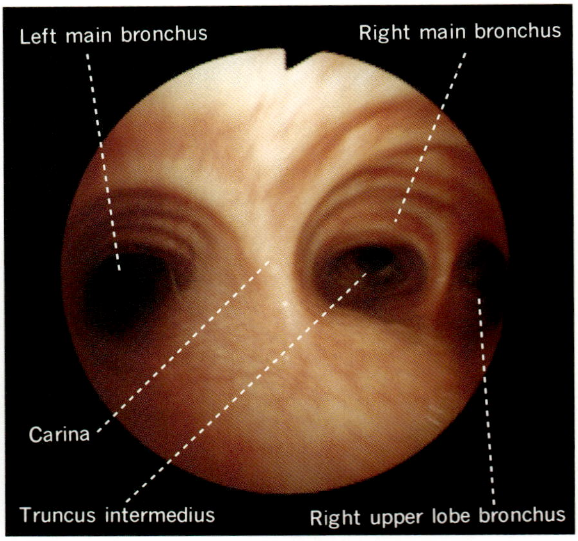

5.20 The carina.

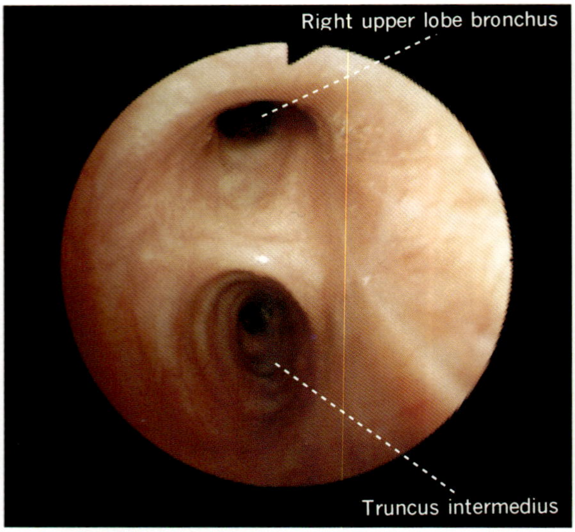

5.21 The right upper lobe bronchus and truncus intermedius.

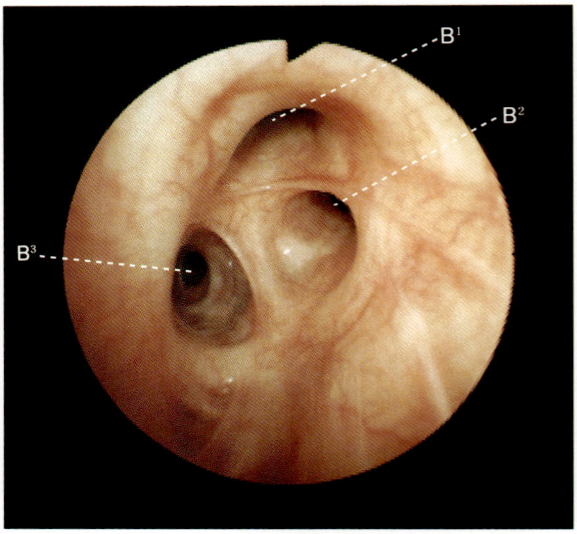

5.22 The right upper lobe bronchus.

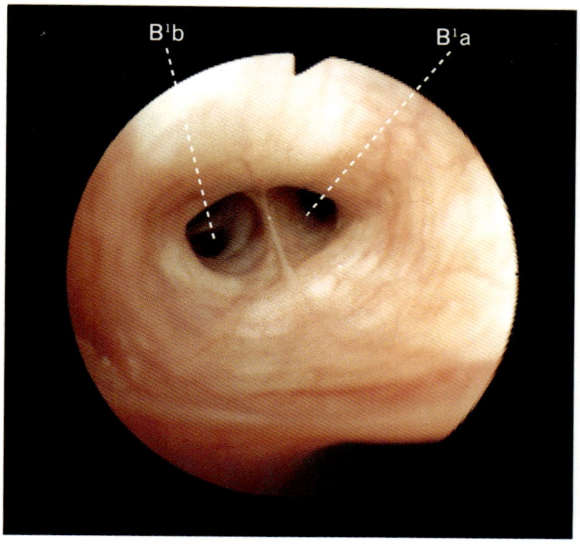

5.23 The orifice of right B^1.

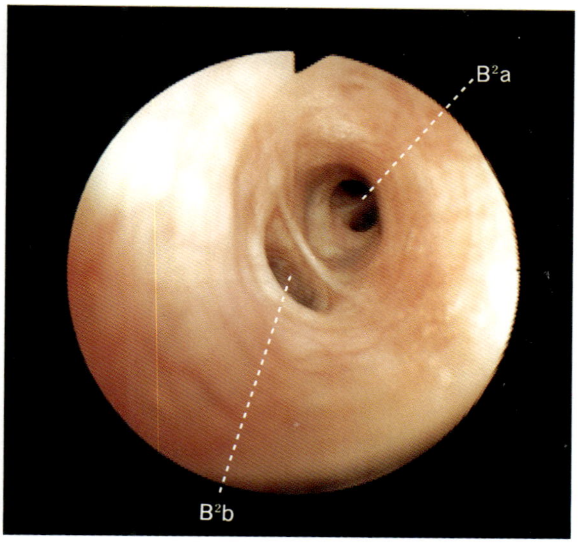

5.24 The orifice of right B^2.

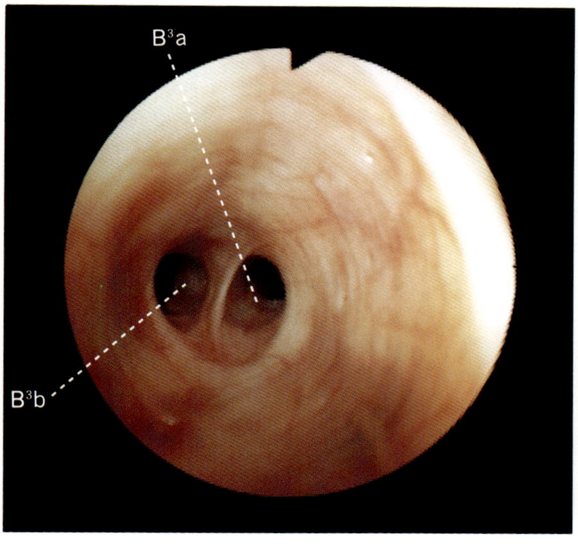

5.25 The orifice of right B^3.

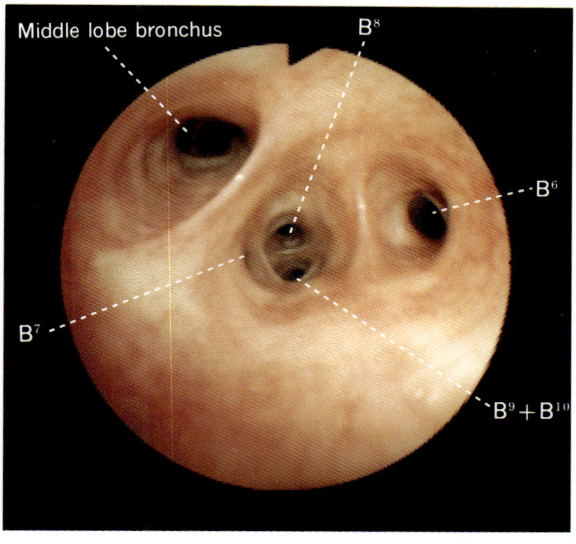

5.26 The orifices of the right middle and lower lobe bronchi.

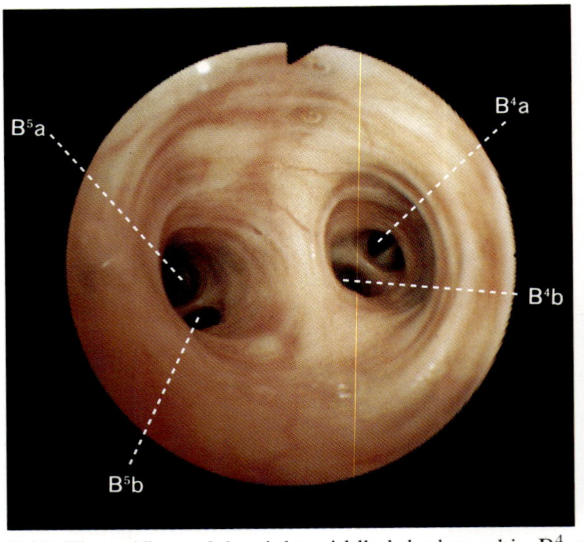

5.27 The orifices of the right middle lobe bronchi, B^4 and B^5.

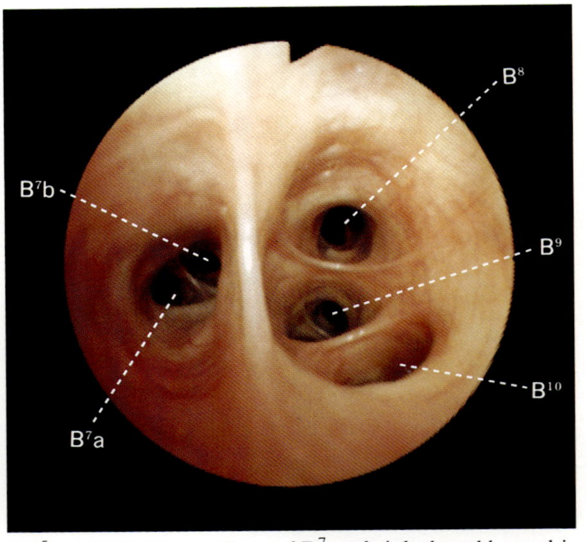

5.28 The orifices of B^7 and right basal bronchi.

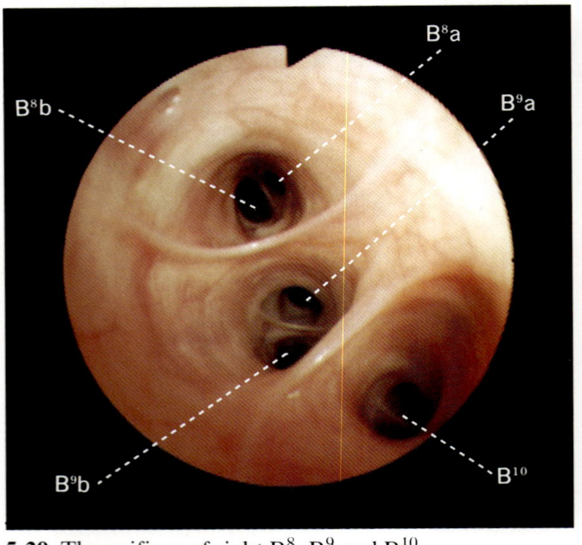

5.29 The orifices of right B^8, B^9 and B^{10}.

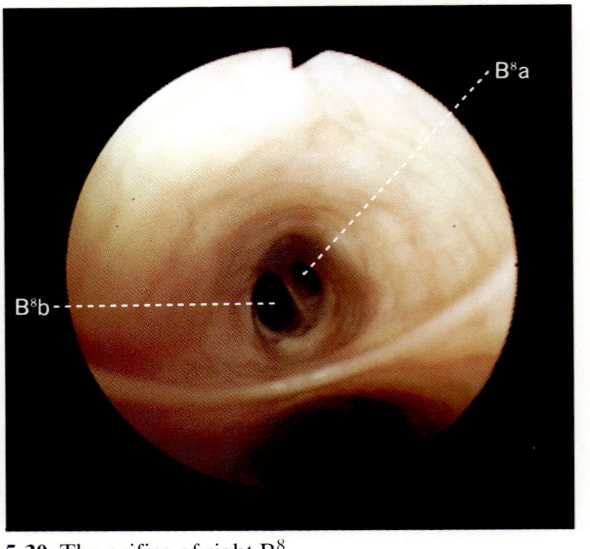

5.30 The orifice of right B^8.

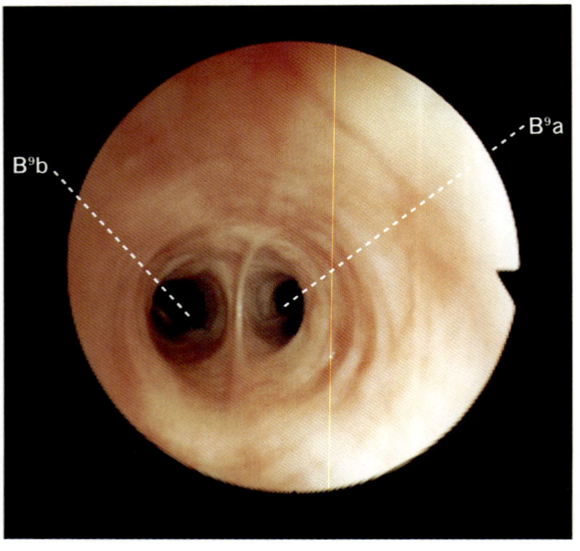

5.31 The orifice of right B^9.

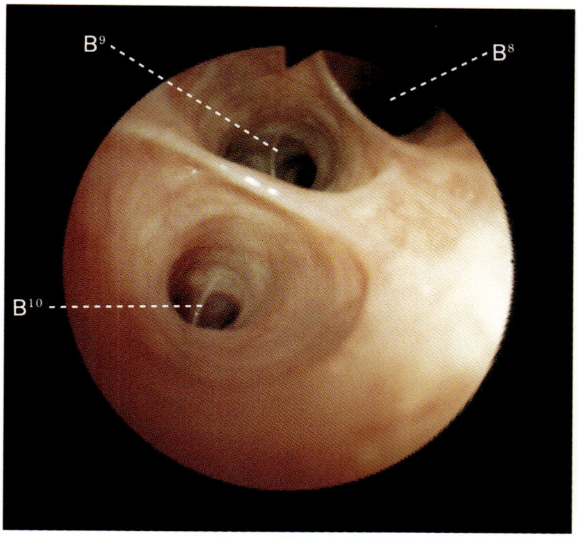

5.32 The orifice of right B^{10}.

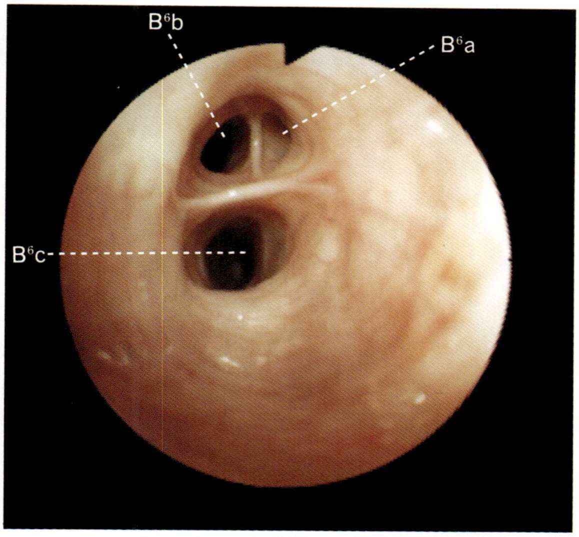

5.33 The orifice of right B^6.

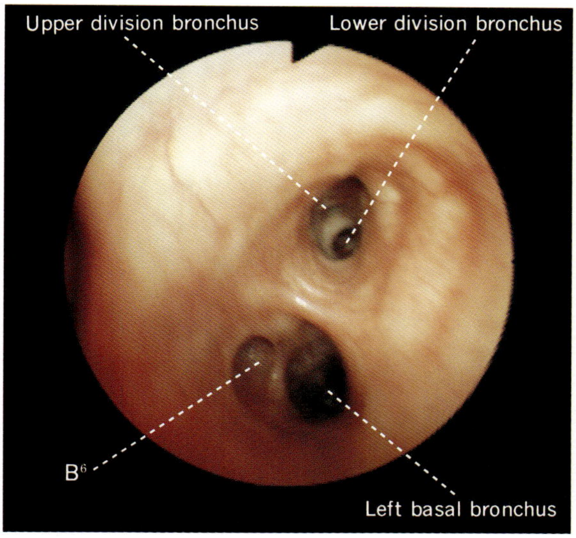

5.34 The bifurcation of the left upper and lower lobe bronchi.

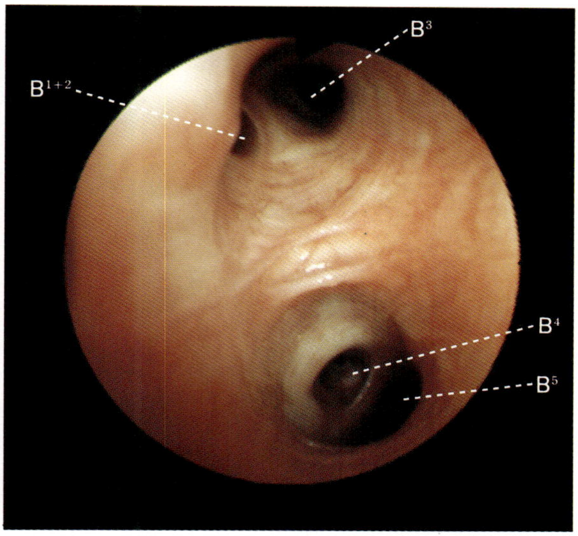

5.35 The orifices of the left upper lobe bronchi.

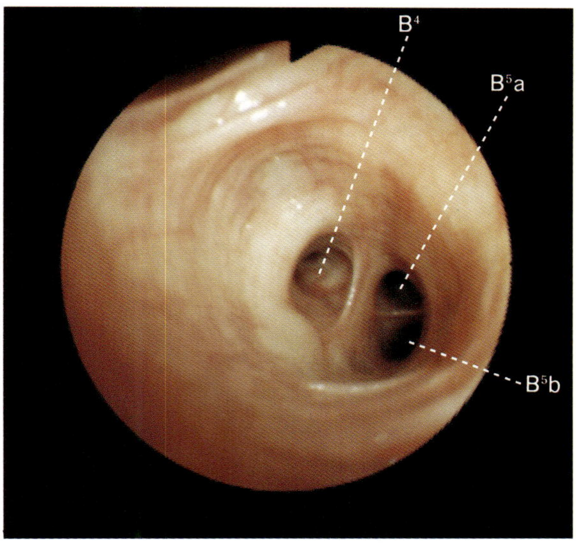

5.36 The orifices of the lower division bronchi, B^4 and B^5.

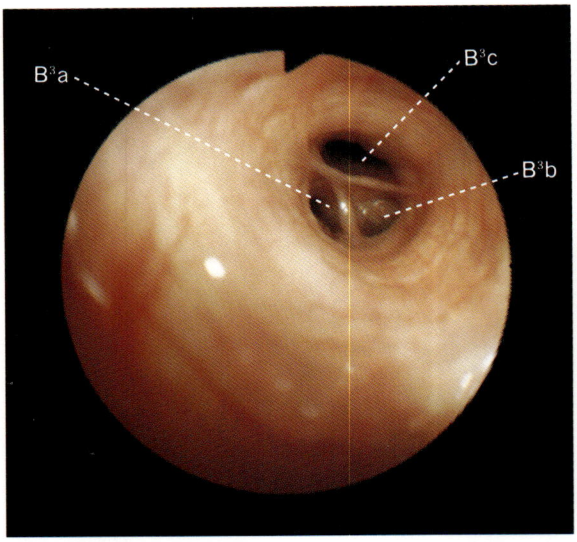

5.37 The orifices of left B^3.

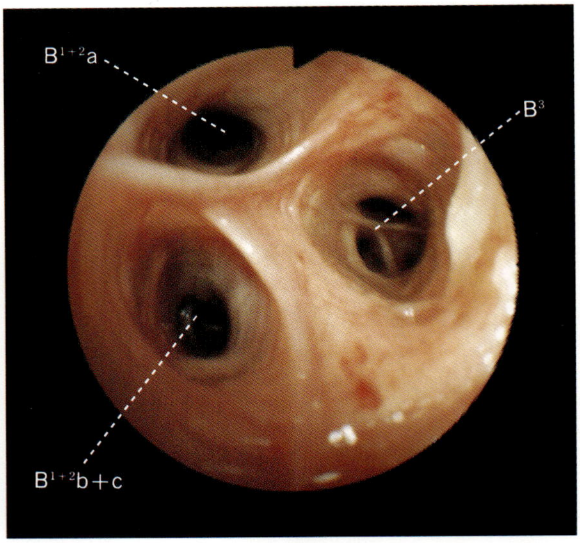

5.38 The orifices of left B^{1+2}.

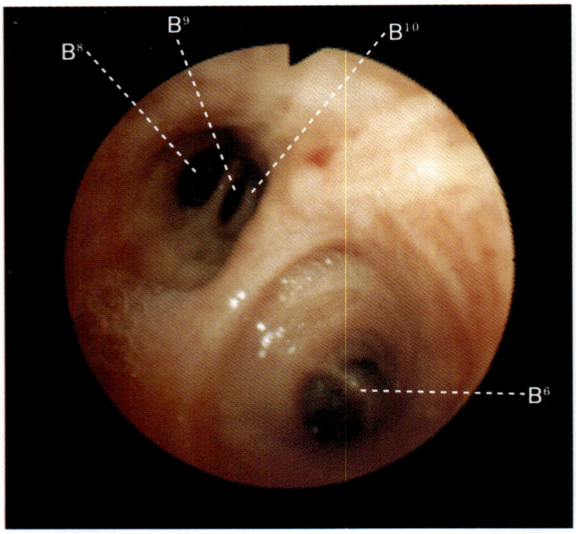

5.39 The orifices of the left lower lobe bronchi. The orifices of B^6 and left basal bronchi are also visible.

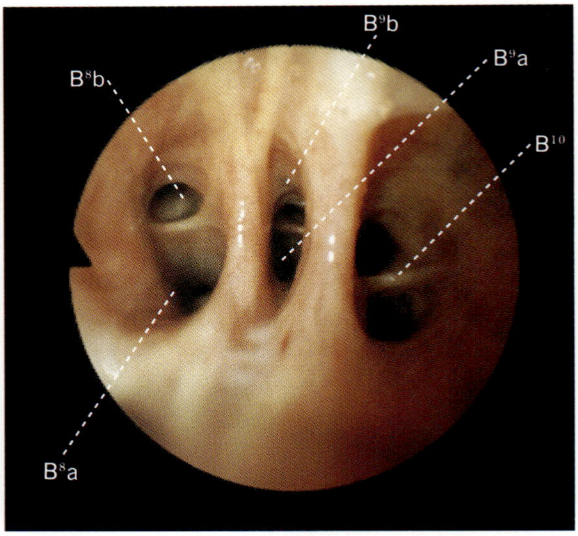

5.40 The orifices of the left basal bronchi, B^8, B^9 and B^{10}.

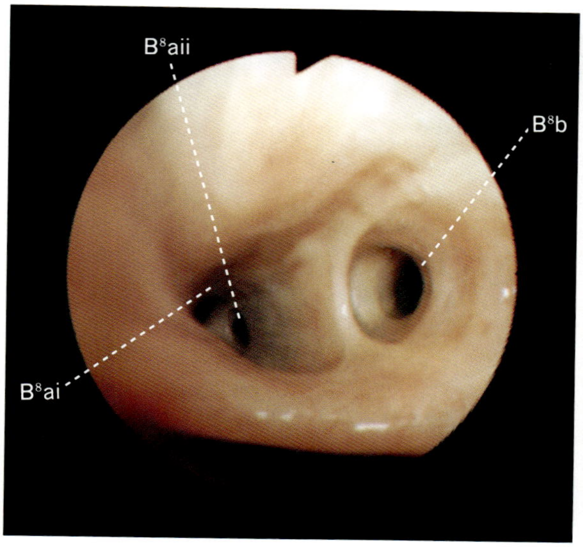

5.41 The orifice of left B^8.

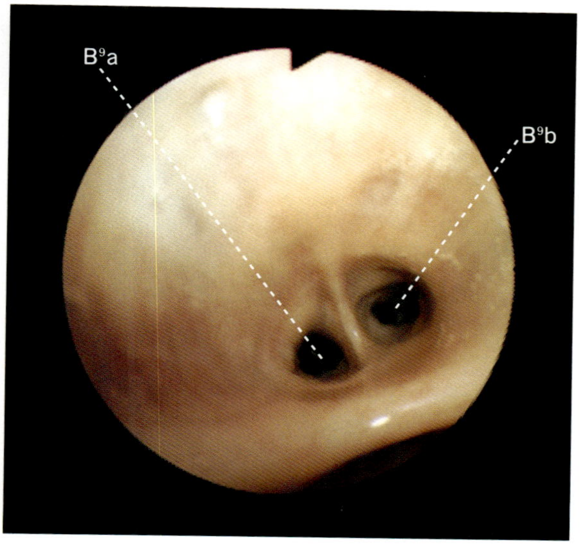

5.42 The orifice of left B^9.

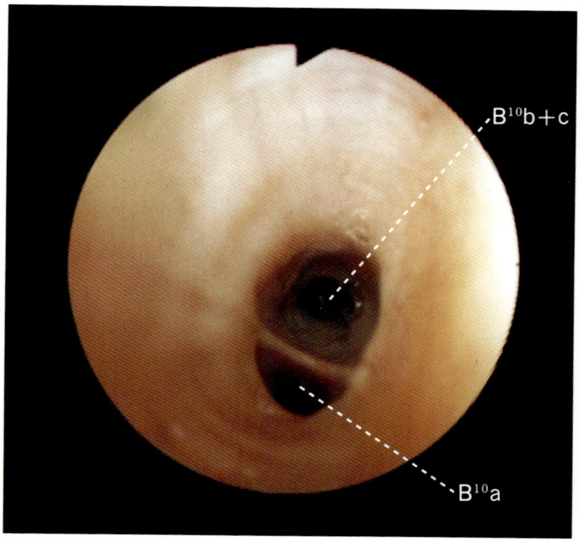

5.43 The orifice of left B^{10}.

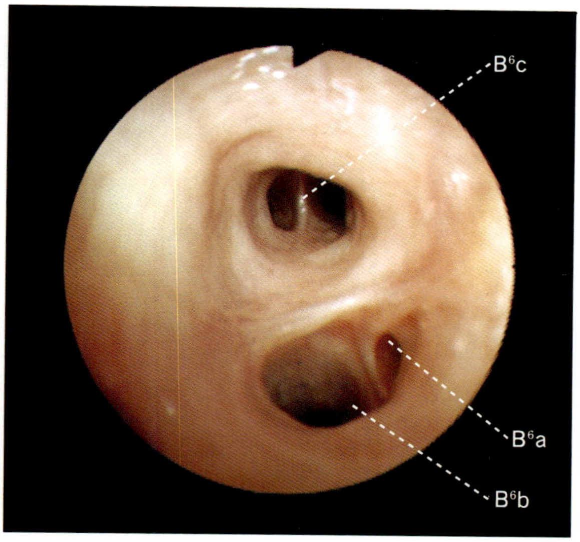

5.44 The orifice of left B^6.

6 The anatomy of the airways and bronchial nomenclature

1 The anatomy of the airways

The airway begins with the oral cavity, nasal cavity, trachea, the right and left main bronchi, lobar bronchi, segmental bronchi and subsegmental bronchi and continues to branch until the 19th division, that is the terminal bronchiole (TB). The areas from the trachea to the terminal bronchioles are called conducting airways, because only air passes through these structures. After this come the respiratory bronchioles (RB), which are divided into three sections—the first, second and third bronchioles (RB^1, RB^2, RB^3), and continue to the alveolar ducts (AD) and terminate at the alveoli.

Conventionally, the conducting airways comprise the trachea, the bronchi, and the non-respiratory bronchioles, including the terminal bronchioles. This omits the obvious fact that respiratory bronchioles also conduct air to more distal respiratory bronchioles, alveolar ducts, and alveoli, but because all these structures participate in gas exchange, they are collectively named as the terminal respiratory units (**6.1**).

The trachea, left and right main bronchi and truncus intermedius have horseshoe-shaped cartilage crescents, usually 16–20 in the trachea, 9–12 in the left main bronchus, 6–8 in the right main bronchus and 4–6 in the truncus intermedius. Each cartilage crescent is connected by ligaments and smooth muscle. The posterior wall of trachea and large bronchi, which is free of cartilage crescents, is referred to as the membranous portion, which has a large amount of smooth muscle.

The main difference between the intrapulmonary bronchus and the extrapulmonary bronchus is the progressive reduction of the cartilage crescents. Figure **6.2** shows how the crescents diminish to intermittent plates of cartilage at the point of transition from the extrapulmonary bronchus to the intrapulmonary bronchus. The layer of elastic fibre between the mucosal epithelium and the submucosa is gradually replaced by smooth muscle, which extends in rings surrounding the entire circumference of the bronchi. Some of the elastic fibre remains consolidated into bundles at intervals between the mucosal epithelium and smooth muscle around the bronchi. These elastic fibre bundles appear as ridges running longitudinally.

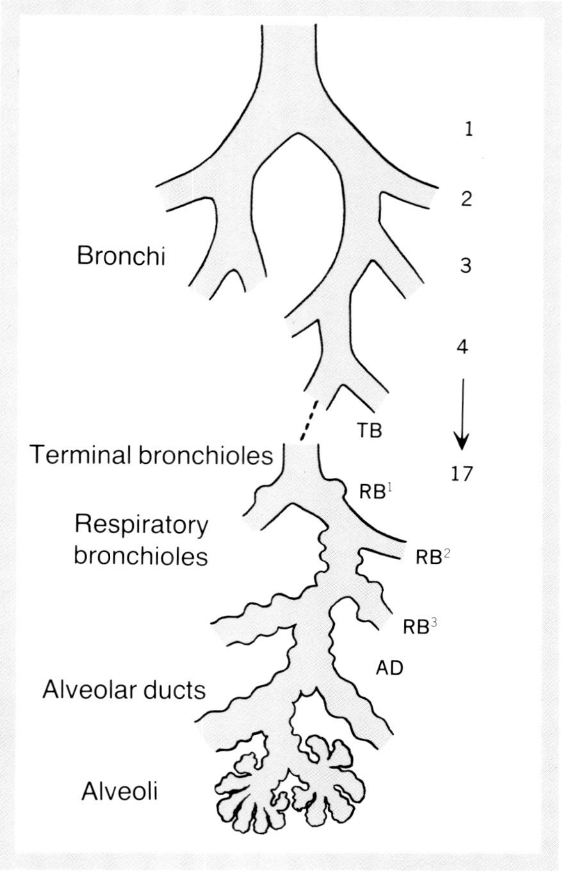

6.1 Bronchial nomenclature commonly used to annotate airways branch network.

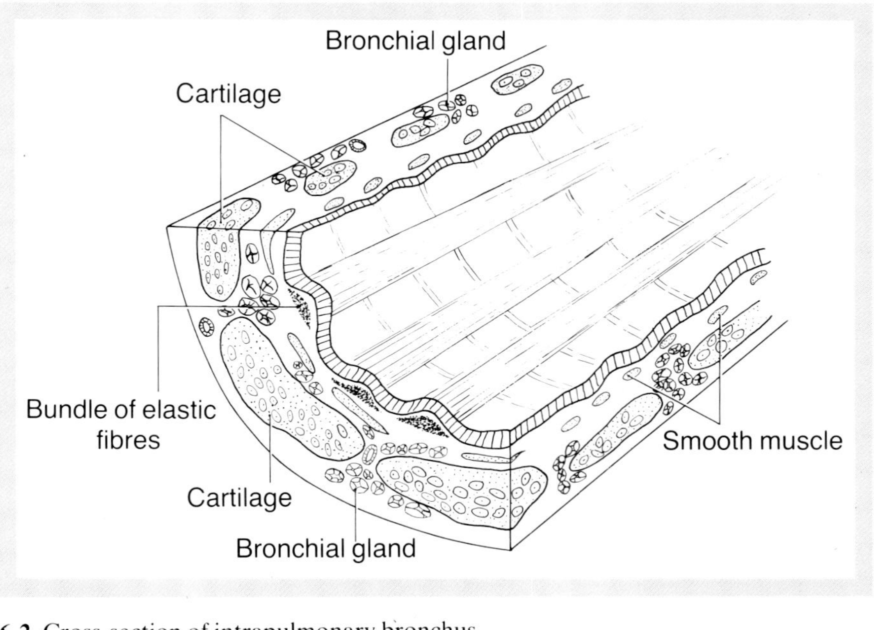

6.2 Cross-section of intrapulmonary bronchus.

2 Bronchial nomenclature

It is very important that general practitioners as well as chest physicians have a thorough knowledge of bronchial nomenclature to pinpoint lesions in chest radiographs.

Jackson's nomenclature (1943[1]) has been used universally. The Japanese Bronchial Nomenclature Committee (1950) widely use a modified version of Jackson's nomenclature. However, this version went up to subsegmental bronchi. The recent progress of fibreoptic bronchoscopy has made it possible to observe from the subsegmental bronchus (IV) to the subsubsegmental bronchus (VI). Therefore, further bronchial nomenclature was necessary.

Figure **6.3**, Table 6.1 and Figure **6.4** show the classification universally used and **6.5** shows the bronchial nomenclature proposed by the Bronchial Nomenclature Committee (Chairman: Prof. Yoshihiro Hayata) at the 1970 annual meeting of the Japan Lung Cancer Society.

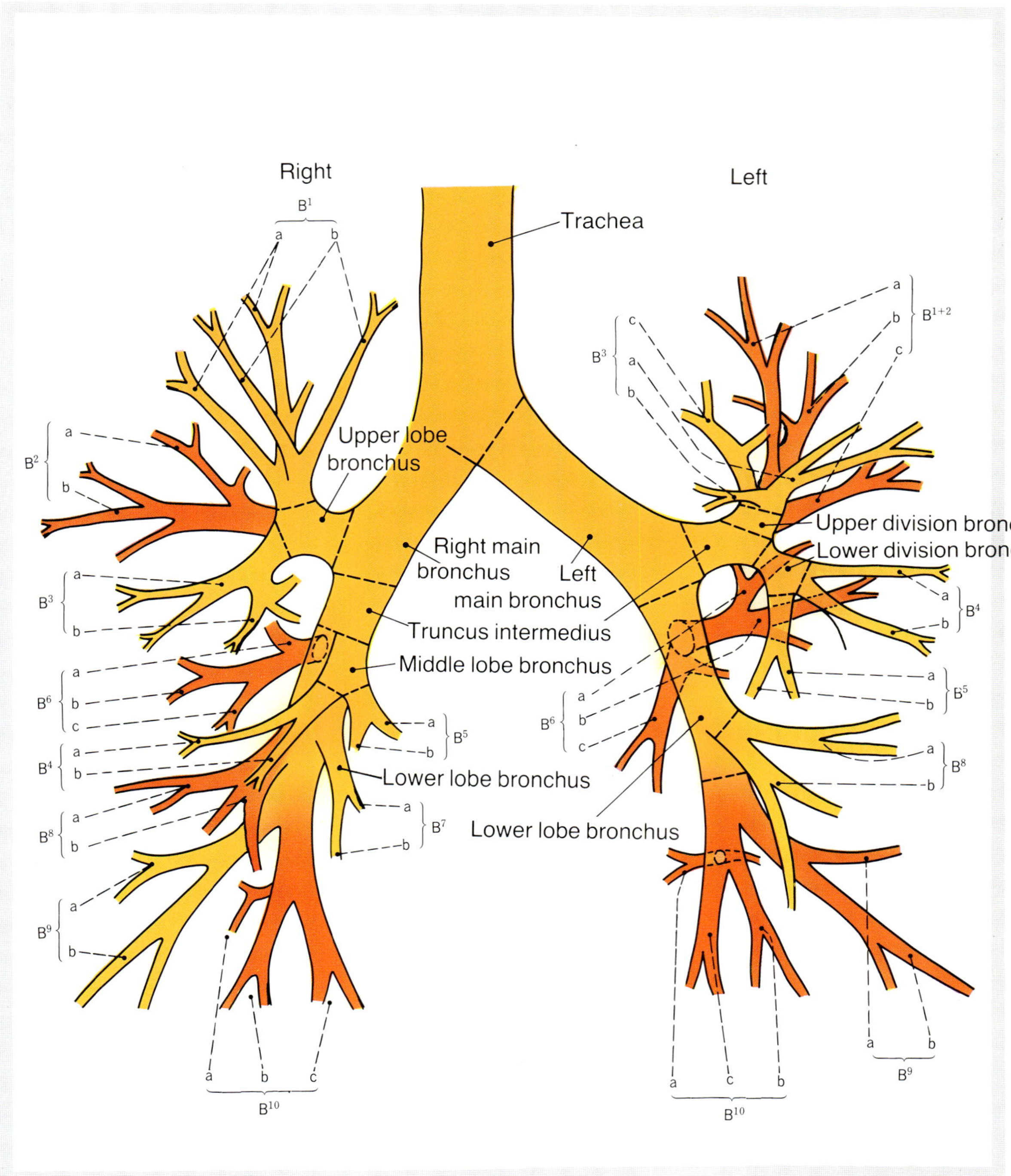

6.3 Bronchial nomenclature universally used.

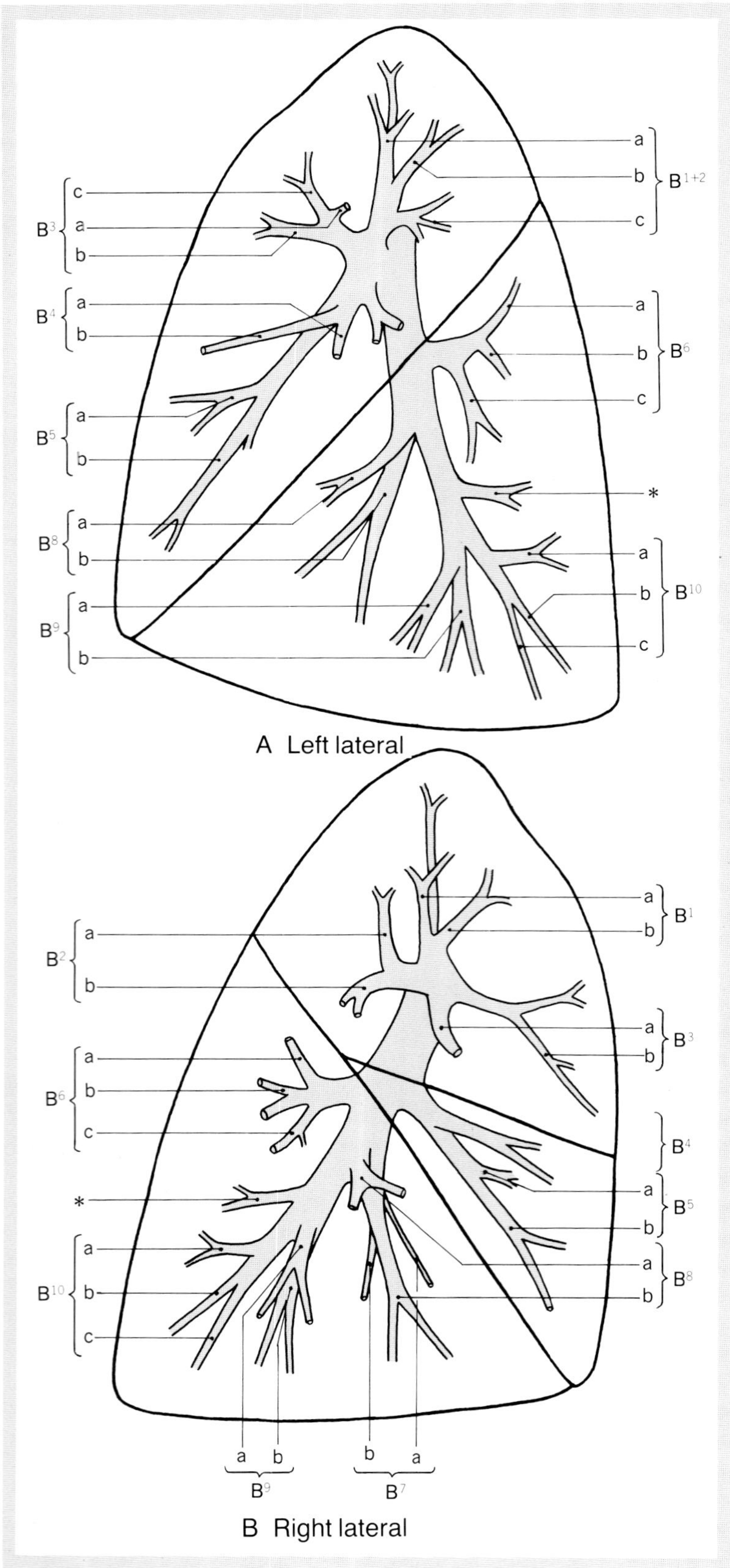

6.4 Nomenclature adopted by the Japanese Committee on Bronchial Nomenclature in 1950.

Table 6.1 Bronchial nomenclature

Right lung			Left lung			
Upper lobe	B^{1}:R. apicalis	a. Rm. apicalis proprius	Upper lobe	upper division bronchus	B^{1+2}: R. apicodorsalis	a. Rm. apicalis
		b. Rm. (subapicalis) ventralis				b. Rm. (subapicalis) dorsalis
	B^{2}: R. (lobi superioris) dorsalis	a. Rm. (subapicalis) dorsalis				c. Rm. (lobi sup.) horizontalis
		b. Rm. (lobi sup.) horizontalis			B^{3}: R. (lobi superioris) ventralis	a. Rm. (lobi sup. ventr.) lateralis
	B^{3}: R. (lobi superioris) ventralis	a. Rm. (lobi sup. ventr.) lateralis				b. Rm. (lobi sup. ventr.) medialis
		b. Rm. (lobi sup. ventr.) medialis				c. Rm. (lobi sup. ventr.) superior
Middle lobe	B^{4}: R. medius lateralis	a. Rm. lateralis		lower division bronchus	B^{4}: R. lingualis superior	a. Rm. lateralis ventralis
		b. Rm. medialis				b. Rm. (lobi sup.) ventralis
	B^{5}: R. medius medialis	a. Rm. lateralis			B^{5}: R. lingualis inferior	a. Rm. superior
		b. Rm. medialis				b. Rm. inferior
Lower lobe	B^{6}: R. (lobi inferioris) superior	a. Rm. superior	Lower lobe		B^{6}: R. (lobi inferioris) superior	a. Rm. superior
		b. Rm. lateralis				b. Rm. lateralis
		c. Rm. medialis				c. Rm. medialis
	B^{*}: R. (lobi inferioris) subsuperior				B^{*}: R. (lobi inferioris) subsuperior	
	B^{7}: R. mediobasalis	a. Rm. dorsalis			superior	
		b. Rm. ventralis				
	B^{8}: R. ventrobasalis	a. Rm. lateralis			B^{8}: R. ventrobasalis	a. Rm. lateralis
		b. Rm. basalis				b. Rm. basalis
	B^{9}: R. laterobasalis	a. Rm. lateralis			B^{9}: R. laterobasalis	a. Rm. lateralis
		b. Rm. basalis				b. Rm. basalis
	B^{10}: R. dorsobasalis	a. Rm. dorsalis			B^{10}: R. dorsalis	a. Rm. dorsalis
		b. Rm. lateralis				b. Rm. lateralis
		c. Rm. medialis				c. Rm. medialis

Reference

[1] Jackson, C.L., Huber, J.F., Correlated applied anatomy of the bronchial tree and lungs with a system of nomenclature. *Dis. Chest*, **9**: 319, 1943.

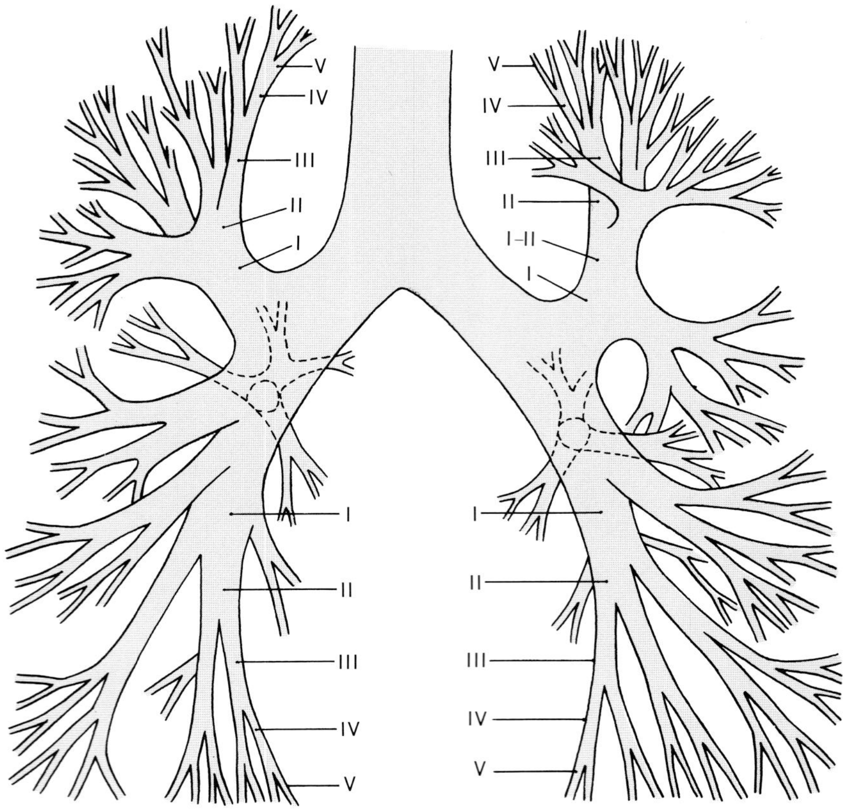

Lobar bronchus	Order I
Division bronchus	Order I-II
Segmental bronchus	Order II B1
Sub-segmental bronchus	Order III . . . . a b
Sub-segmental bronchus	Order IV . . . . . i ii
	Order V . . . *a* β

6.5 Bronchial nomenclature. Proposal made by the Bronchial Nomenclature Committee (Chairman: Prof. Yoshihiro Hayata) to the 1970 annual meeting of the Japan Lung Cancer Society.

7 Normal bronchoscopic findings

1 Bronchoscopic findings in the tracheal and bronchial mucous membrane

When bronchoscopy is carried out, it is essential to note with utmost care the condition of lumina, especially their colour, shape and movement. In the normal bronchus, white cartilage rings alternate with reddish mucous membrane. The trachea has 16 to 20 cartilage rings, which do not extend to the posterior wall, which is the membranous portion. During a cough, this membranous portion protrudes into the lumen. The trachea divides into two main bronchi, the right and left main bronchus, and these undergo further subdivision into primary, secondary and tertiary bronchi. With each progressive division, the cartilage rings become less distinct. During a cough the entire lumen becomes smaller. Especially in the left main bronchus and in the vicinity of the opening into the left upper lobe bronchus, the pulsation of the heart and the aorta is transmitted to the bronchial walls.

When the surface of the bronchial mucous membrane is observed with a bronchofibrescope, the light penetrates the tissue to a depth of 0.5 mm, the thickness of the lamina propria mucosae. Usually the colour of the bronchial mucous membrane is that of the lamina propria mucosae seen through the mucous epithelium and basement membrane and in which exist white elastic fibres, small vessels and anthracosis. Especially, the vascular findings reflect the condition of the subepithelial mucous membrane and provide information useful for analysing the various bronchoscopic findings[1].

The bronchoscopic appearance of the mucous membrane naturally varies according to age and sex, and is also influenced by environmental factors. The contours of the folds of the mucous membrane are distinct in young people and visible in segmental and subsegmental bronchi. With advancing age, the contours become obscure as a result of a decrease of elastic fibres and an increase of collagen fibres. The cartilage becomes more prominent as a result of atrophy of the lamina propria mucosae and the smooth mucle fibres. In smokers or people who have worked for many years in a dusty environment, the bronchial mucous membrane exhibits deposits of inhaled substances and may become blackish. The bronchial mucous membrane of a young person is reddish overall and the cartilage rings are not so prominent.

Figures **7.1–7.8** show bronchoscopic findings in the orifices of the right upper lobe segmental bronchi, demonstrating differences of age and sex.

7.1 The overall colour is red and the cartilage is not very prominent (23-year-old male).

7.2 The cartilage has begun to be prominent and circular folds of mucous membrane can be seen in B^1 and B^3 (40-year-old male).

7.3 Shows marked atrophy of the lamina propria mucosae and the smooth muscle layer. The circular folds have disappeared, leaving only the cartilaginous component. The surface of the mucous membrane is yellowish and anthracosis is present (74-year-old male).

7.4 The mucous membrane exhibits an overall reddish colour and the upper region is moist and oedematous. Such bronchoscopic findings are especially common in young women during menstruation, because of an increase of goblet cells in the mucosal epithelium[2] (23-year-old female).

7.5 The lamina propria mucosae shows a slight atrophy and the cartilaginous component has begun to be prominent (48-year-old female).

7.6 The findings are similar to those of the 74-year-old male in **7.3**: atrophy of the lamina propria mucosae and the smooth muscle layer is evident, the circular folds have completely disappeared and the cartilaginous component remains (75-year-old female).

(Illustrations to above captions on next page)

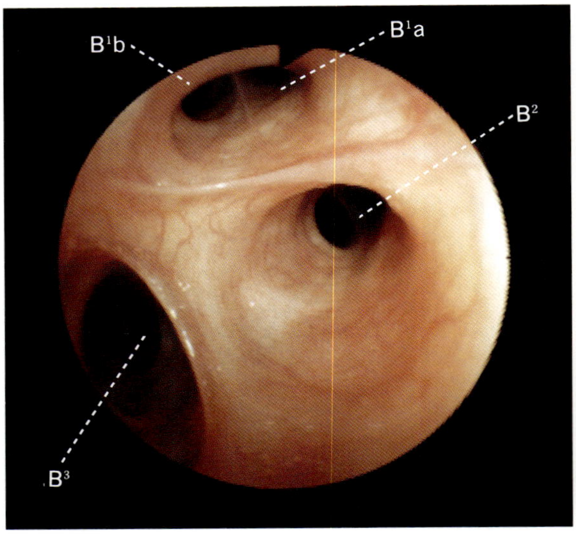

7.1

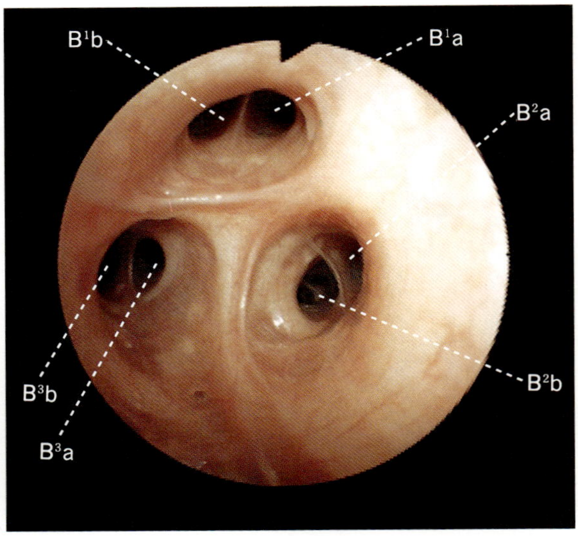

7.2

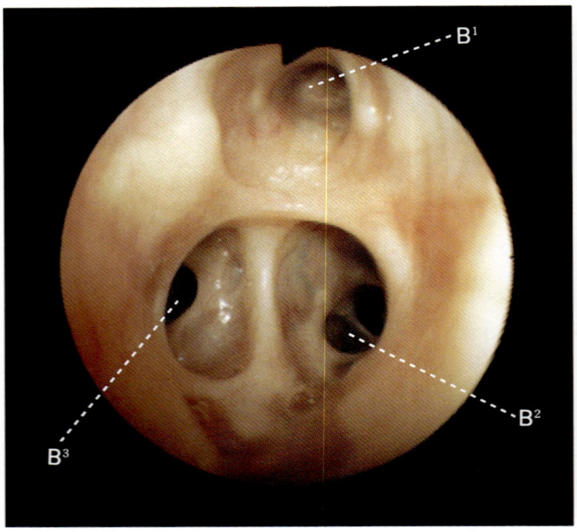

7.3

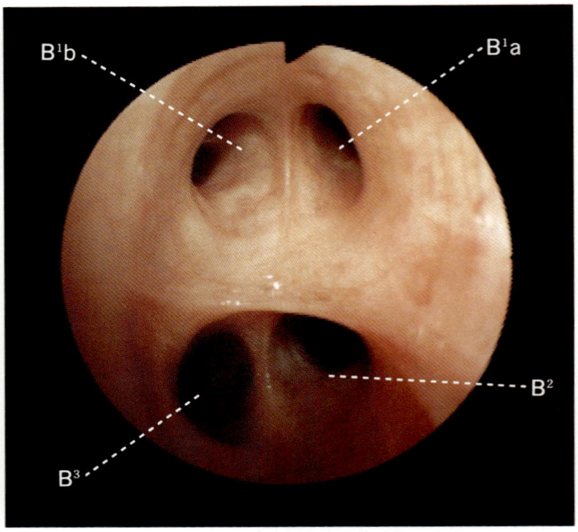

7.4

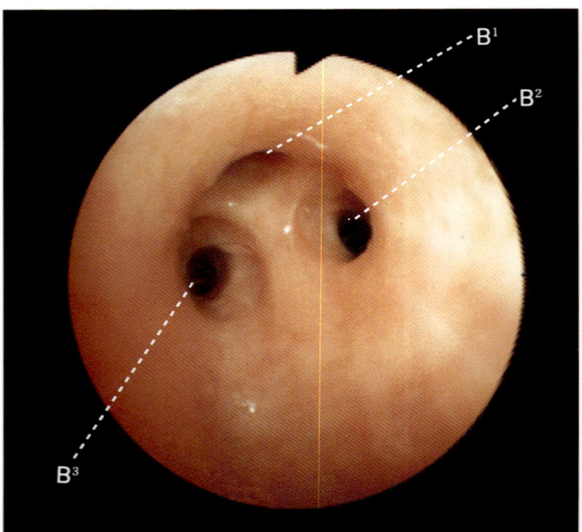

7.5

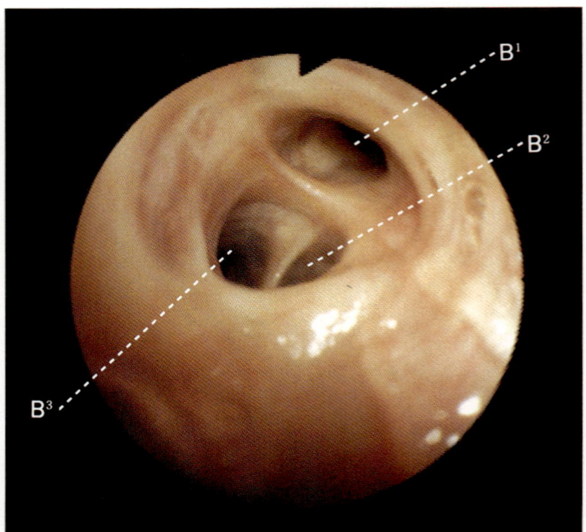

7.6

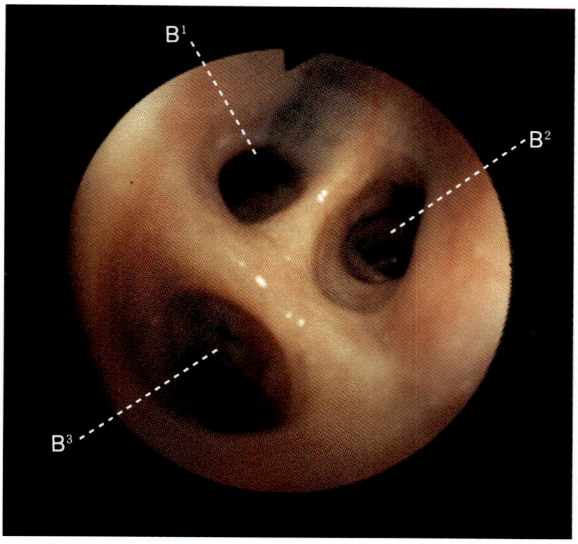

7.7 Anthracosis is evident at the orifices to B^1 and B^3 (75-year-old female smoker).

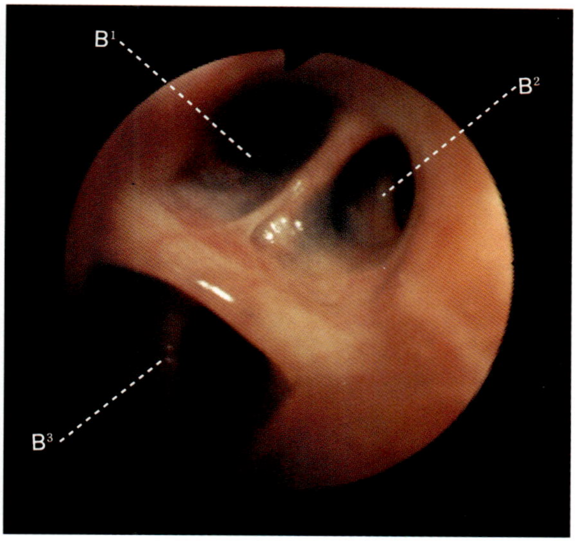

7.8 Anthracosis is evident at the orifices to B^2 (75-year-old female, who is a non-smoker but who was engaged in agriculture for several years).

2 Nomenclature of the branching of the right upper lobe bronchi

Branching anomalies of the bronchi are seen routinely in a daily practice. Because these branching anomalies are usually associated with branching anomalies of vasculature, a clear understanding of these branching patterns is absolutely essential before surgery is undertaken.

There are several variations of bronchial branching in the right upper lobe, so that the complete trifurcation pattern, the so-called standard, is found in at most 38 per cent of cases[3]. Various patterns of branching anomalies of the right upper lobe bronchi are shown in **7.9**. A is the standard pattern. In B, the apical bronchus (B^1) is divided into two branches, one arising from B^3 and the other from B^2. This pattern is present in a fairly high percentage (30 per cent), but it is extremely difficult to identify by fibreoptic bronchoscopy. In C, the horizontal branch (B^{2b}) of the posterior branch (B^2) is dislocated anteriorly, and arises opposite to the apical bronchus (B^1), resulting in four-way branching of the upper lobe bronchus. This pattern is found in about 16 per cent. In D, the apical bronchus (B^1) arises close to the origin of the anterior bronchus (B^3); this pattern is seen in about 10 per cent[3, 4].

Figure **7.10** presents schematic diagrams of these branching patterns of the right upper lobe bronchi as they appear through a bronchoscope (based on the author's modification of the classification of Professor Kenkichi Oho[1]). Diagrams A-E show the branching pattern of complete trifurcation (figures in parentheses indicate the incidence of each subgroup): A, 'standard' trifurcation (about 60 per cent); B, Y-shaped trifurcation (about 25 per cent); C, inverted Y-shaped trifurcation (about 10 per cent); D, parallel trifurcation (about 10 per cent), and E, I-shaped trifurcation (very rare). Diagrams F-L show the other branching patterns: F $B^1 + B^2$, B^3 division; G complete anteroposterior bifurcation ($B^1 + B^2$, B^3); H B^1, $B^2 + B^3$ division; I complete vertical bifurcation (B^1, $B^2 + B^3$); J $B^1 + B^3$, B^2 division, and K and L four-way division. Patterns F and H are the next most common to complete trifurcation, with an incidence of about 20 per cent each.

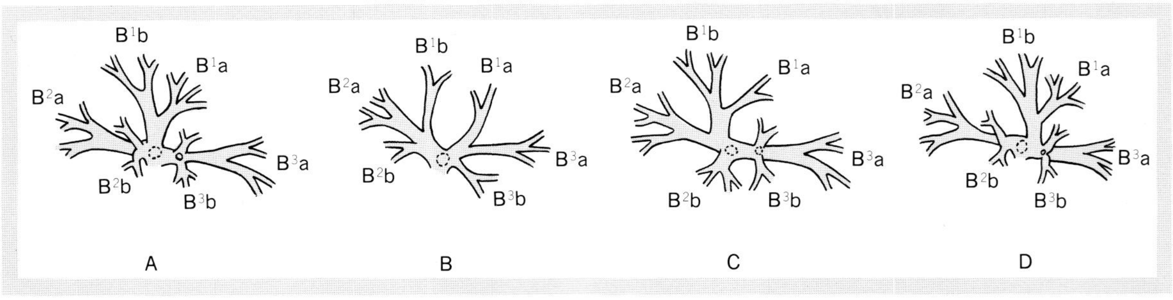

7.9 Various patterns of branching anomalies of the right upper lobe bronchi (lateral view).

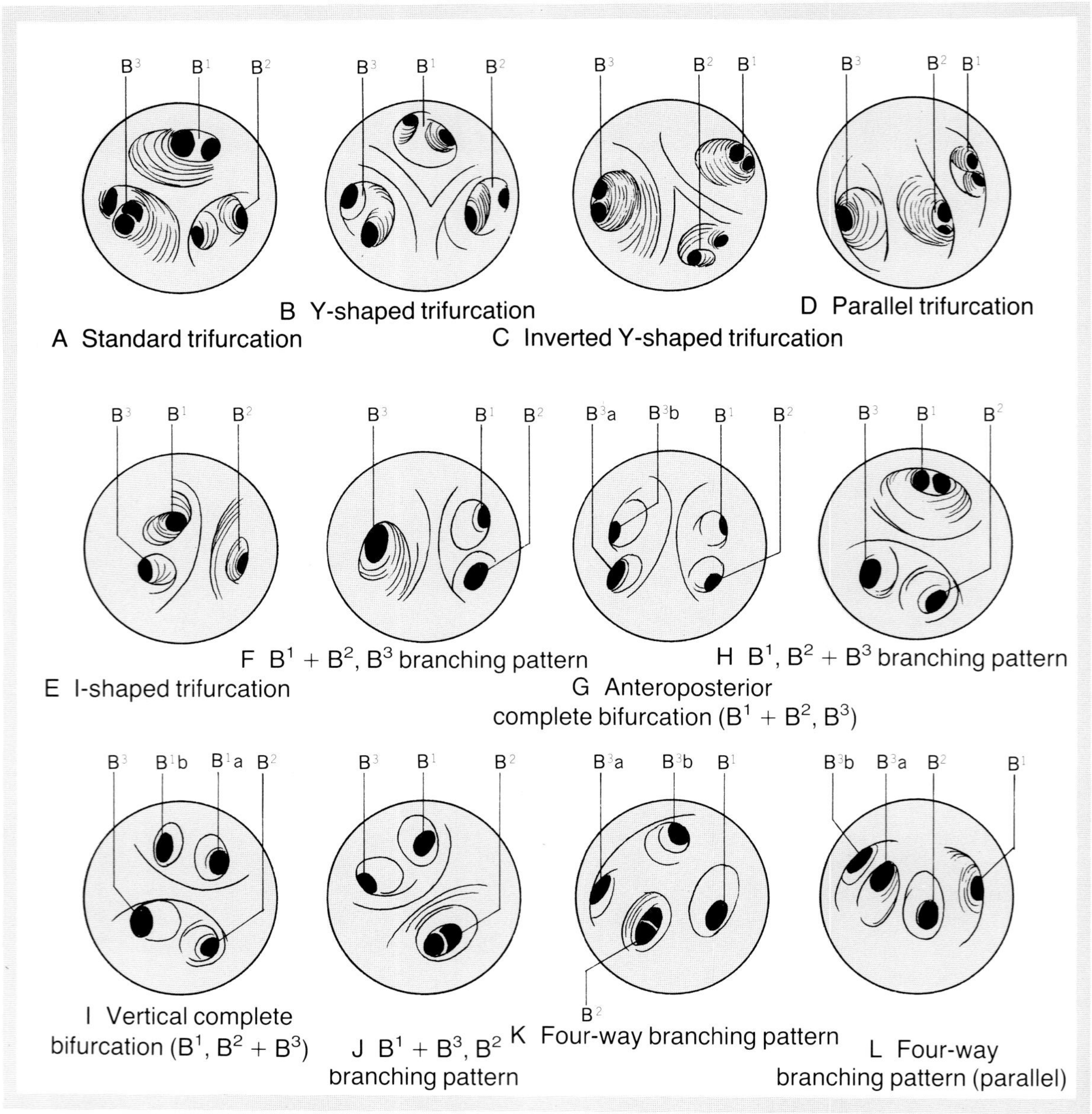

7.10 Branching patterns of the right upper lobe bronchi: A standard trifurcation; B Y-shaped trifurcation; C inverted Y-shaped trifurcation; D parallel trifurcation; E I-shaped trifurcation; F B^{1+2}, B^3 branching pattern; G anteroposterior complete bifurcation (B^{1+2}, B^3) H B^1, B^{2+3} branching pattern; I vertical complete bifurcation (B^1, B^{2+3}); J B^{1+3}, B^2 branching pattern; K four-way branching pattern; L four-way branching pattern (parallel).

3 Nomenclature of the branching of the right middle lobe bronchi

The right middle lobe bronchus divides into two segmental bronchi, B^4 laterally (to the right) and B^5 mediastinally. The nomenclature of the middle lobe bronchi in **7.11** is that of Dr Oho[1]. In the case of a branching pattern such as seen in diagram A, the bronchi are named B^4a, B^4b, B^5b in the zigzag order pattern. In the case of a branching pattern such as that in diagram B, the bronchi are named B^4a, B^4b, B^5a, and B^5b from right to left. Vertical complete bifurcation and trifurcation branching patterns are occasionally seen in the middle lobe bronchi. The branching pattern of middle lobe bronchi is illustrated in **7.12**.

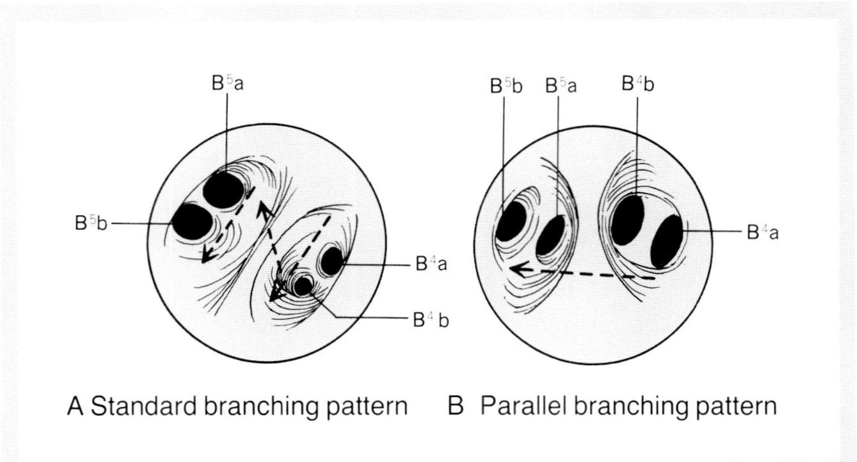

7.11 Nomenclature of the right middle lobe:
A standard branching pattern; B parallel branching pattern.

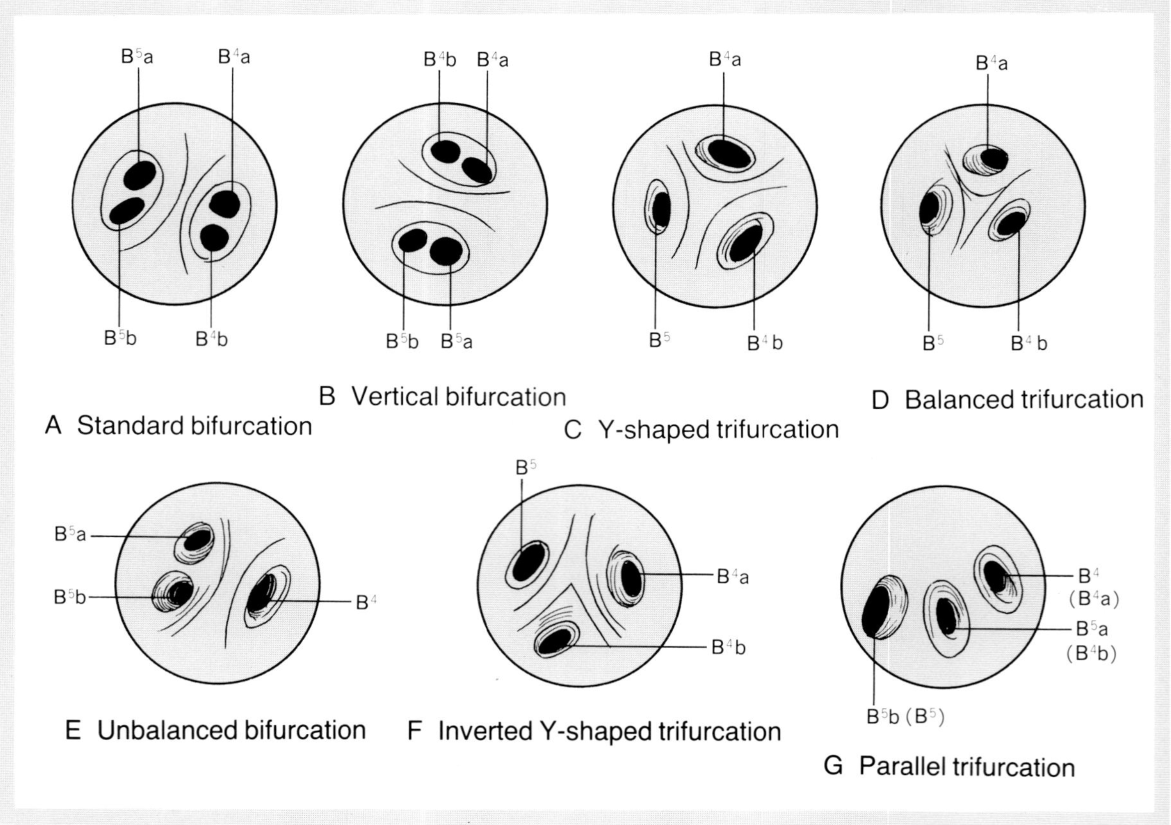

7.12 Branching patterns of the right middle lobe bronchi: A standard bifurcation; B vertical bifurcation; C Y-shaped trifurcation; D balanced trifurcation; E unbalanced bifurcation; F inverted Y-shaped trifurcation; G parallel trifurcation.

4 Nomenclature of the branching of the right lower lobe bronchi

There are several variations of the segmental bronchi of the right lower lobe, and these are shown in Figure **7.13** with the nomenclature of Dr Oho. In A the overall view of the bronchi of the right lower lobe is shown, and the bronchi are named starting at B^6 and moving spirally in a clockwise direction: B^6, B^7a, B^7b, B^8, B^9, B^{10}. B shows the nomenclature of the subsegmental bronchi of right B^6 and B^{10}, and the letters a, b, and c named in an anti-clockwise direction starting at the most central branching, B^6a or B^{10}a. In C the nomenclature of the right B^8 and B^9 is shown, and the letters a and b named from lateral to mediastinal subsegmental bronchi.

Figure **7.14** presents schematic diagrams of the branching patterns of the right lower lobe bronchi through a fibreoptic bronchoscope. In the linear pattern shown in A, B^8, B^9, and B^{10} are named in a straight lateral to medial (mediastinal), and there is a thick mucosal fold between B^8 and B^9. The linear pattern in B is similar, but there is no thick mucosal fold. In C B^8, B^9, and B^{10} are named in a left-curving line, D shows a linear pattern; a thick mucosal fold is visible between B^9 and B^{10}. In E B^8, B^9, and B^{10} are named in a right-curving line.

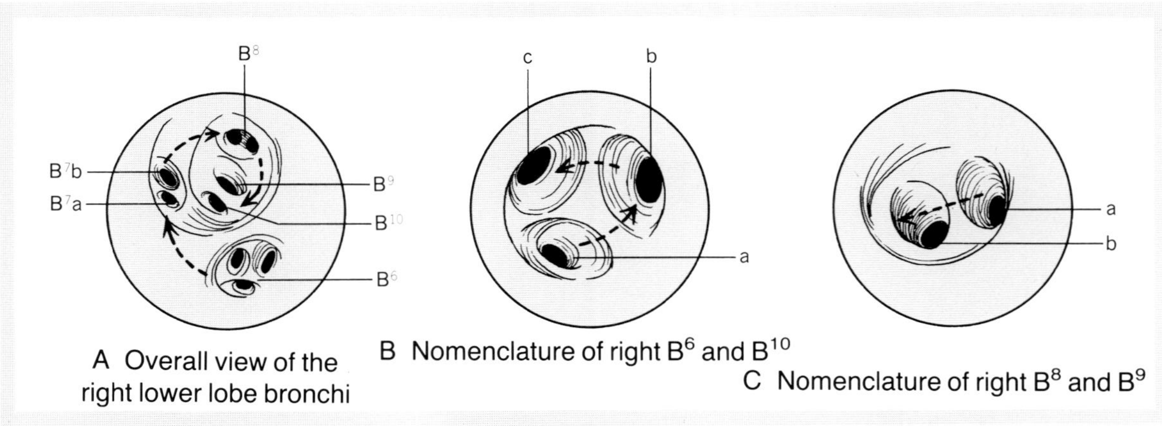

7.13 Nomenclature of the right lower lobe bronchi: A overall view of the right lower lobe bronchi; B nomenclature of right B^6 and B^{10}; C nomenclature of right B^8 and B^9.

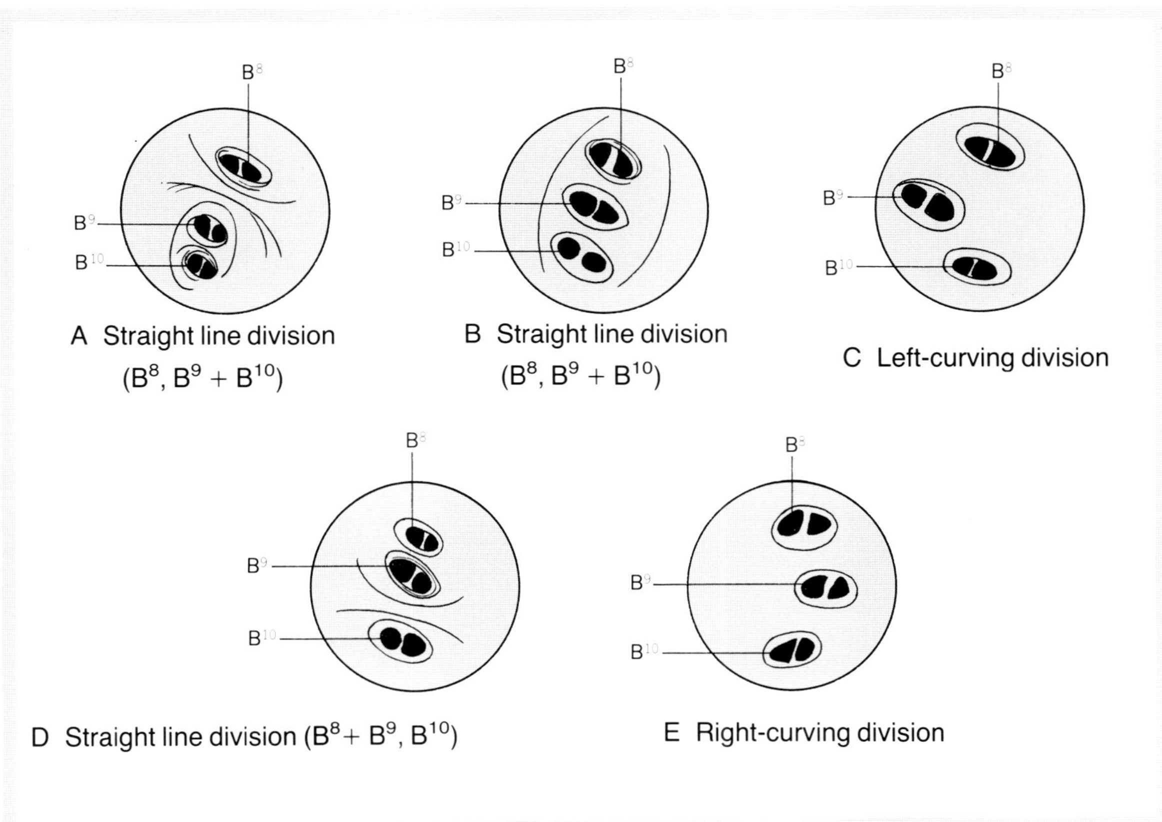

7.14 Branching patterns of the right lower lobe bronchi: A Straight line division (B^8, B^{9+10}); B Straight line division (B^8, B^9, B^{10}); C left-curving division; D Straight line division (B^{8+9}, B^{10}); E right-curving division.

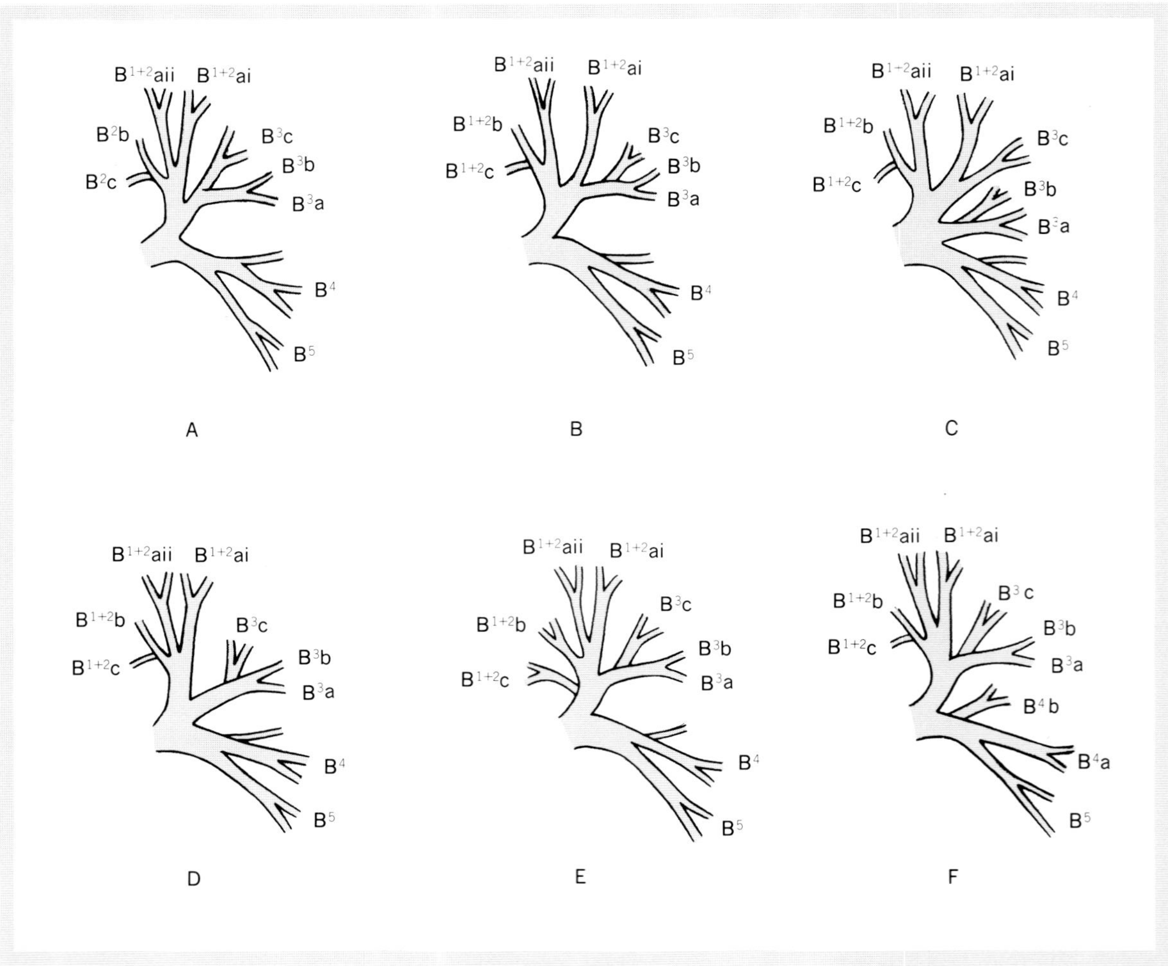

7.15 Various patterns of branching anomalies of the left upper lobe bronchi (oblique view I).

5 Nomenclature of the branching of the left upper lobe bronchi

The left upper lobe bronchi, especially the upper division bronchus, exhibit numerous variations, and it is difficult to specify the nomenclature of this region. The patterns illustrated in **7.15** are modifications of those described by Boyden[3,4]. A shows the 'standard' branching pattern. In B, the apical bronchus divides into two bronchi; this pattern is seen in 38 per cent. A trifurcation is found in 27 per cent of left upper lobe bronchi: the pattern shown in C, in which the apical bronchus is divided, accounts for 21 per cent. In the remaining 6 per cent B^3 forms the central branch (D). In E the horizontal branch of the posterior segmental bronchus (B^{1+2}) is dislocated inferiorly, and the apicoposterior bronchus is trifurcated superiorly. In F B^4b is dislocated superiorly, and arises directly from the lingular bronchus, creating a mediolateral pattern similar to that of the right middle lobe. This branching pattern is found in 15 per cent.

Figure **7.16** shows Dr Oho's nomenclature of the upper division bronchus, which depends on where B^{1+2} arises. The pattern of

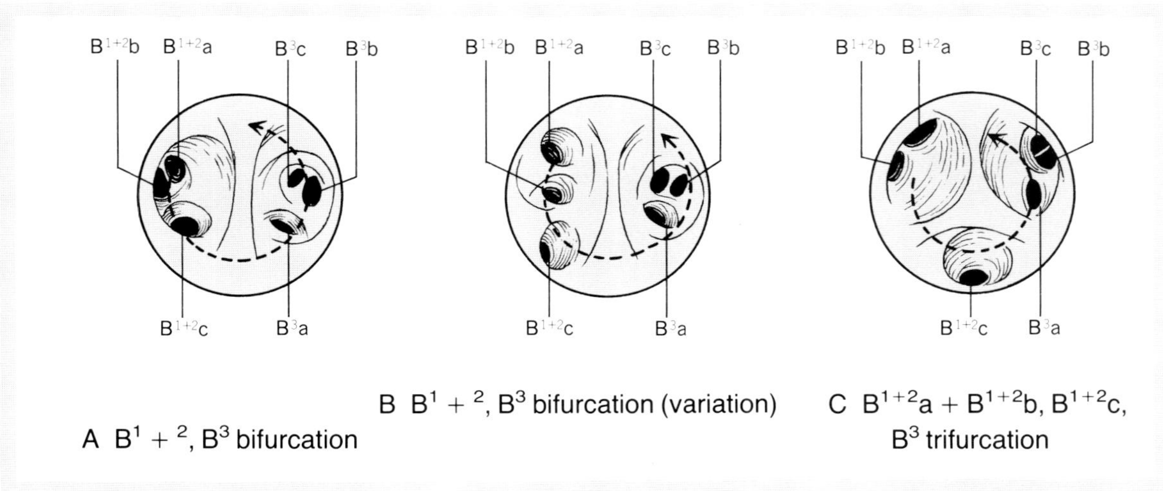

7.16 Nomenclature of the upper division bronchus of the left upper lobe: A B^{1+2}, B^3 bifurcation; B B^{1+2}, B^3 bifurcation (variation); C $B^{1+2}a + B^{1+2}b$, $B^{1+2}c$, B^3 trifurcation.

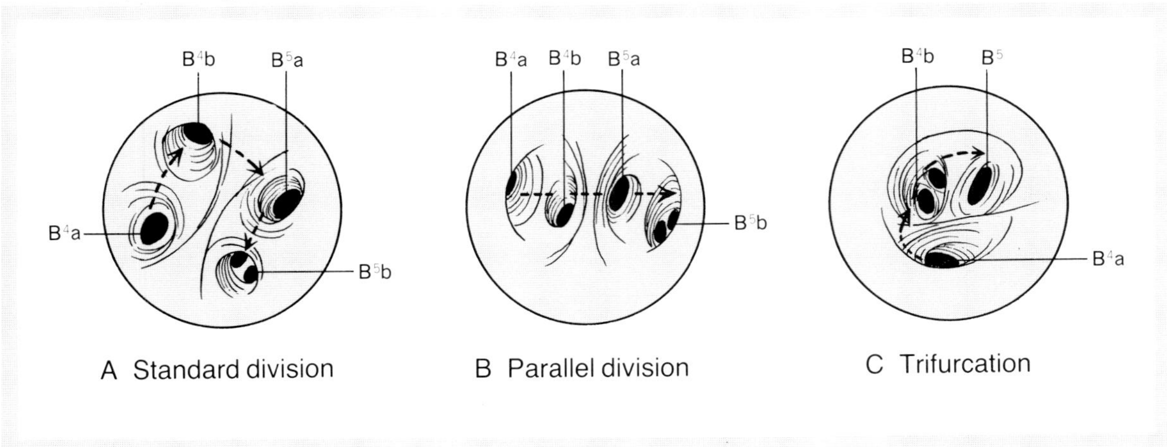

7.17 Nomenclature of the lower division bronchus: A standard division; B parallel division; C trifurcation.

bifurcation into B^{1+2} and B^3 occurs in 72 per cent. In the remainder, B^{1+2} branches directly from the upper division bronchus. A shows a pattern of bifurcation into B^{1+2} and B^3, with B^{1+2} branching peripherally. B shows bifurcation into B^{1+2} and B^3, with B^{1+2} branching from central portion. C shows trifurcation into $B^{1+2}a + B^{1+2}b$, $B^{1+2}c$, and B^3.

The nomenclature of the lower division bronchus of the left upper lobe is shown in **7.17**. Diagrams A and B belong to Dr Oho, while diagram C has been added by the author. The lingular segmental bronchi B^4 and B^5 branch parallel or at an angle slightly laterally. B^4a is the most lateral and branches dorsally, and is usually designated as the starting point in a clockwise direction: B^4a, B^4b, B^5a, and B^5b. A shows the 'standard' pattern. B is a pattern of parallel division, and its incidence is low. C shows a trifurcation, the next most common to the 'standard' pattern.

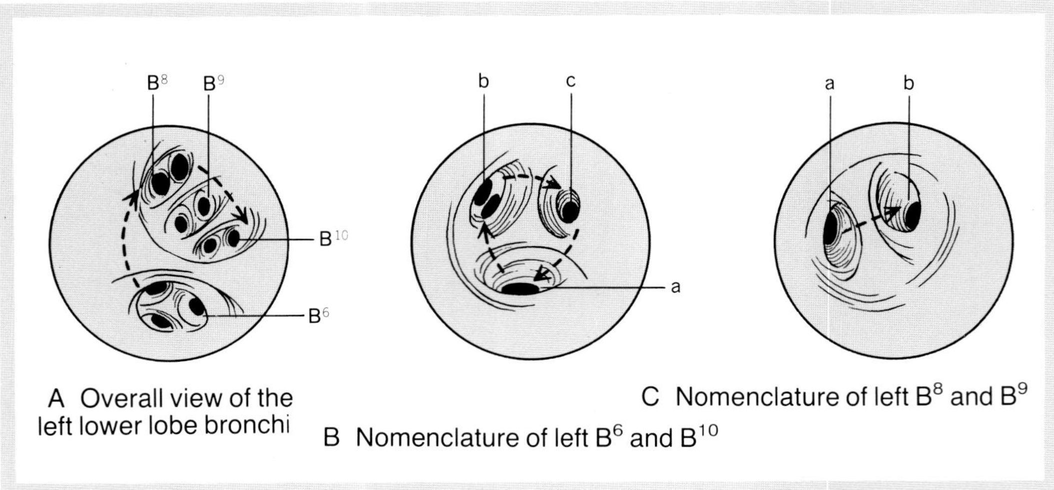

7.18 Nomenclature of left lower lobe bronchi:
A overall view of the left lower lobe bronchi; B nomenclature of left B^6 and B^{10}; C nomenclature of left B^8 and B^9.

References

[1] K. Oho and R. Amemiya, *Practical Fibreoptic Bronchoscopy*. Igaku-Shoin, Tokyo, 1981.

[2] Chalon, J., Leow, D.A.Y., Orkin, L.R. Tracheobronchial cytologic change during the menstrual cycle. *JAMA,* **218**: 1928, 1971.

[3] Boyden, E.A., *Segmental Anatomy of the Lungs*. A Study of the Patterns of the Segmental Bronchi and Related Pulmonary Vessels, McGraw-Hill, New York, 1955.

[4] Boyden, E.A., Developmental anomalies of the lungs. *Am. J. Surg.,* **89**: 79, 1955.

[5] Yamashita, H., *Roentgenologic Anatomy of the Lung*. Igaku-Shoin, Tokyo & New York, 1978.

6 Nomenclature of the branching of the left lower lobe bronchi

Branching anomalies of the left lower lobe bronchi are relatively rare. But a branch corresponding to the right B^7, or a B^* near the opening to the basal bronchus are occasionally seen. Figure **7.18** shows Dr Oho's nomenclature. A shows the overall nomenclature of the left lower lobe bronchi, and the bronchi are named starting at B^6 and moving in a clockwise direction: B^6, B^8, B^9, and B^{10}. B shows the nomenclature of the subsegmental bronchi of left B^6 and B^{10}, and the letters a, b, and c are positioned in a clockwise direction starting at the most central branch, B^6a or B^{10}a. In C the nomenclature of left B^8 and B^9 is shown, and the letters a and b are positioned from the lateral to the mediastinal. Trifurcation of B^6 is found occasionally.

Figures **7.19–7.149** show normal bronchoscopic findings.

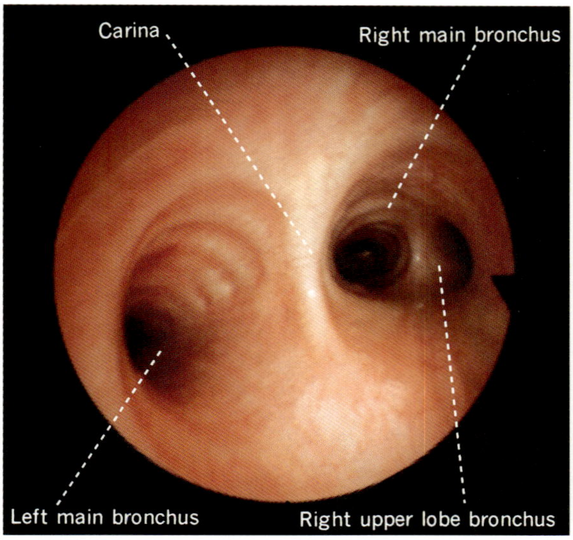

7.19 Carina (23-year-old female). This bronchoscopic photograph shows the most common type of carina, presenting as a sharp line. The trachea divides at the carina into the right and left main bronchi; about 2 cm below the carina the right upper bronchus branches from the right main bronchus. The folds of the membranous part divide into the right and left main bronchi. The left upper bronchus branches from the left main bronchus about 4 cm below the carina.

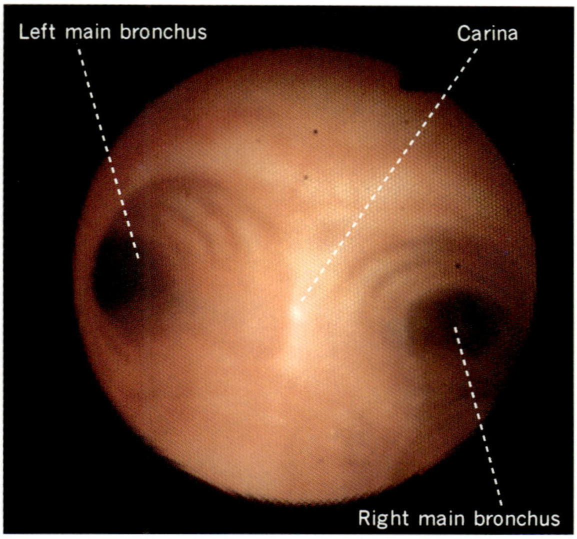

7.20 Carina (49-year-old female). The bifurcation angle is relatively wide. A distinct, linear structure is not visible at the carina.

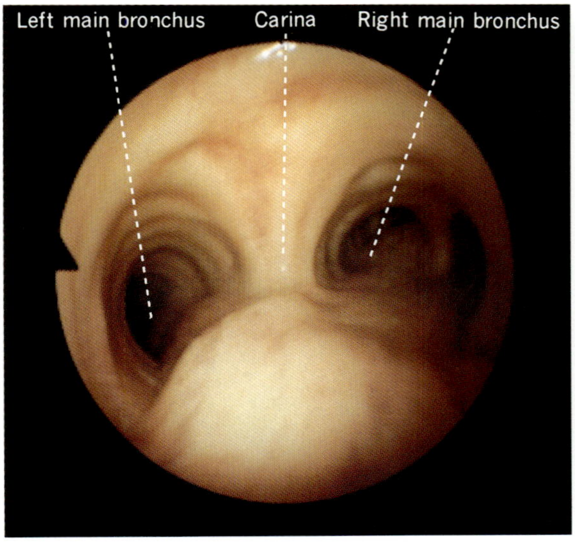

7.21 Carina (79-year-old male). The carina is thick and broad. The bifurcation angle is sharp. The openings into right and left bronchi are visible. Atrophy of mucous membrane is marked and cartilage rings are prominent. The folds of the membranous part are indistinct.

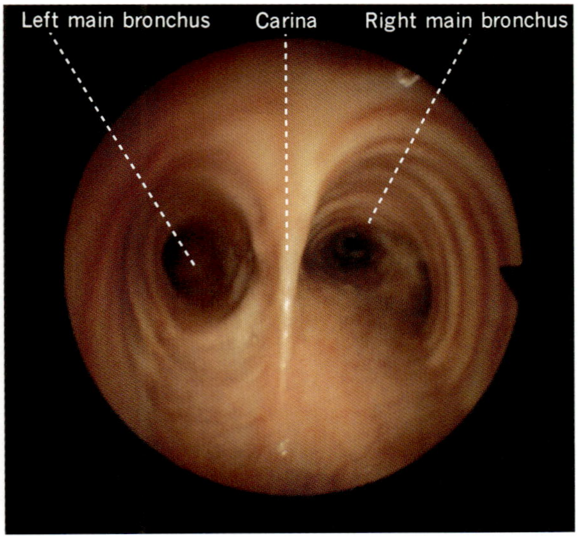

7.22 Carina (70-year-old male). The carina is thin and linear and the bifurcation angle is relatively sharp. The cartilage rings are prominent and result from atrophy of the mucous membrane.

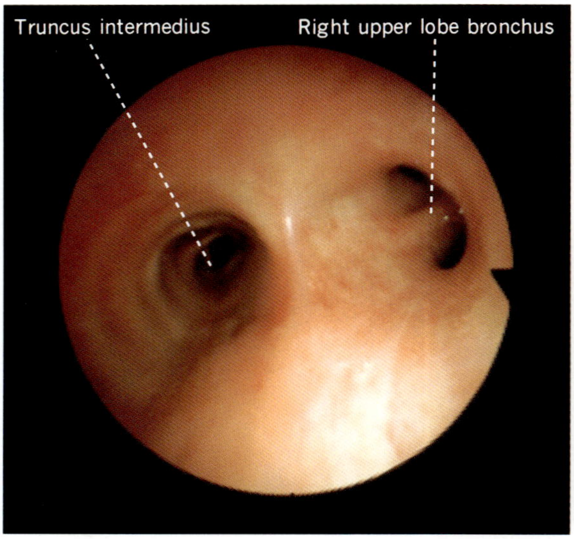

7.23 Right main bronchus: the bifurcation into the truncus intermedius and right upper lobe bronchus. The right upper lobe bronchus arises from the lateral side of the thick right main bronchus about 2 cm from the carina. The bifurcation angle is relatively wide. The longitudinal mucosal folds divide to the truncus intermedius and upper lobe bronchus.

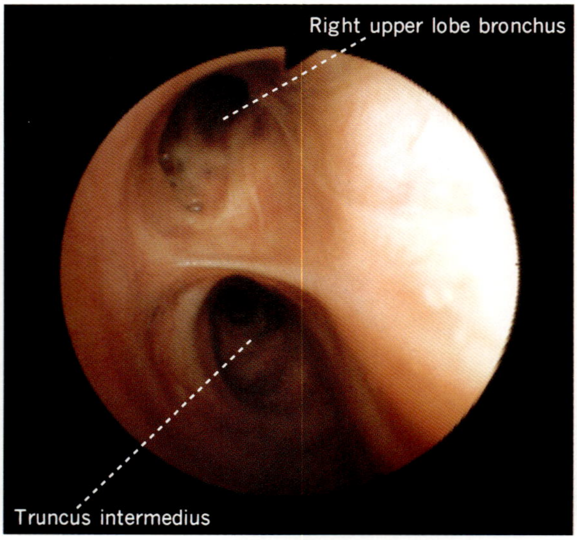

7.24 Right main bronchus: bifurcation into the truncus intermedius and right upper lobe bronchus. The right upper lobe bronchus diverges laterally from the main bronchus at an angle of 90 degrees. The bifurcation angle is sharp and linear. The membranous part of the posterior wall of the upper lobe bronchus continues from the main bronchus; four thick longitudinal folds continue into the right upper lobe bronchus.

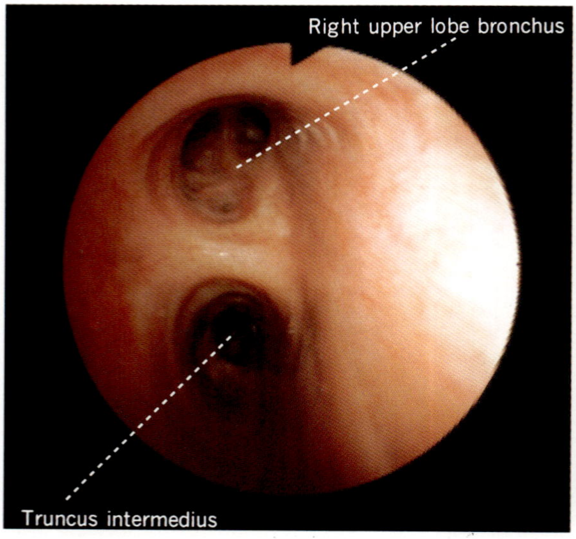

7.25 Right main bronchus: bifurcation into the truncus intermedius and right upper lobe bronchus. The longitudinal folds divide into right and left from the membranous part of the right main bronchus and continue to the truncus intermedius and right upper lobe bronchus. The bifurcation angle between the truncus intermedius and right upper lobe bronchus is wide.

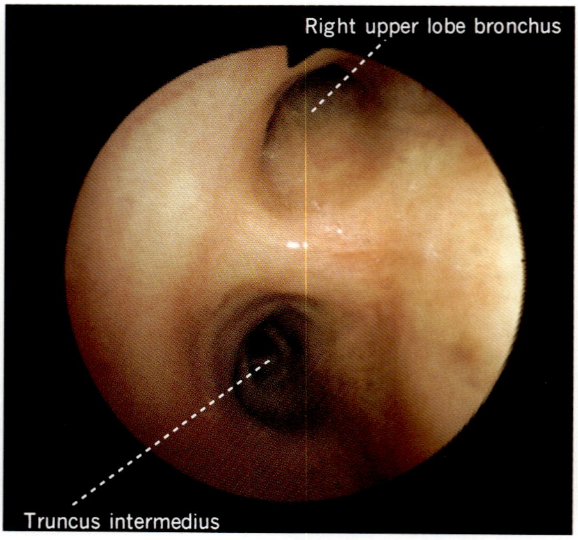

7.26 Right main bronchus: bifurcation into the truncus intermedius and right upper lobe bronchus. Longitudinal folds are not clearly visible. The right upper lobe bronchus makes a relatively obtuse angle with the truncus intermedius and the bifurcation site is oedematous. These findings suggest chronic bronchitis.

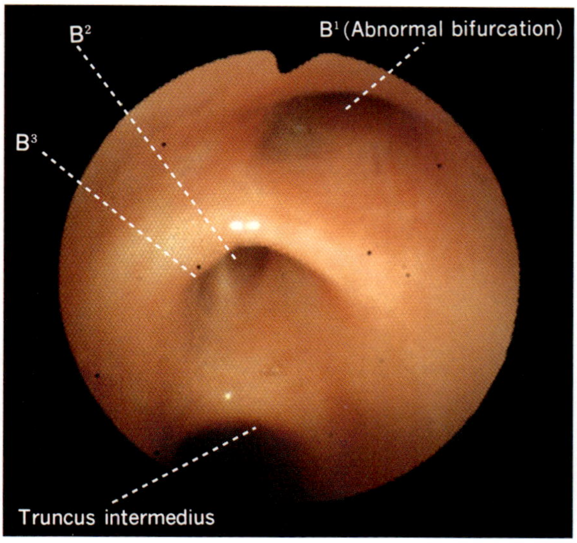

7.27 Bifurcation of the right upper lobe bronchus: abnormal bifurcation. The right upper lobe bronchus arises from the level of the bifurcation of the trachea. From a site 5 mm below, B^1 arises laterally from the right upper lobe bronchus. B^2 and B^3 arise from the original dividing site of the upper lobe bronchus.

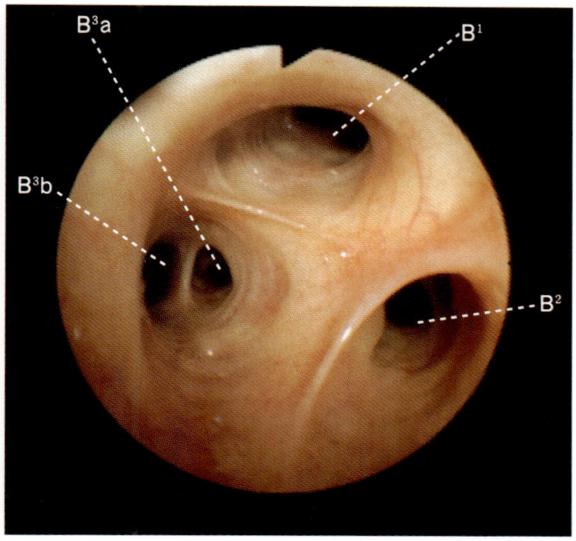

7.28 Right upper lobe bronchus: standard trifurcation type (B^1, B^2, B^3). The right upper lobe bronchus trifurcates equally into three segmental bronchi.

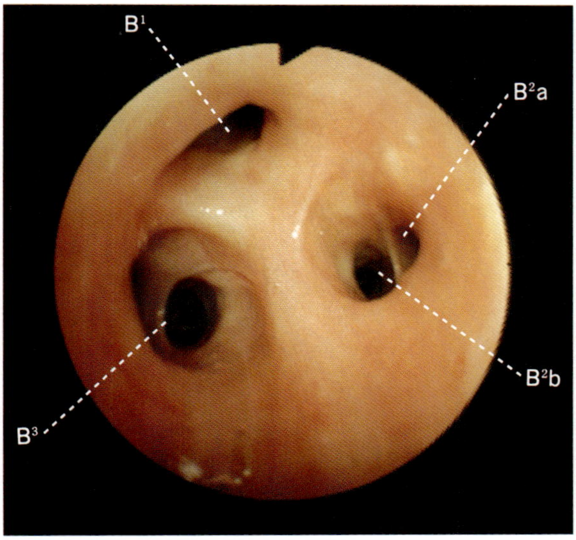

7.29 Right upper lobe bronchus: standard trifurcation type (B^1, B^2, B^3). Each orifice is located at each apex of an equilateral triangle, showing equal trifurcation.

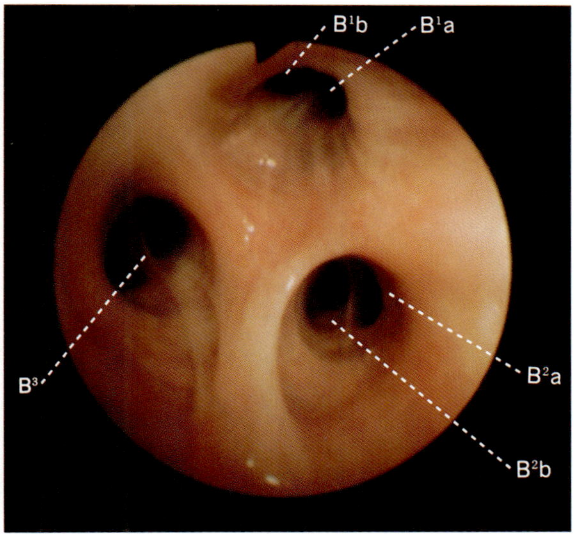

7.30 Right upper lobe bronchus: trifurcation type (B^1, B^2, B^3). This is a Y-shaped trifurcation and a sub-type of complete trifurcation of the right upper lobe bronchus. A thick longitudinal mucosal fold divides into two in a Y-shape.

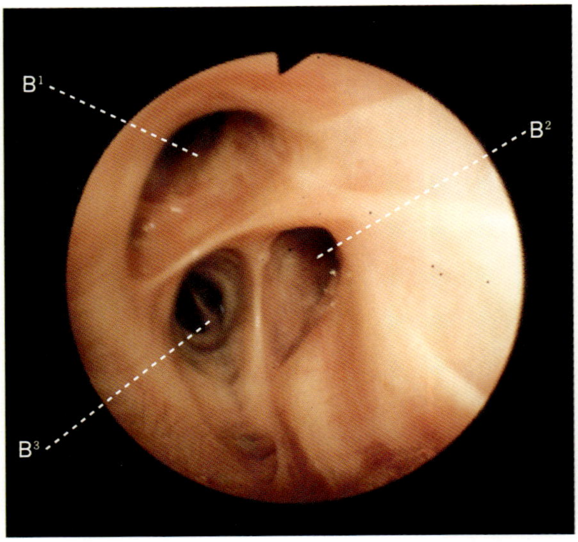

7.31 Right upper lobe bronchus: trifurcation type (B^1, B^2, B^3). This is a sub-type of complete trifurcation of the right upper lobe bronchus. The Y-shape lies on its side.

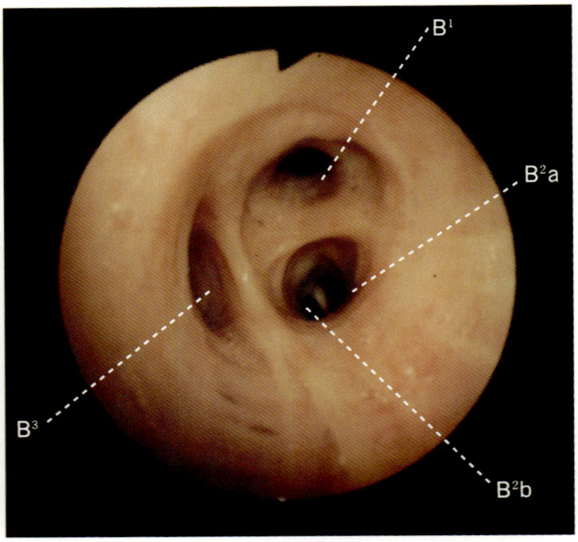

7.32 Right upper lobe bronchus: trifurcation type (B^1, B^2, B^3). This is a sub-type of the Y-shaped complete trifurcation of the right upper lobe bronchus. The thick longitudinal mucosal fold divides into two in a Y-shape, but the right branch runs far to the right.

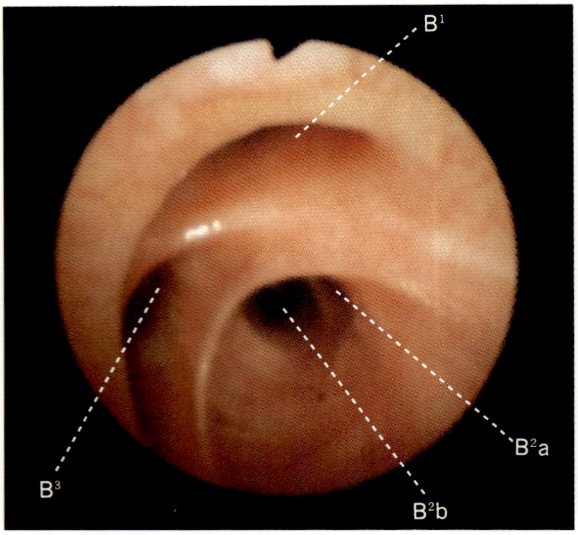

7.33 Right upper lobe bronchus: trifurcation type (B^1, B^2, B^3). A sub-type of the Y-shaped trifurcation. The left branch runs far to the left.

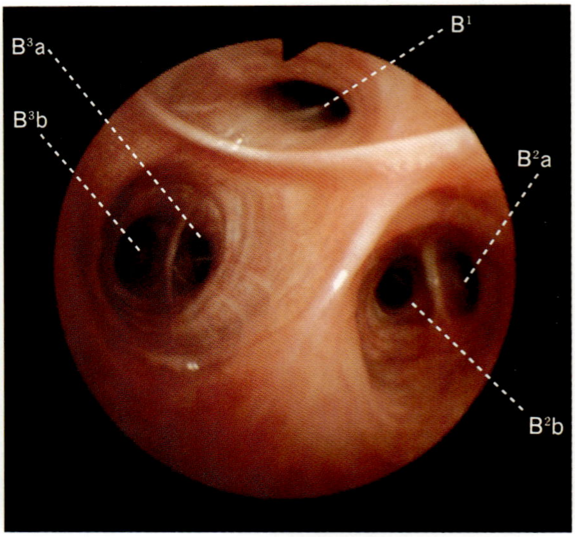

7.34 Right upper lobe bronchus: trifurcation type (B^1, B^2, B^3). The horizontal Y-shaped trifurcation. B^1 is located above, B^2 on the right, and B^3 on the left of the horizontal Y-shape.

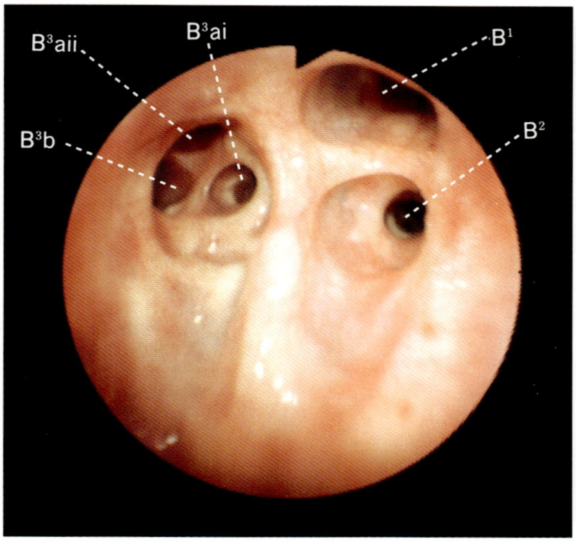

7.35 Right upper lobe bronchus: trifurcation type (B^1, B^2, B^3). I-shaped trifurcation. A thick longitudinal mucosal fold extends upward; B^1 and B^2 are located on its right and B^3 on its left. The orifice of each branch is almost at each apex of an equilateral triangle.

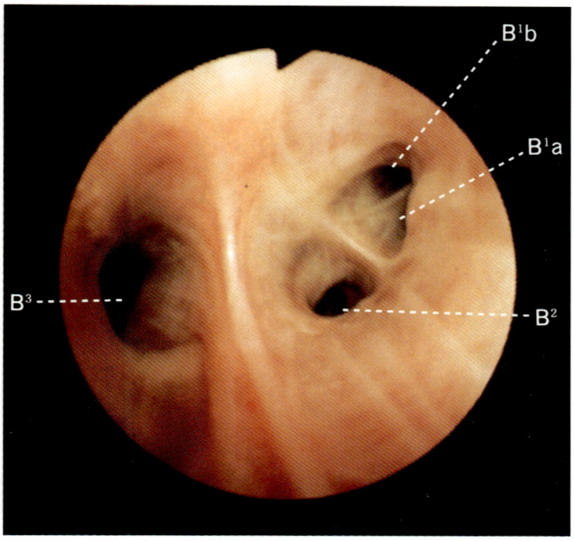

7.36 Right upper lobe bronchus: trifurcation type (B^1, B^2, B^3). A subtype of the I-shaped trifurcation. B^1 and B^2 are situated closely on the right side of the I-shape.

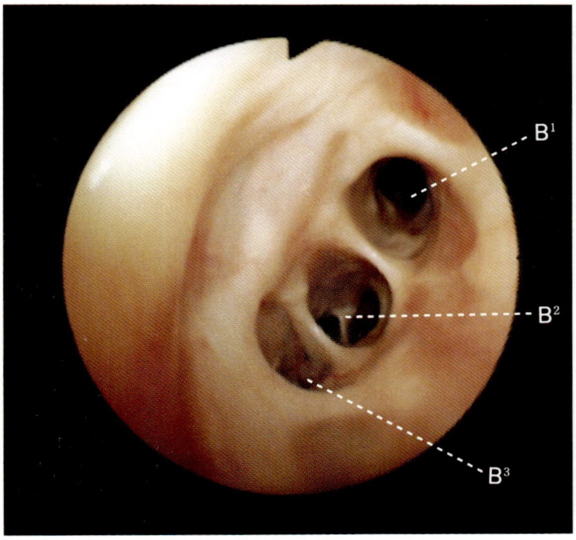

7.37 Right upper lobe bronchus: parallel trifurcation type (B^1, B^2, B^3). The most uncommon type of trifurcation of the right upper lobe bronchus.

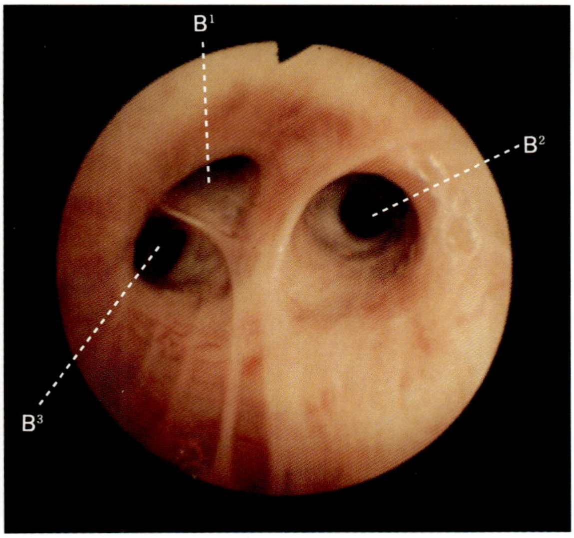

7.38 Right upper lobe bronchus: bifurcation type ($B^1 + B^3$ and B^2). Any two of B^1, B^2, and B^3 are common-stem bronchi. In this case, B^1 and B^3 are common-stem bronchi.

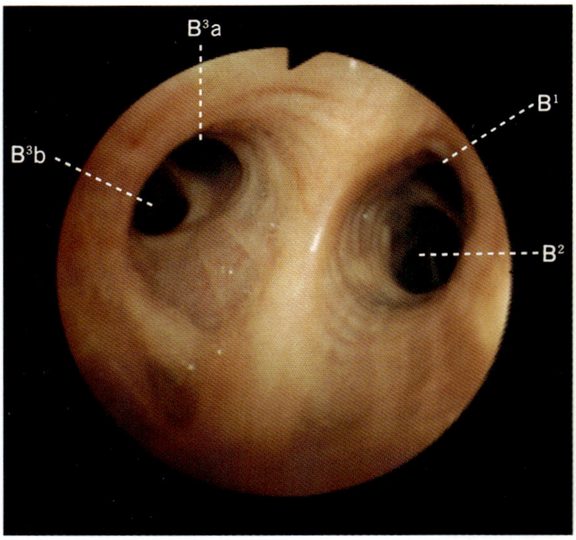

7.39 Right upper lobe bronchus: anteroposterior complete bifurcation type ($B^1 + B^2$ and B^3). The right upper lobe branch completely bifurcates into anterior and posterior. The diameter of $B^1 + B^2$ is similar to that of B^3.

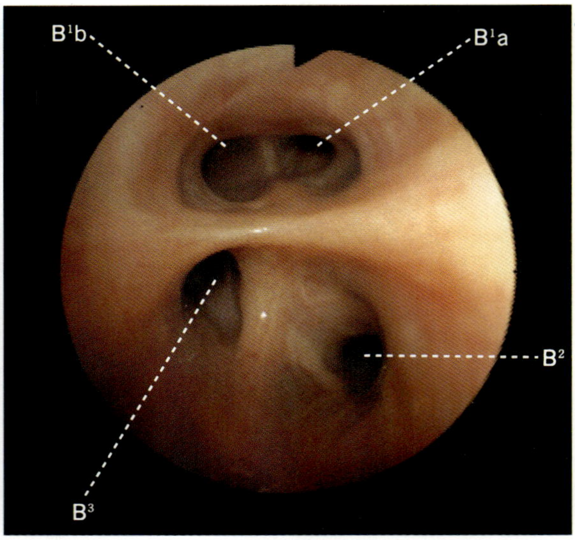

7.40 Right upper lobe bronchus: bifurcation type (B^1 and $B^2 + B^3$). The right upper lobe bronchus bifurcates to B^1 and $B^2 + B^3$. The diameters of the segmental bronchi are similar.

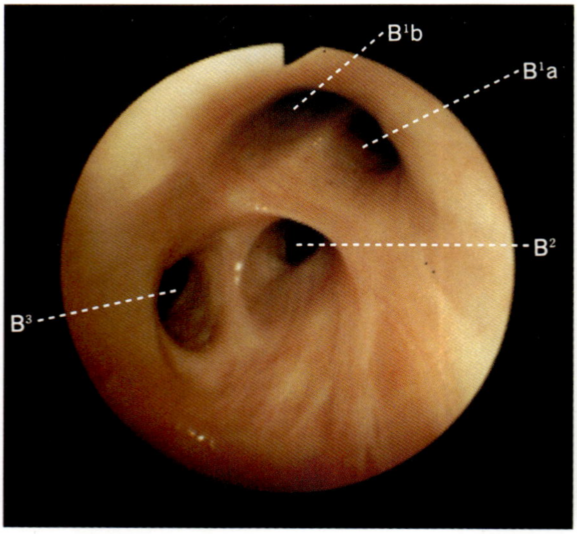

7.41 Right upper lobe bronchus: superior-inferior complete bifurcation type. The right upper lobe bronchus bifurcates completely into superior and inferior divisions. The diameter of B^1 is similar to that of $B^2 + B^3$.

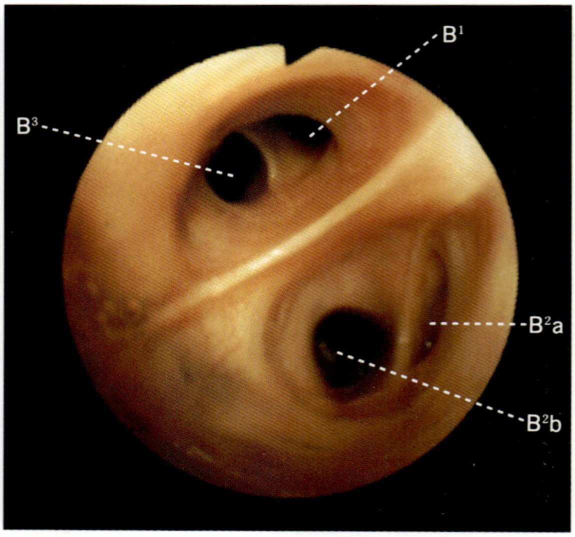

7.42 Right upper lobe bronchus: bifurcation type ($B^1 + B^3$ and B^2). The incidence of bifurcation into $B^1 + B^3$ and B^2 was reported to be 10 per cent by Boyden[3].

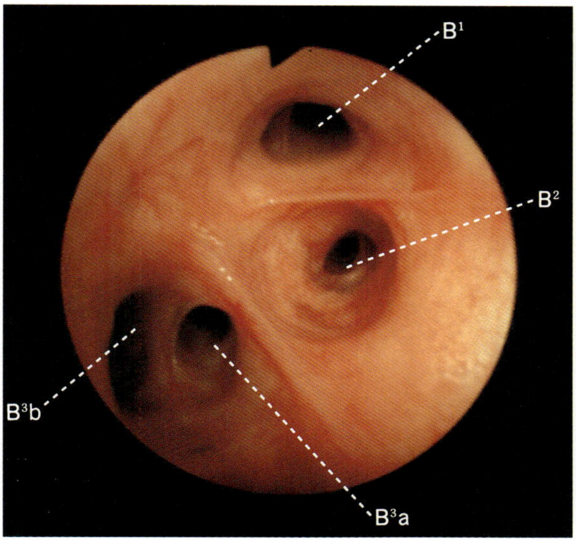

7.43 Right upper lobe bronchus: quadrifurcation type (B^1, B^2, B^3a, and B^3b). The incidence of quadrifurcation was reported to be 14 per cent by Boyden and 4 per cent by Oho *et al*[1]. Identification of the segmental bronchi is sometimes difficult and usually done by bronchography. In this case B^1, B^2, B^3a and B^3b are observed.

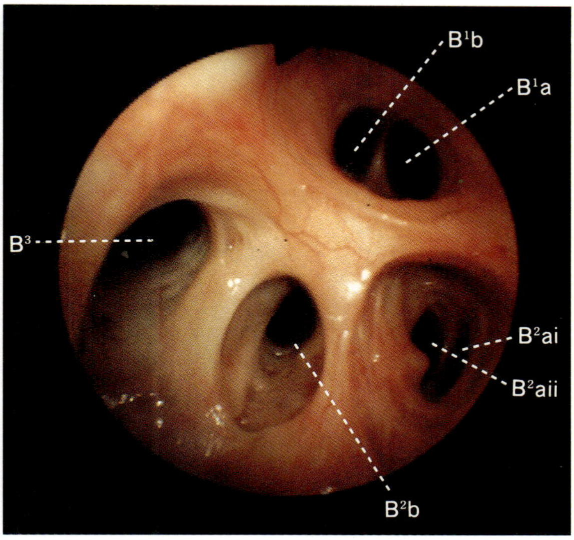

7.44 Right upper lobe bronchus: quadrifurcation type (B^1, B^2a, B^2b, B^3). A sub-type of quadrifurcation of the right upper lobe bronchus. Yamashita[5] reported that the incidence of B^1, B^2, B^3a, B^3b is 8 per cent and that of B^1, B^2a, B^2b, B^3 is 5 per cent. This case is the B^1, B^2a, B^2b and B^3 type.

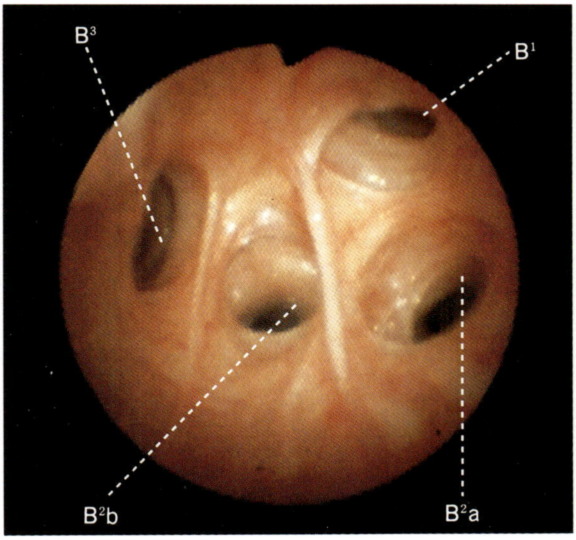

7.45 Right upper lobe bronchus: quadrifurcation type (B^1, B^2a, B^2b, B^3). A sub-type of quadrifurcation of the right upper lobe bronchus. Boyden's nomenclature[3] of this type is B^1, B^2a, B^2b and B^3 or B^1a + B^2b, B^1b, B^2b and B^3. This case is B^1, B^2a, B^2b and B^3 type.

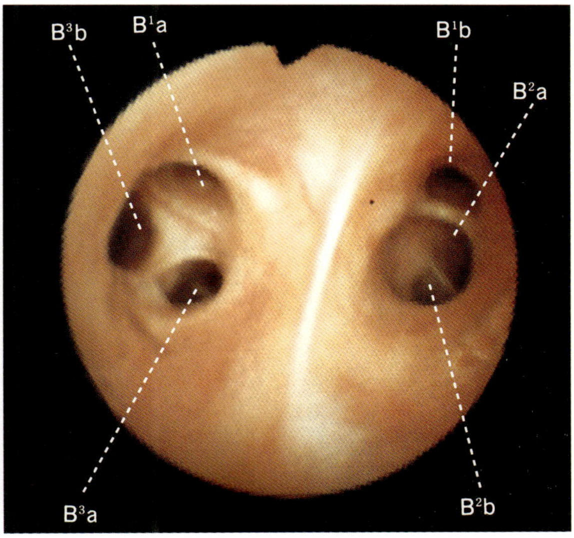

7.46 Right upper lobe bronchus: anteroposterior complete bifurcation type (B^1b + B^2a + B^2b and B^1a + B^3a + B^3b. This is basically classified as the anteroposterior complete bifurcation type. This case is B^1b + B^2a + B^2b and B^1a + B^3a + B^3b.

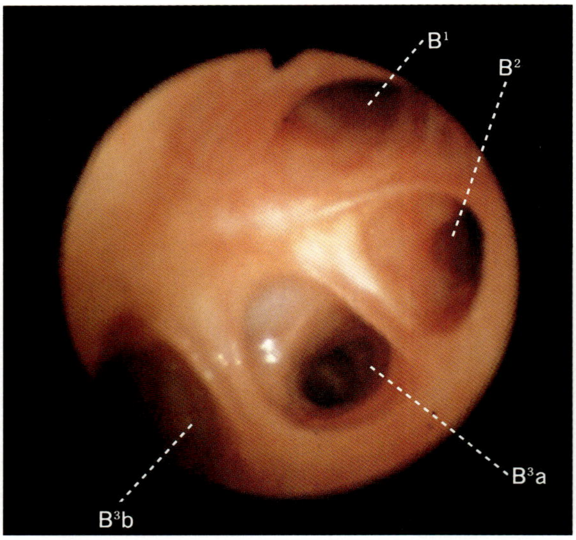

7.47 Right upper lobe bronchus: parallel quadrifurcation type. A sub-type of the quadrifurcation type of the right upper lobe bronchus. Segmental bronchi B^1 and B^2 and subsegmental bronchi B^3a and B^3b with similar size orifice are located almost linearly. In this case, B^1 is located slightly above the linear arrangement. This type is rare among quadrifurcation types.

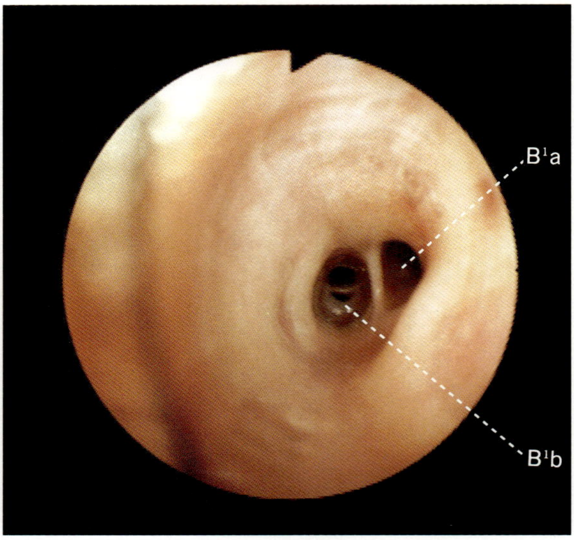

7.48 Right upper lobe segmental bronchus B^1: standard type. The right upper lobe segmental bronchus B^1 usually bifurcates to B^1a and B^1b at its orifice.

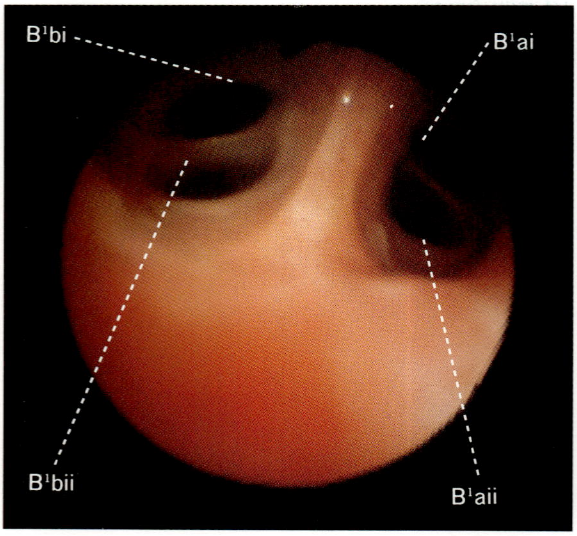

7.49 Right upper lobe segmental bronchus B^1: (B^1ai, B^1aii, B^1bi, B^1bii). In this case, B^1a and B^1b bifurcate to B^1ai and B^1aii and B^1bi and B^1bii at the orifice.

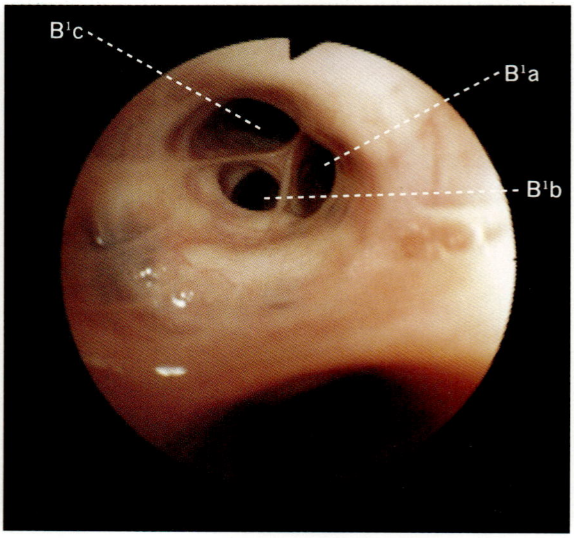

7.50 Right upper lobe segmental bronchus: trifurcation type (B^1a, B^1b, B^1c). The right upper lobe segmental bronchus B^1 trifurcates into B^1a, B^1b and B^1c at its orifice.

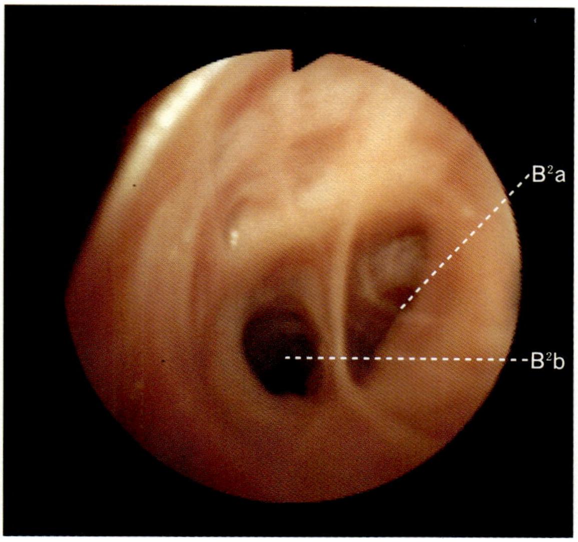

7.51 Right upper lobe segmental bronchus B^2: standard type. The right upper lobe segmental bronchus B^2 bifurcates into B^2a and B^2b. Each diameter at its orifice is similar.

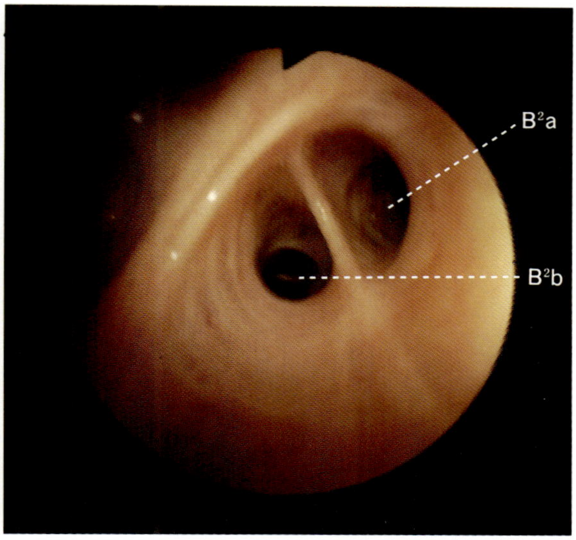

7.52 Right upper lobe segmental bronchus B^2: standard type. The right upper lobe segmental bronchus B^2 bifurcates into B^2a and B^2b. B^2a makes a right angle with B^2b at its orifice.

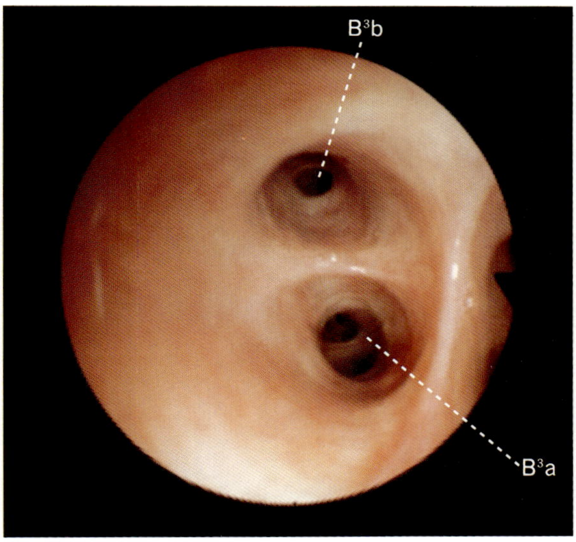

7.53 Right upper lobe segmental bronchus B^3: standard type. The right upper lobe segmental bronchus B^3 bifurcates into B^3a and B^3b at its orifice. The bifurcation is sharp.

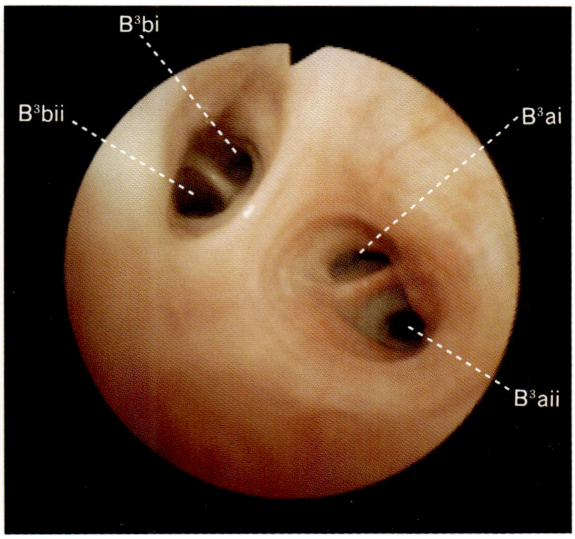

7.54 Right upper lobe segmental bronchus B^3: standard type. The right upper lobe segmental bronchus B^3 bifurcates into B^3a and B^3b at its orifice. The bifurcation is obtuse. Each of B^3a and B^3b bifurcates further.

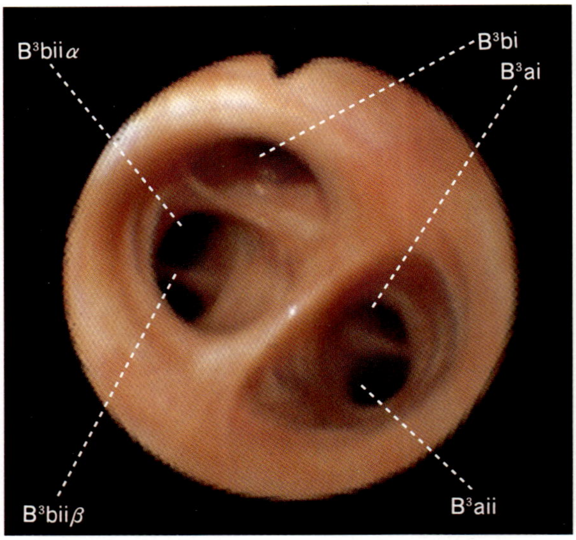

7.55 Right upper lobe segmental bronchus B^3 trifurcation. It bifurcates at its orifice into right (B^3a) and left (B^3b); B^3b bifurcates into B^3bi and B^3bii, and B^3bii bifurcates into B^3bii α and β. B^3a bifurcates into B^3i and B^3ii.

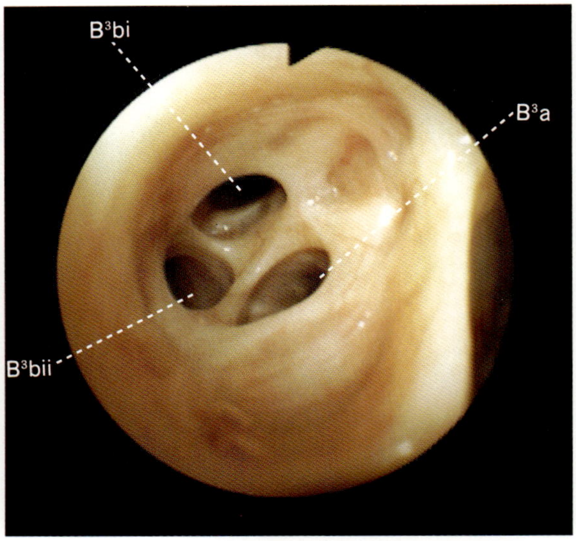

7.56 Right upper lobe segmental bronchus B^3: trifurcation type. The right upper lobe segmental bronchus B^3 trifurcates equally into B^3bi, B^3bii and B^3a.

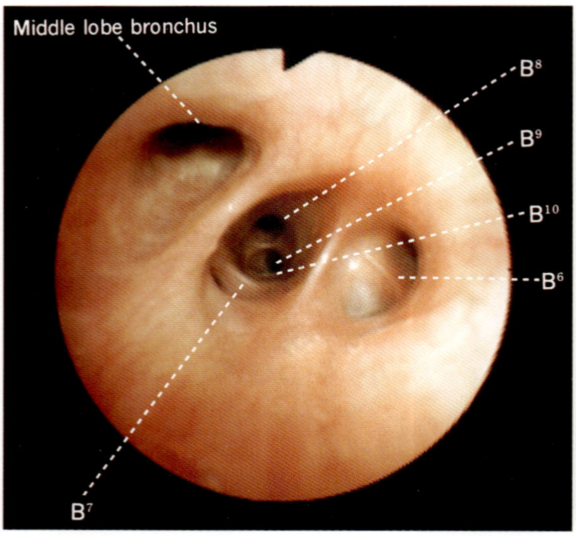

7.57 Truncus intermedius. This is a peripheral view from the truncus intermedius. Three large bronchial orifices are seen linearly from the left upper to right lower area. Longitudinal mucosal folds of the truncus intermedius continue to the basal bronchus.

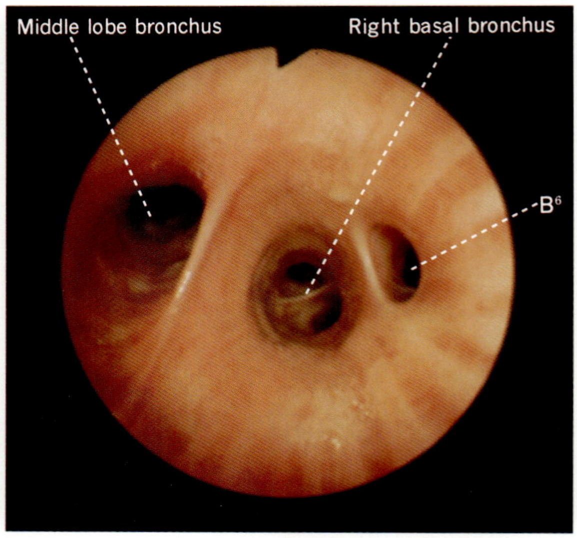

7.58 Truncus intermedius. This is also a peripheral view from the truncus intermedius. The orifice of B^6 is smaller than that of the middle lobe bronchus or basal bronchus.

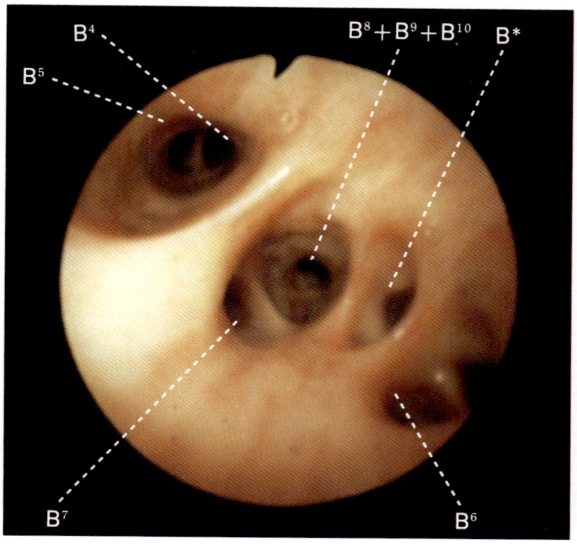

7.59 Truncus intermedius. This peripheral view from the truncus intermedius shows quadrification. From the top, the orifices of the middle lobe bronchus, basal bronchus, B*, and B^6 are seen.

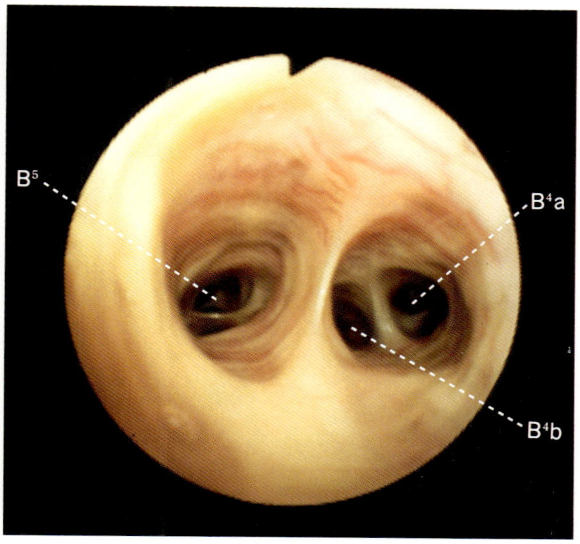

7.60 Middle lobe bronchus: bifurcation type. The most common bifurcation of the right middle lobe bronchus. B^4 makes an angle of 45 degrees with B^5. Subsegmental bronchi run in different directions.

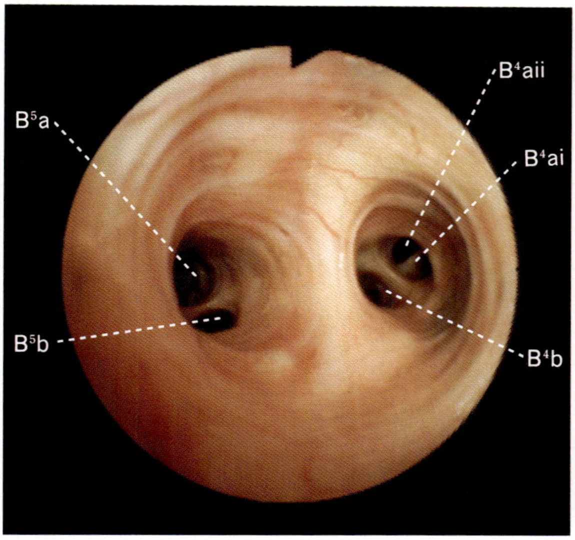

7.61 Middle lobe bronchus: bifurcation type. This is a common bifurcation of the right middle lobe bronchus. B^4 and B^5 arise laterally and medially (mediastinal site). The subsegmental bronchi arise superiorly and inferiorly.

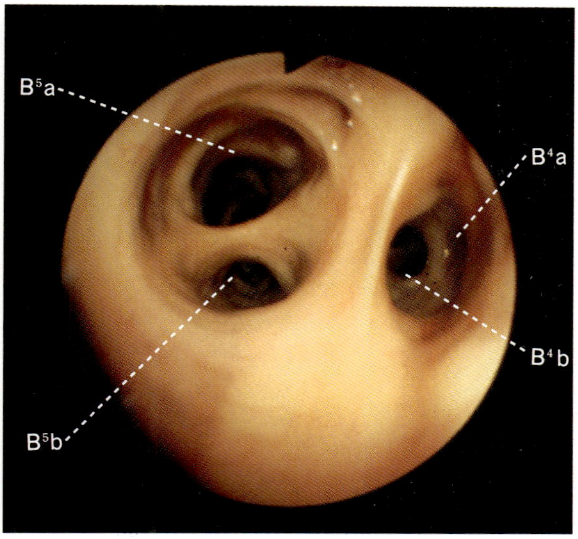

7.62 Middle lobe bronchus: bifurcation type. B^4 and B^5 bifurcate. B^5 bifurcates at its orifice and B^4 at an inner site.

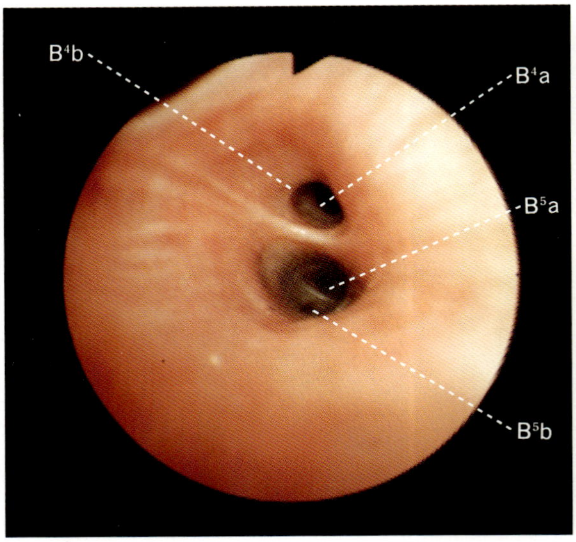

7.63 Middle lobe bronchus: bifurcation type. The middle lobe bronchus bifurcates superiorly into B^4a and B^4b, and inferiorly into B^5a and B^5b.

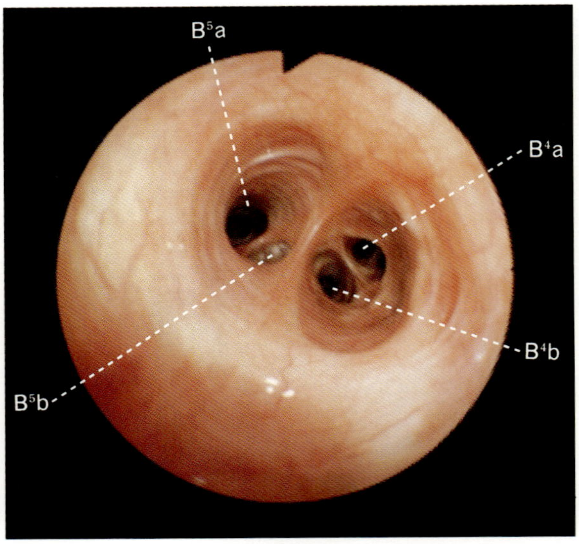

7.64 Middle lobe bronchus: bifurcation type. The middle lobe bronchus bifurcates superiorly into B^4a and B^4b and inferiorly into B^5a and B^5b.

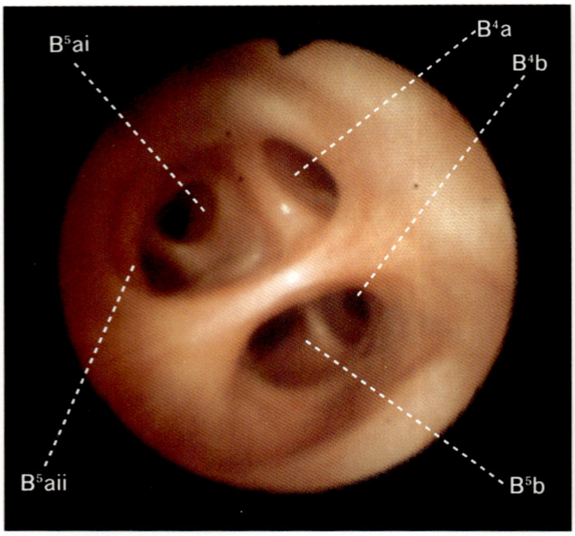

7.65 Middle lobe bronchus: bifurcation type. The middle lobe bronchus bifurcates superiorly into B^4a and B^4b, and inferiorly into B^5a and B^5b.

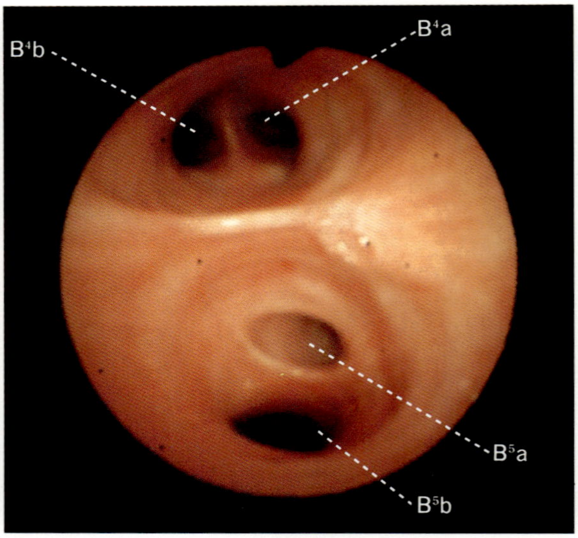

7.66 Middle lobe bronchus: bifurcation type. The middle lobe bronchus bifurcates superiorly into B^4a and B^4b, and inferiorly into B^5a and B^5b.

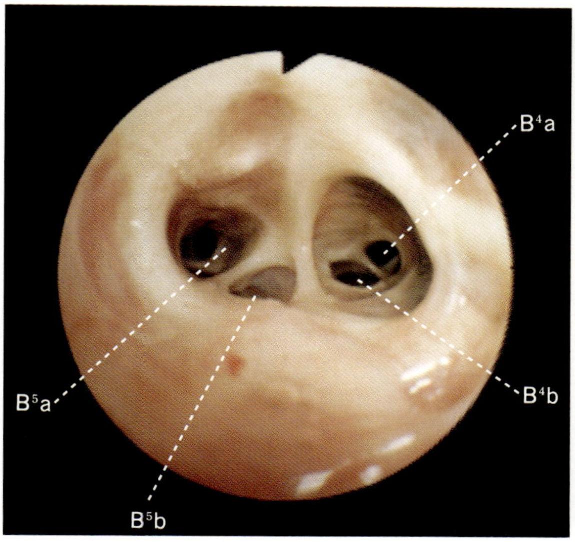

7.67 Middle lobe bronchus: inverted Y-shaped trifurcation. B^4 arises medially and B^5 laterally. B^4 further divides to right and left, and B^5 superiorly and inferiorly into subsegmental bronchi. This type is observed in 20 per cent.

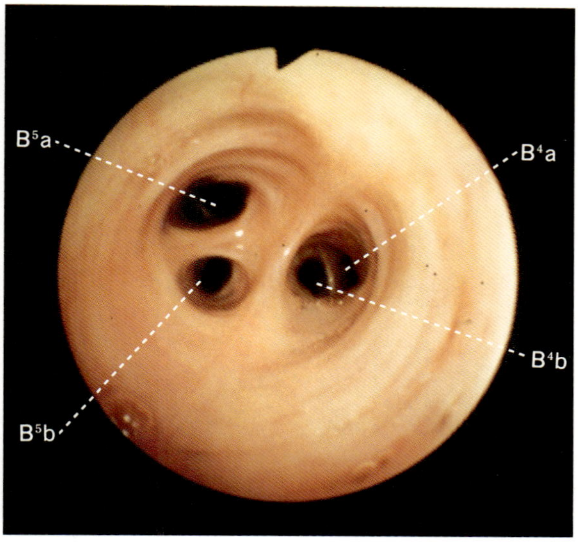

7.68 Middle lobe bronchus: equal trifurcation type. B^5a, B^5b, and B^4 are located at an each apex of an equilateral triangle.

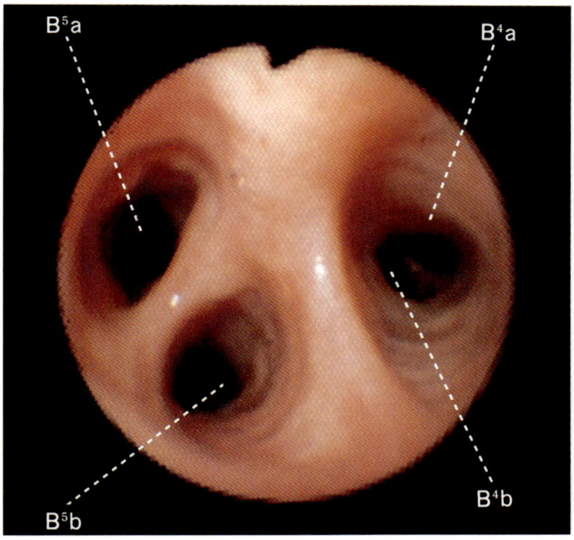

7.69 Middle lobe bronchus: inverted Y-shaped trifurcation. B^5a is observed on the left, B^5b between the short limbs, and B^4 on the right.

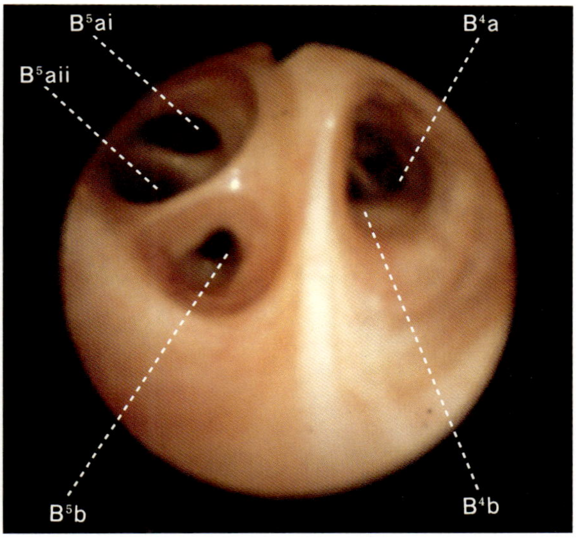

7.70 Middle lobe bronchus: a variation of the trifurcation type. The middle lobe bronchus trifurcates, though initially dividing to the right (B^4) and left (B^5a, B^5b).

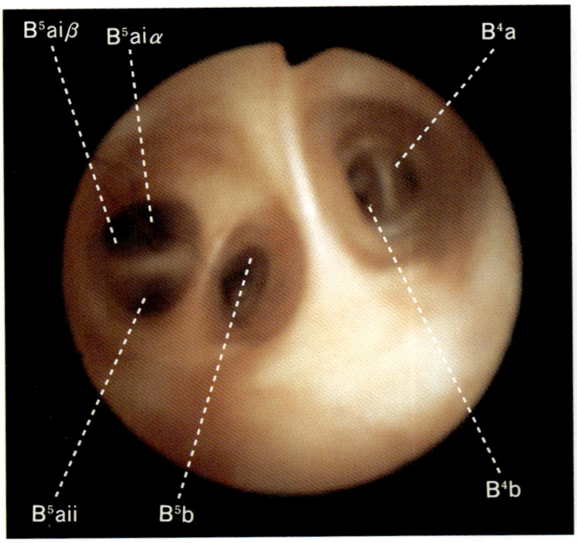

7.71 Middle lobe bronchus: parallel trifurcation type. From the left, B^5a, B^5b and B^4 are almost parallel.

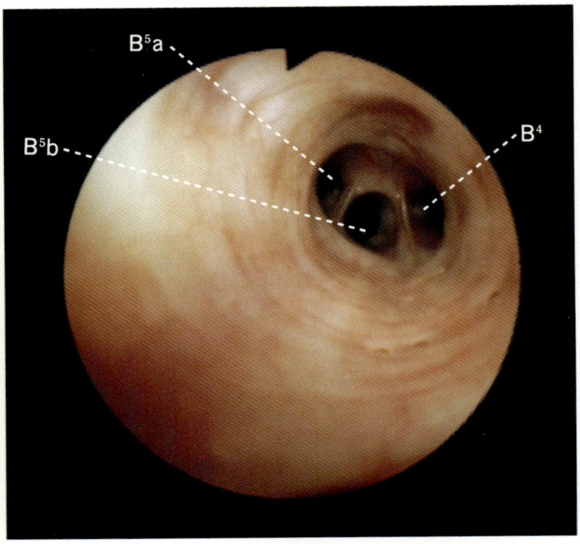

7.72 Middle lobe bronchus: a variation of the trifurcation type. From the left, B^5a, B^5b and B^4 arise with orifices of similar diameters.

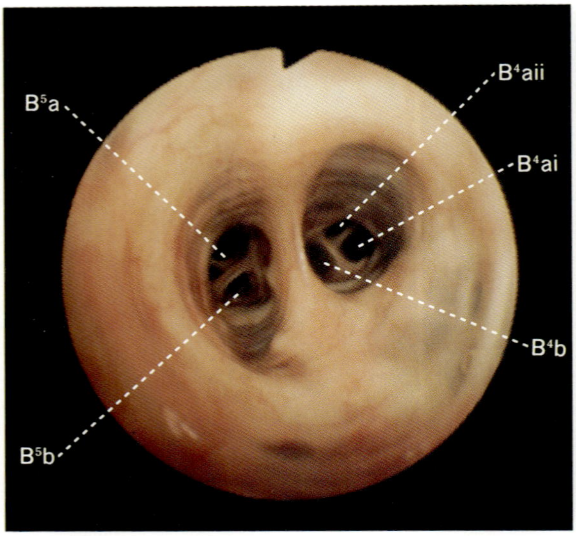

7.73 Middle lobe bronchus: bifurcation type. The middle lobe bronchus bifurcates into B^4 and B^5. Each bronchus divides into three subsegmental bronchi.

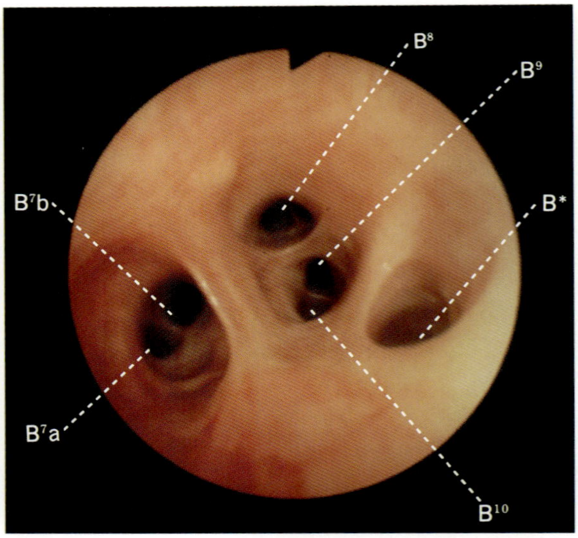

7.74 Right basal bronchus. B^7 arises on the posterior mediastinal aspect at an angle of about 45 degrees with the line connecting B^8, B^9 and B^{10}. B^* is present opposite B^7.

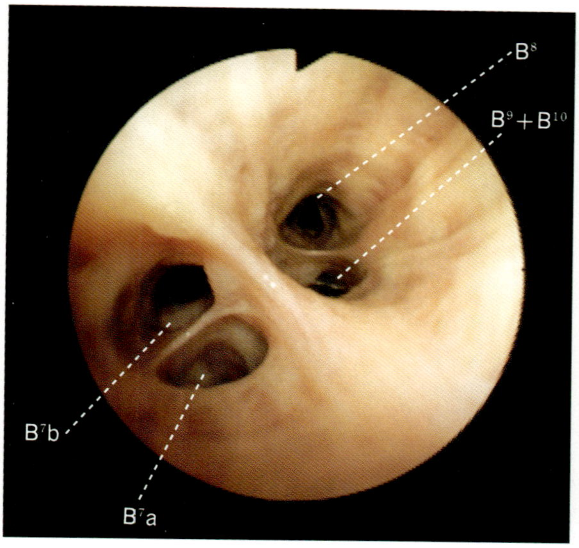

7.75 Right basal lobe bronchus. B^7 arises at an angle of about 45 degrees with the line connecting B^8, B^9 and B^{10}. Subsegmental bronchi of B^7 are observed.

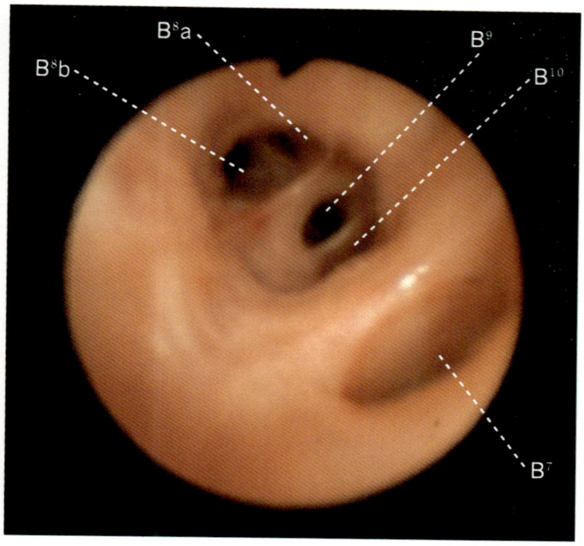

7.76 Right basal lobe bronchus. B^7, B^8, B^9 and B^{10} are almost linear. B^7 arises in the mediastinal direction, and its subsegmental bronchi are not observed.

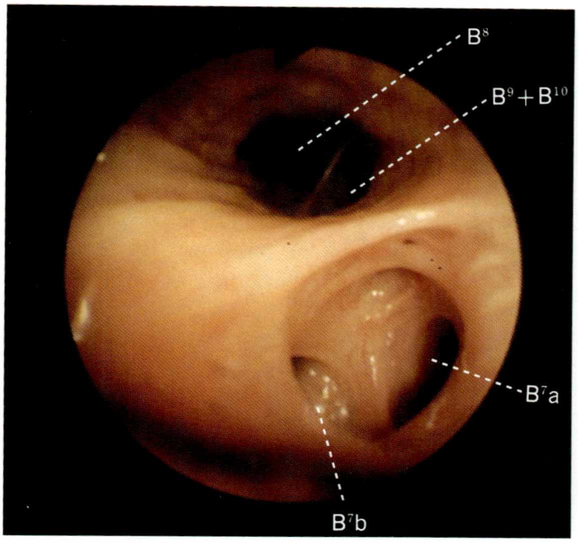

7.77 Right B^7. Subsegmental bronchi branch off from B^7 in opposite directions at an acute angle.

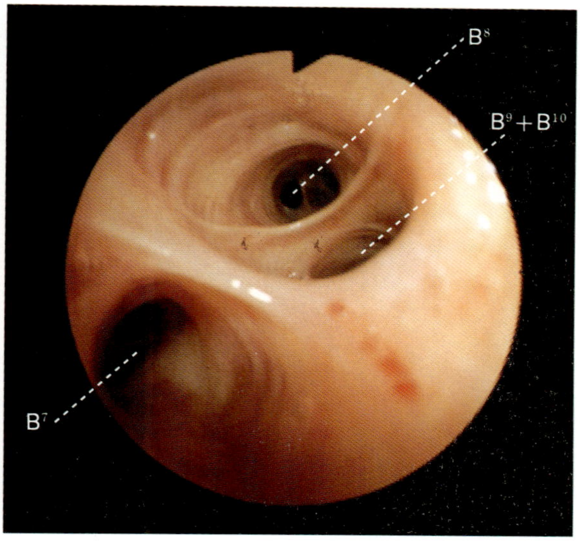

7.78 Right B^7. B^7 bifurcates to subsegmental bronchi at an inner site.

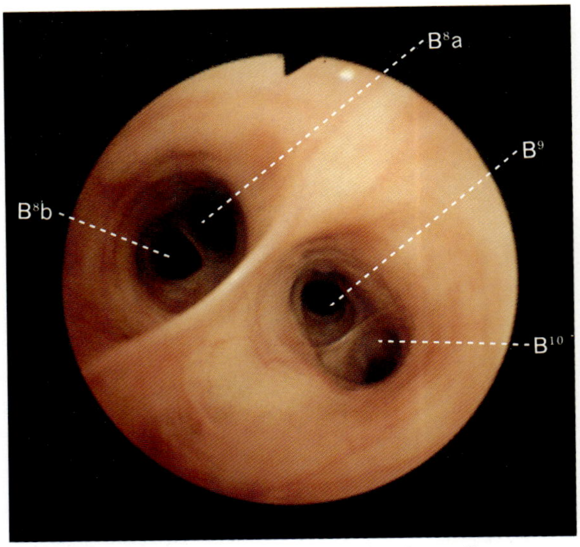

7.79 Right basal lobe bronchus: B^8, $B^9 + B^{10}$. The bronchial orifices in the right basal segments are observed. From the top, B^8a, B^8b, B^9a, B^9b and B^{10} are observed.

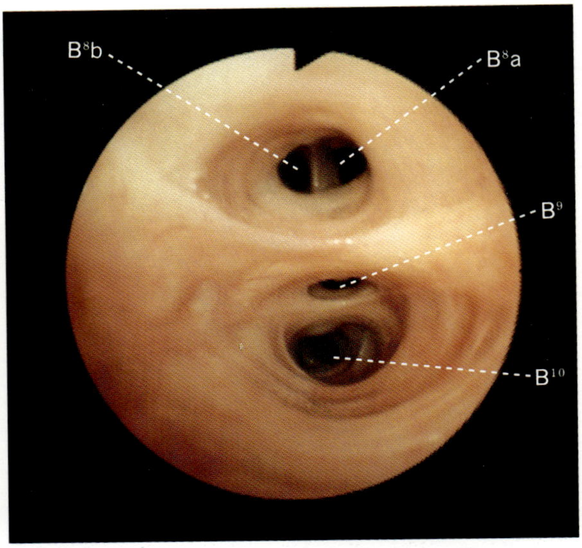

7.80 Right basal lobe bronchus: B^8, $B^9 + B^{10}$. The orifice of B^9 is smaller than that of B^8 or B^{10}.

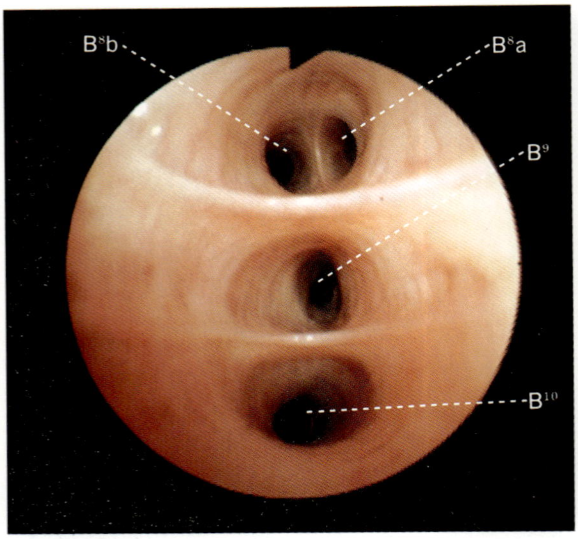

7.81 Right basal lobe bronchus: B^8, B^9, B^{10}. B^8, B^9 and B^{10} are situated on a vertical line with similar size orifices.

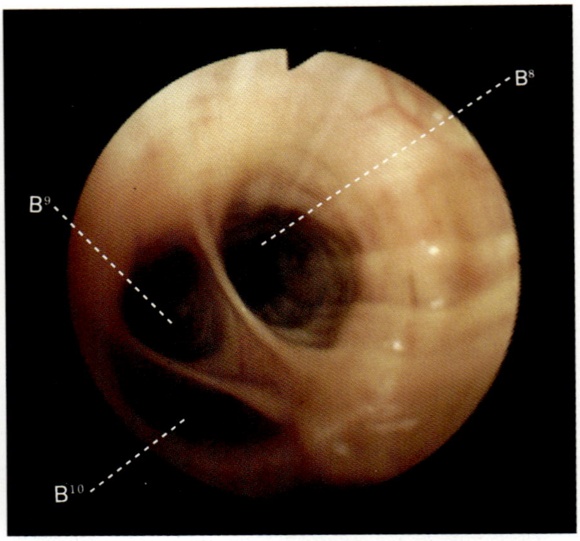

7.82 Right basal lobe bronchus: B^8, B^9, B^{10}. B^8, B^9 and B^{10} are situated on a curve that is convex towards the left with similar size orifices.

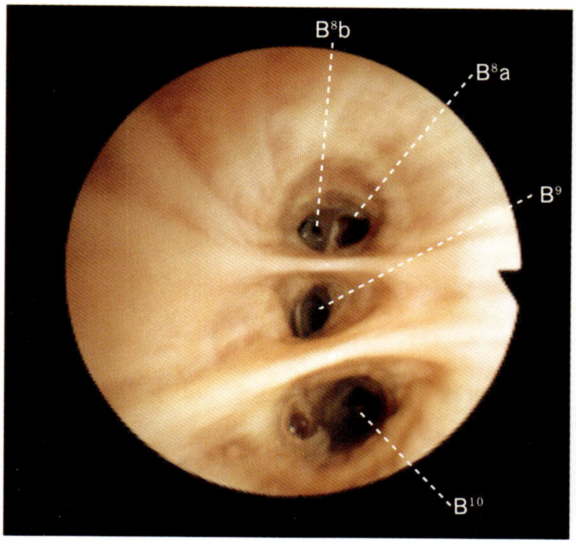

7.83 Right basal lobe bronchus: $B^8 + B^9$, B^{10}. From the top, B^8, B^9 and B^{10} are present on a line. There is a thick mucosal fold between B^9 and B^{10}.

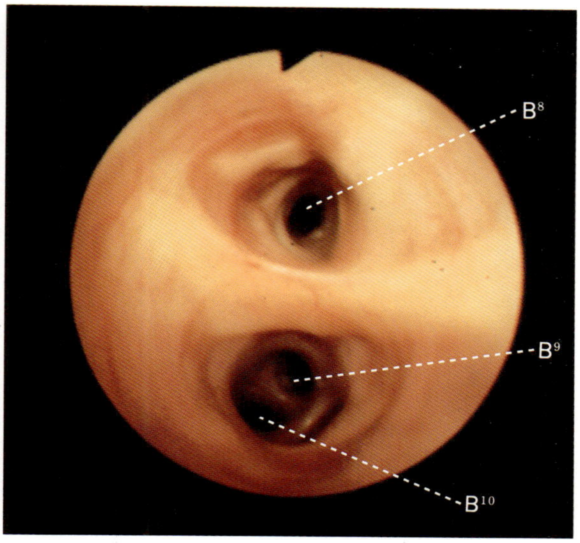

7.84 Right basal lobe bronchus: B^8, $B^9 + B^{10}$. B^8, $B^9 + B^{10}$ are linear. B* is present above $B^9 + B^{10}$.

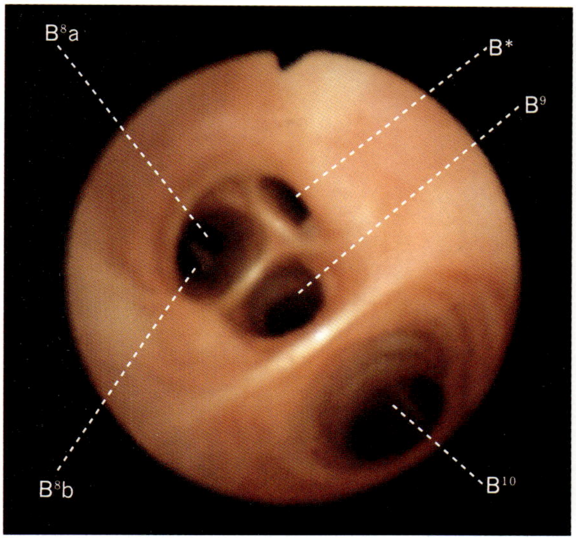

7.85 Right basal lobe bronchus: $B^8 + B^9$, B^{10}. B^8, B^9 and B^{10} are linear. B^{10} is observed beyond a thick mucosal fold. B* is observed in the lateral wall of the orifices of $B^8 + B^9$.

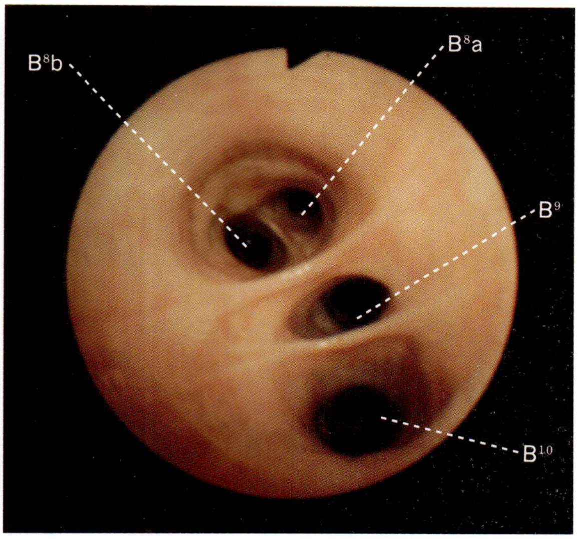

7.86 Right basal lobe bronchus: B^8, B^9, B^{10}. B^8, B^9 and B^{10} are located on a curve that is convex towards the right.

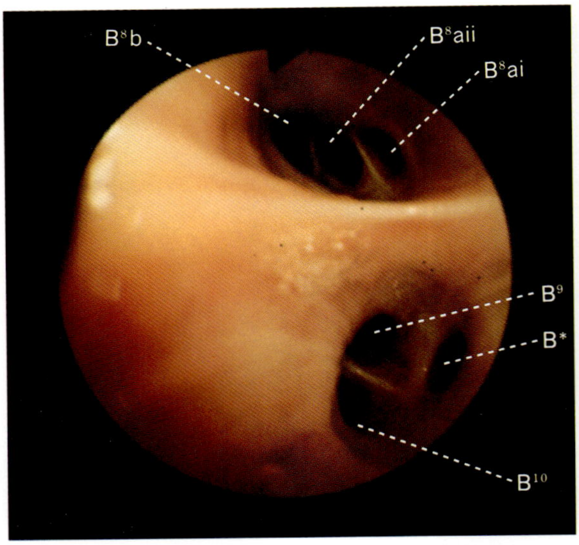

7.87 Right basal lobe bronchus: B^8, $B^9 + B^{10}$. B^8 trifurcates, B* is observed above $B^9 + B^{10}$.

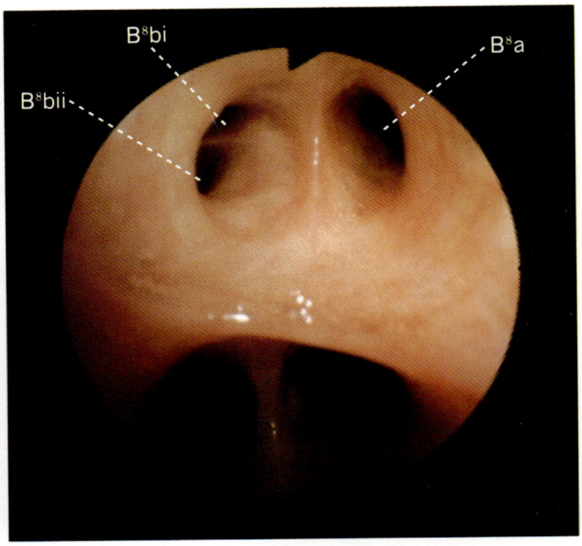

7.88 Right basal lobe bronchus: B^8. B^8 bifurcates to the right (B^8a) and left (B^8b). This is the most common type of bifurcation.

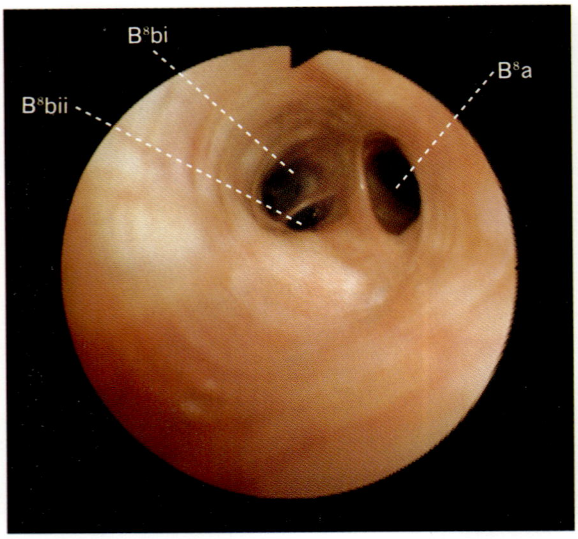

7.89 Right basal lobe bronchus: B^8. B^8 bifurcates to the right (B^8a) and left (B^8b). B^8b further bifurcates into B^8bi and B^8bii.

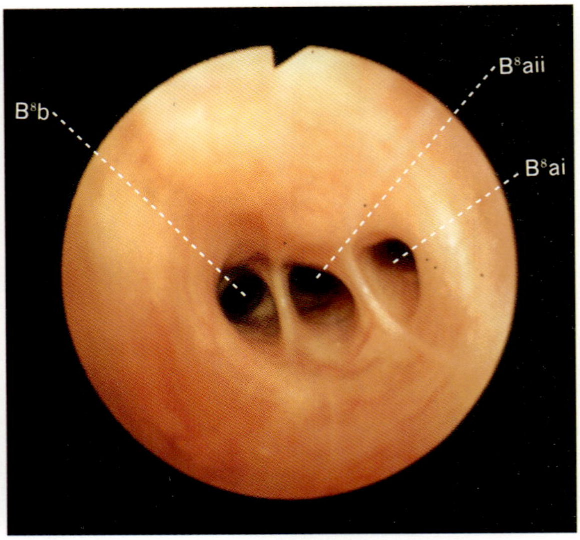

7.90 Right basal lobe bronchus: B^8. B^8 trifurcates into B^8ai, B^8aii, and B^8b.

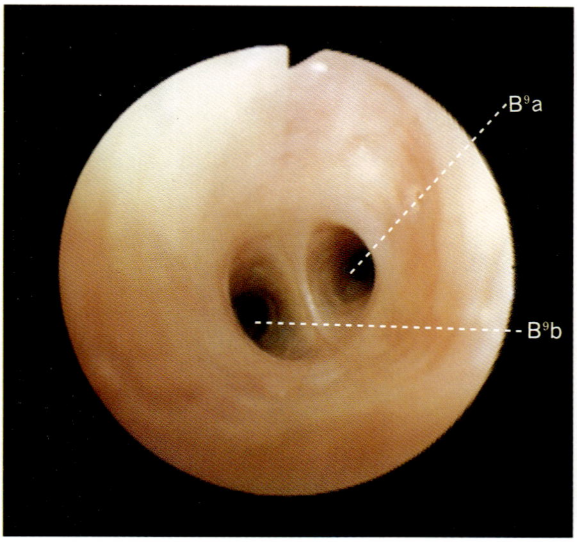

7.91 Right basal lobe bronchus: B^9. B^9 bifurcates to the right (B^{9}a) and left (B^{9}b).

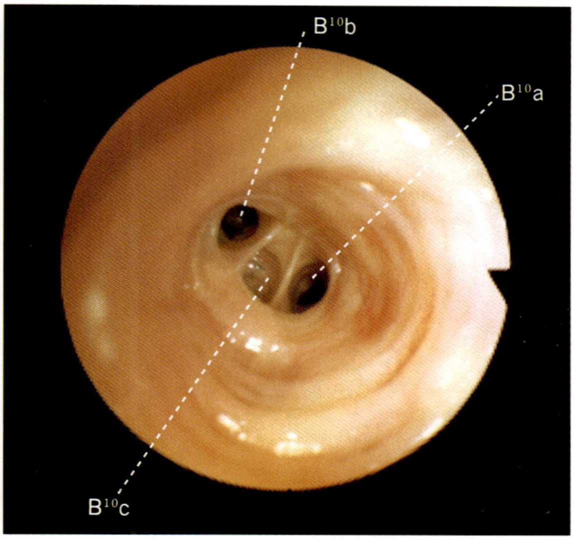

7.92 Right basal lobe bronchus: B^{10}. B^{10} trifurcates counterclockwise into B^{10}a, B^{10}b and B^{10}c.

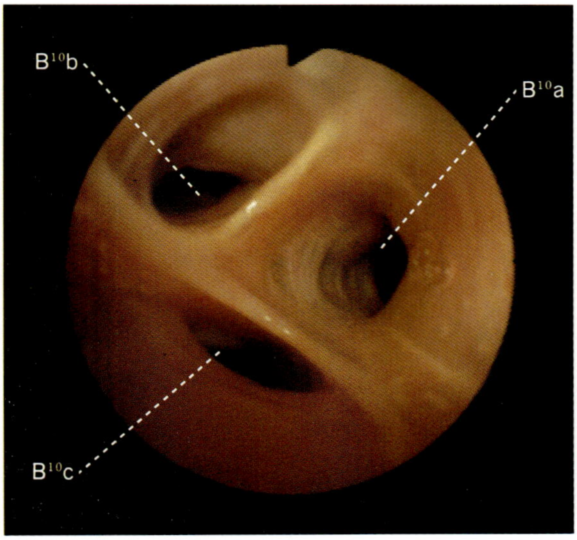

7.93 Right basal lobe bronchus: B^{10}. B^{10} trifurcates anticlockwise into subsegmental bronchi B^{10}a, B^{10}b and B^{10}c.

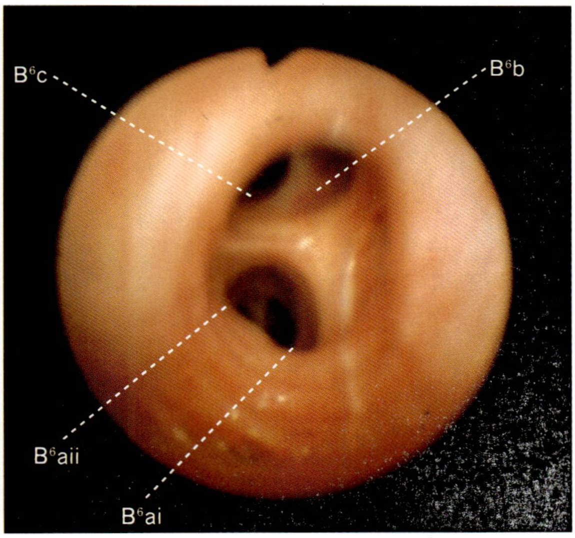

7.94 Right B^6: B^{6}a, B^{6}b + B^{6}c. There are variations in the division of B^6 into three subsegmental bronchi. In this case, B^{6}a arises posteriorly (dorsally), B^{6}b laterally, and B^{6}c medially (mediastinal direction).

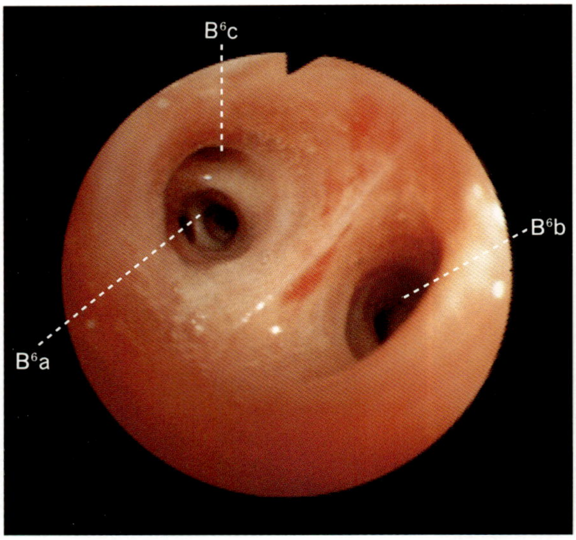

7.95 Right B^6: $B^6a + B^6c$, B^6b. $B^6a + B^6c$ and B^6b types are the most common in the right lung. The incidence of these types is reported to be 79 per cent by Boyden[3] and 53 per cent by Oho[1].

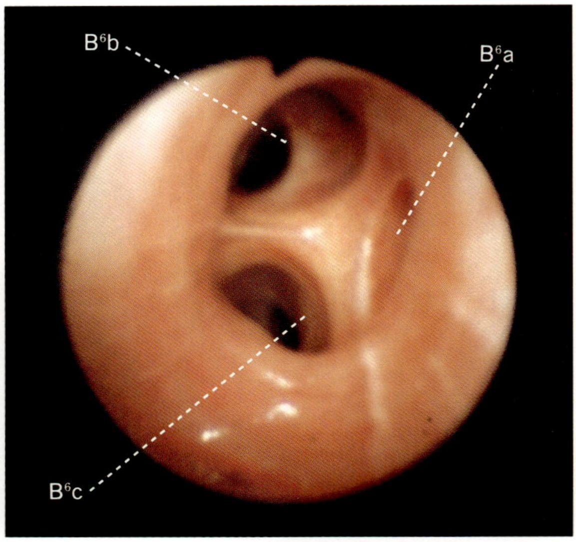

7.96 Right B^6: B^6a, B^6c, B^6b. This is a common type. The subsegmental bronchi from B^6 frequently arise at an acute angle.

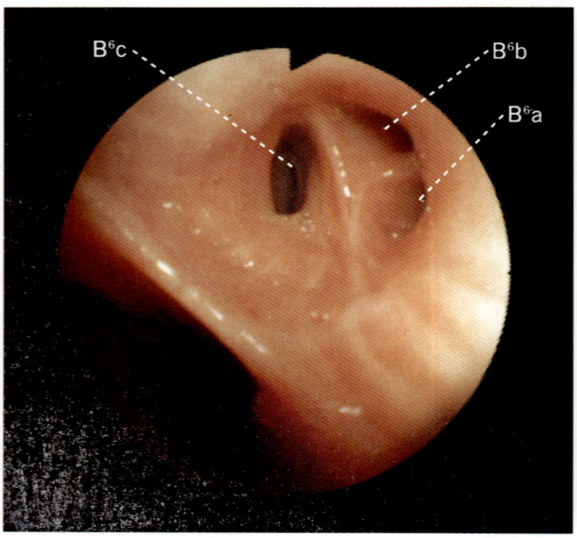

7.97 Right B^6: $B^6a + B^6b$, B^6c. The incidence of this type was reported to be 4 per cent by Boyden[3] and 23 per cent by Oho[1].

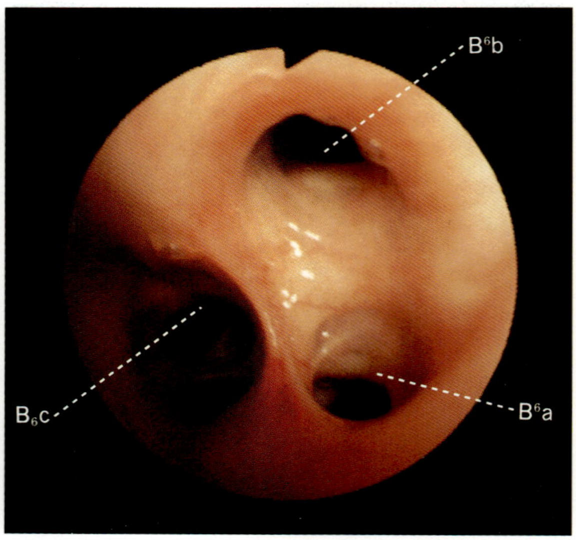

7.98 Right B^6: a variation of $B^6a + B^6b$, B^6c. B^6 trifurcates because the orifices of B^6a and B^6b are widely separated.

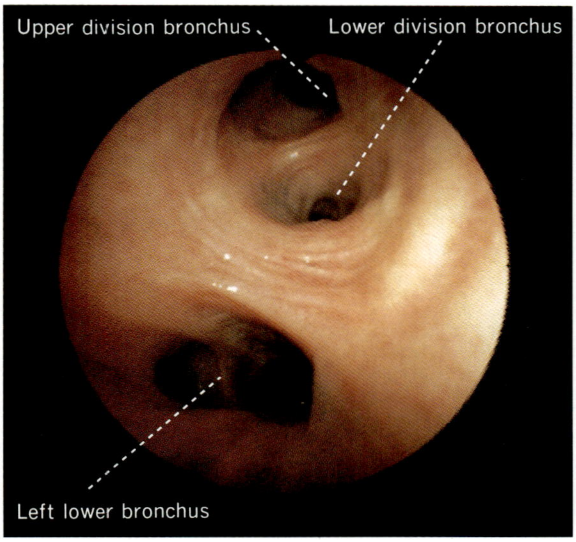

7.99 Site of bifurcation into the left upper and lower lobe bronchi. The bifurcation angle between the left upper and lower lobe bronchi is sometimes obtuse as in this photo.

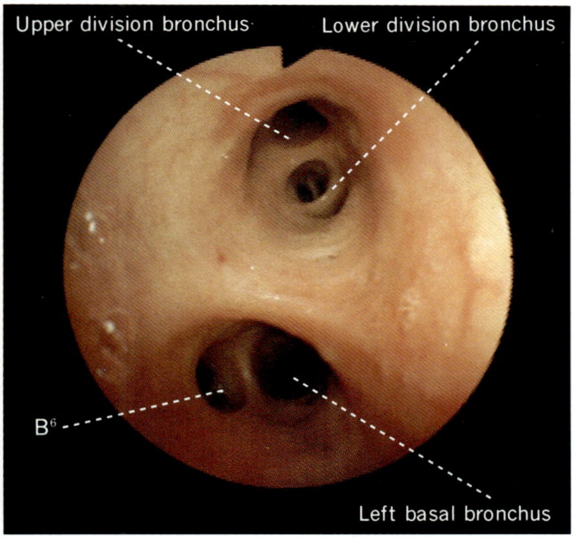

7.100 Site of bifurcation into the left upper and lower lobe bronchi. The left upper lobe bronchus bifurcates into the upper division bronchus and lower division bronchus. The bifurcation angle between the upper lobe and lower lobe bronchus is relatively sharp. In the left lower lobe bronchus there is the orifice of B^6, into which longitudinal mucosal folds enter.

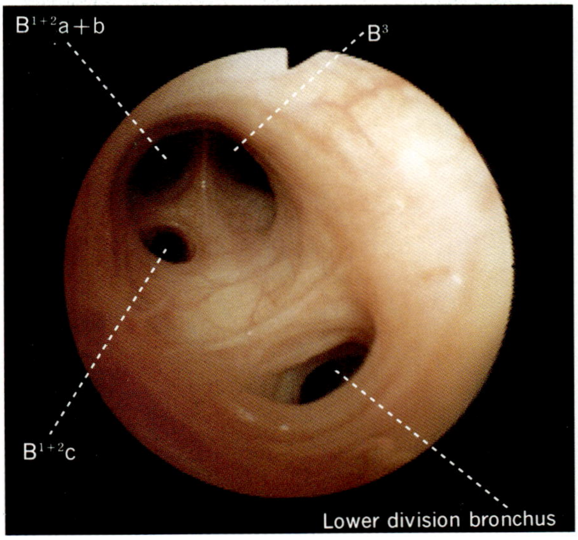

7.101 Left upper lobe bronchus (division into the upper and lower division bronchi): bifurcation type. The upper division bronchus and lower division bronchus separate and the upper division bronchus trifurcates into B^{1+2} and B^3.

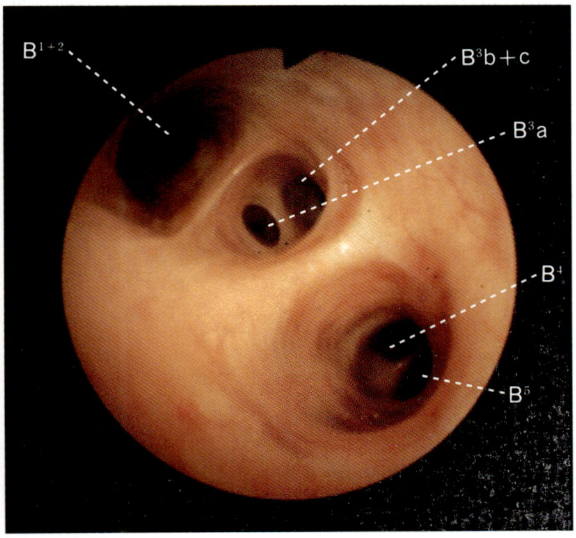

7.102 Trifurcation type. Usually the left upper lobe bronchus bifurcates. Trifurcation into B^{1+2}, B^3, and the lower division bronchus is observed in 2 per cent. Two clear longitudinal folds running to B^{1+2} are observed.

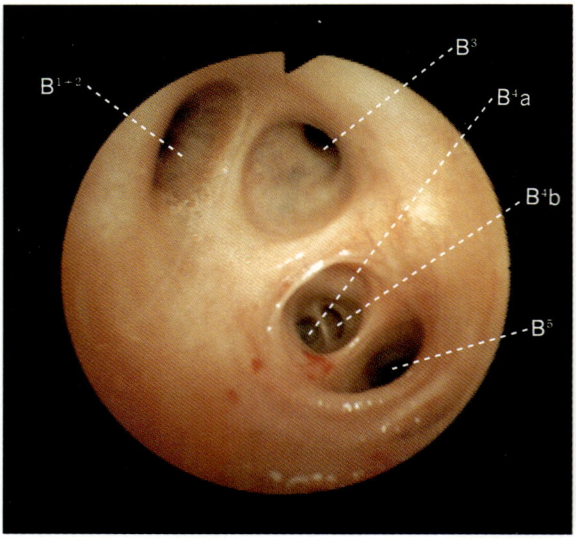

7.103 Left upper lobe bronchus (division into the upper and lower division bronchi): quadrifurcation type. The left upper lobe bronchus quadrifurcates into B^{1+2}, B^3, B^4 and B^5.

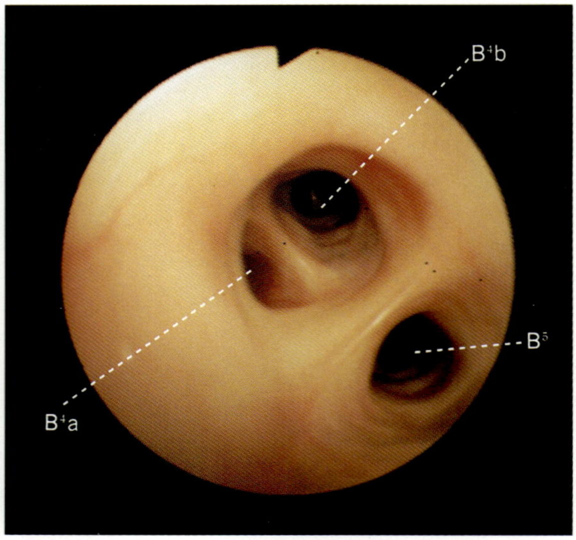

7.104 Lower division bronchus (lingular bronchus): bifurcation type. B^4 branches off near the orifice and B^5 more peripherally. This type is relatively common.

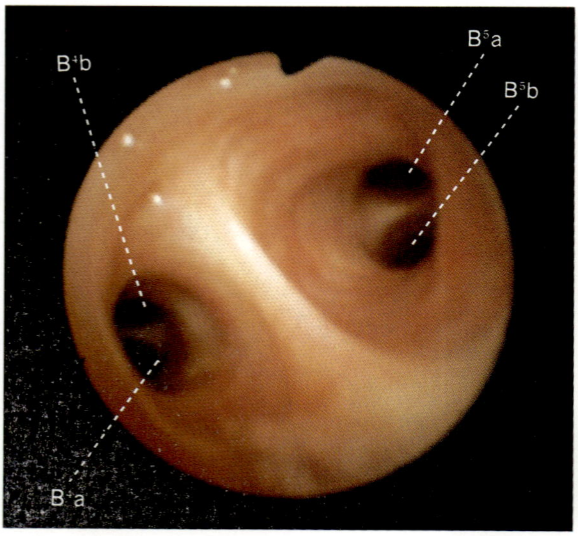

7.105 Lower division bronchus: bifurcation type. The lower division bronchus is divided into lateral and medial bronchi by a thick mucosal fold. At the peripheral site, subsegmental bronchi arise superiorly and inferiorly. The incidence of this type is about 33½ per cent.

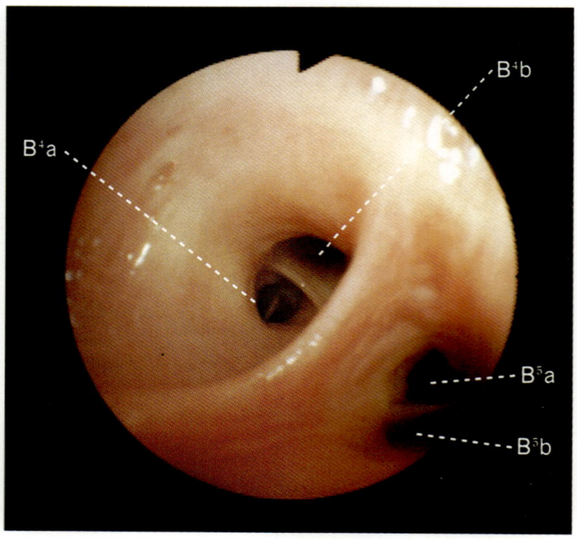

7.106 Lower division bronchus: bifurcation type. B^4 and B^5 bifurcate near the orifice into superior and inferior divisions. The incidence of this type is about 20 per cent.

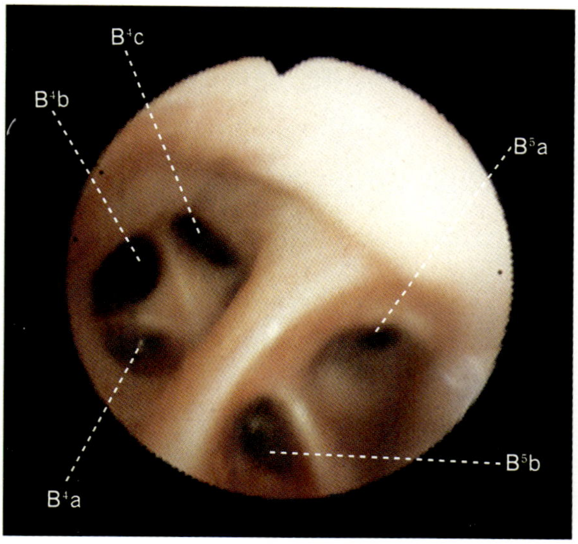

7.107 Lower division bronchus (lingular bronchus): bifurcation type. B^4 and B^5 trifurcate and bifurcate, respectively, near the orifice into the subsegmental bronchi.

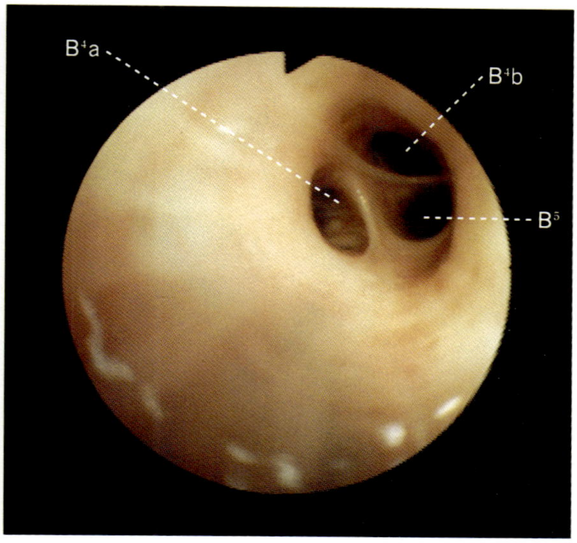

7.108 Lower division bronchus (lingular bronchus): complete trifurcation type. The lower division bronchus completely trifurcates. From the left, B^4a, B^4b, and B^5 are observed. The diameters of the orifices of the subsegmental bronchi of B^4 are similar to that of B^5.

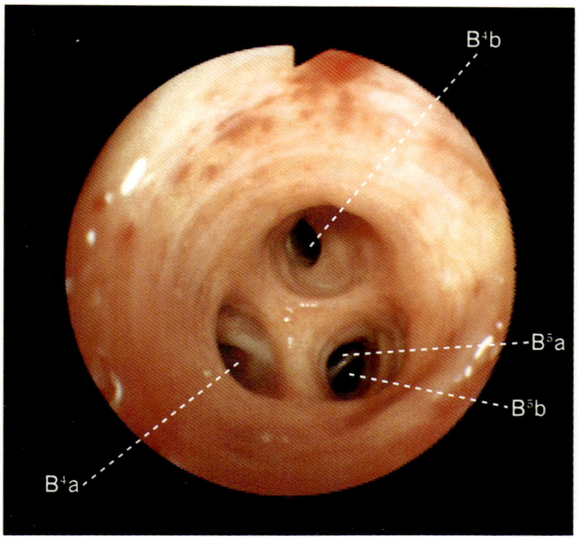

7.109 Lower division bronchus (lingular bronchus): complete trifurcation type. The lower division bronchus completely trifurcates into B^4a, B^4b and B^5 with similar size orifices.

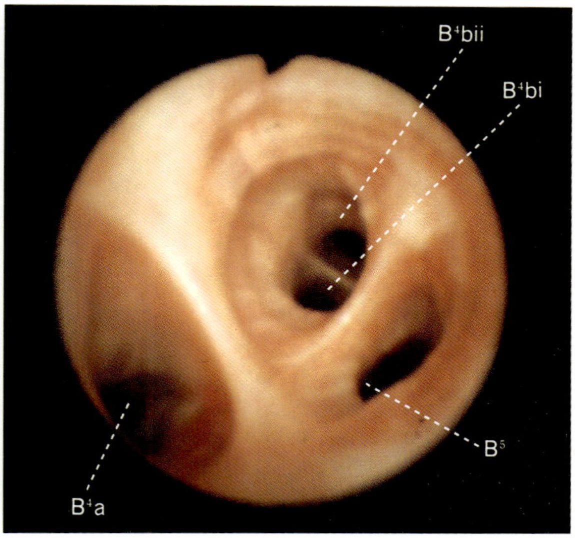

7.110 Lower division bronchus (lingular bronchus): incomplete trifurcation type. The lower division bronchus is divided into two by a thick mucosal fold. B^4a arises on the left side, and B^4b and B^5 on the right side.

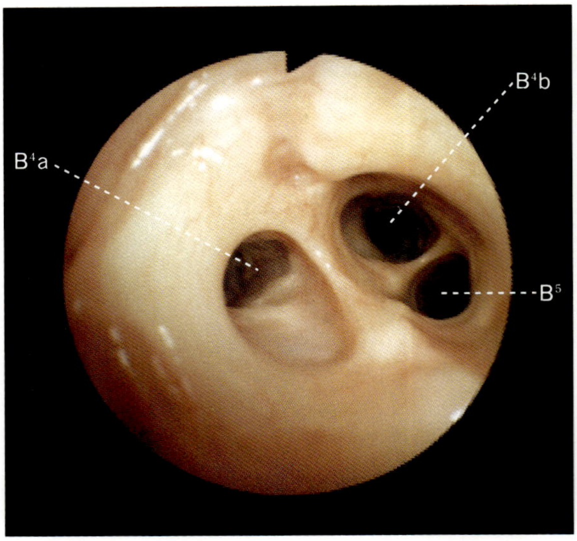

7.111 Lower division bronchus (lingular bronchus): complete trifurcation type. Initially, B^4a branches off laterally and then B^4b and B^5 arise. This is B^4a, and B^4b + B^5 type.

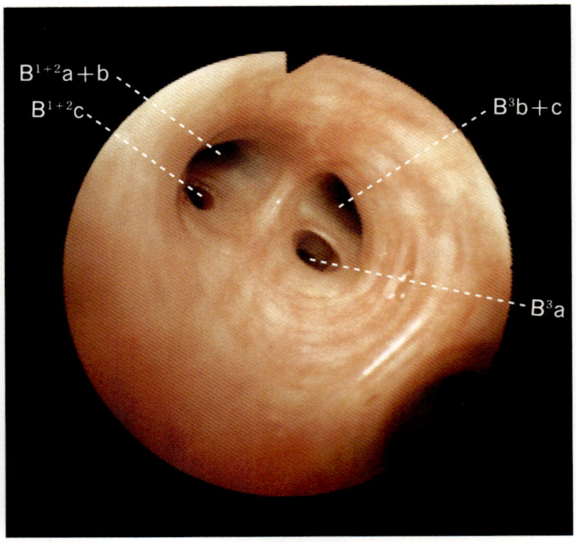

7.112 Upper division bronchus (B^3, B^{1+2}). B^3 is directly visible, and B^{1+2} is difficult to observe unless the scope is further advanced with its tip up.

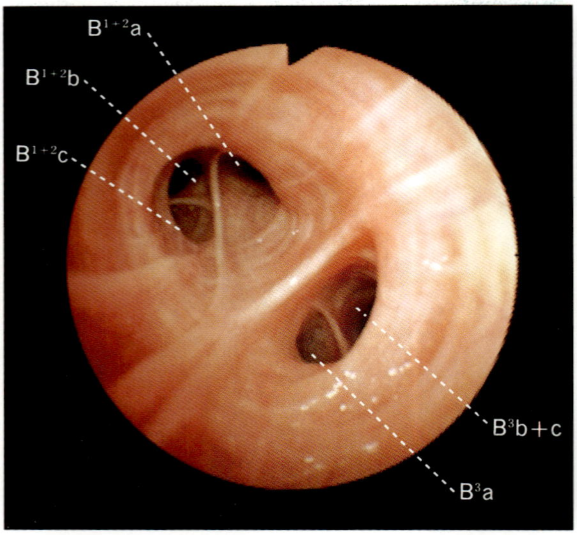

7.113 Upper division bronchus (B^3, B^{1+2}). B^{1+2} and B^3 are on the same level and visible directly. This type is relatively rare. B^{1+2} and B^3c distribute in the direction of the lung apex, B^{1+2} dorsally, B^3b anteriorly, and B^{1+2}c and B^3a in the left lateral direction.

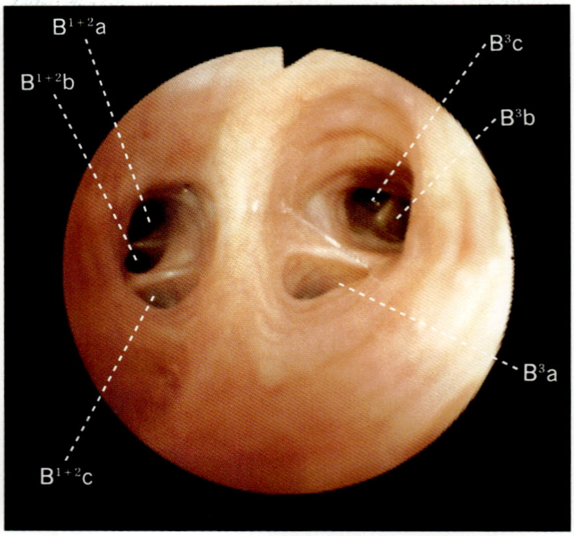

7.114 Upper division bronchus (B^3, B^{1+2}). B^{1+2}a, B^{1+2}b, and B^{1+2}c are observed on the lateral side. B^3 is also observed.

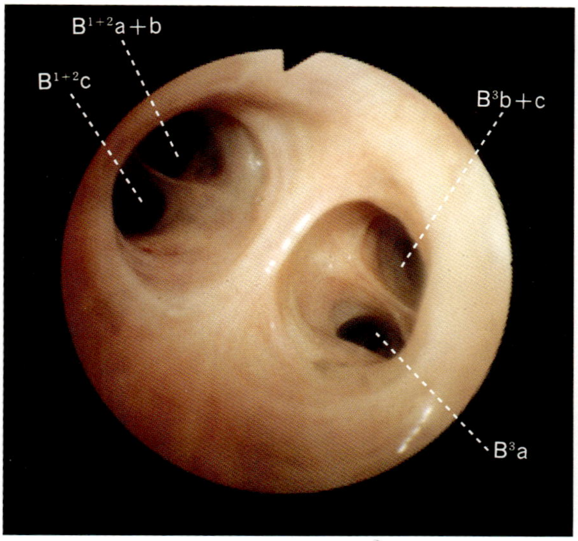

7.115 Upper division bronchus (B^3, B^{1+2}). Both B^{1+2} and B^3 bifurcate at the orifice. The orifice of the upper division bronchus is surrounded with circular folds consisting of smooth muscle.

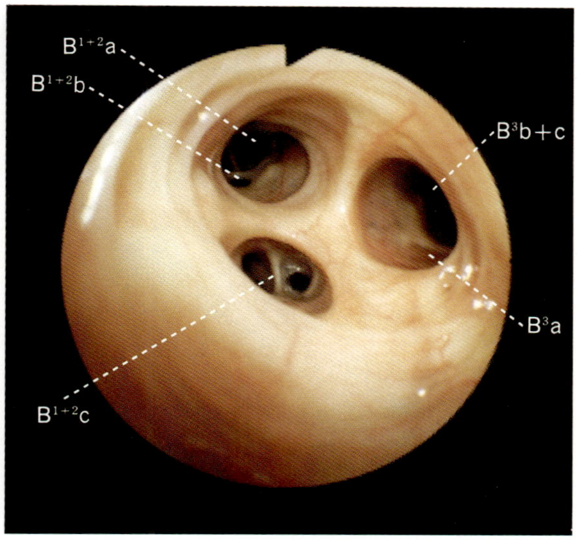

7.116 Upper division bronchus: trifurcation type (B^3, B^{1+2}). This is a type of trifurcation of the upper division bronchus. The diameters of the orifice are similar among $B^{1+2}c$, B^3, $B^{1+2}a + B^{1+2}b$.

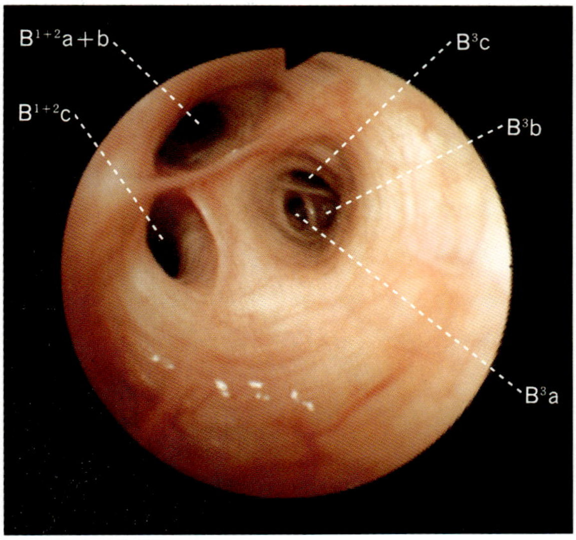

7.117 Upper division bronchus: trifurcation type (B^3, B^{1+2}). The orifices of $B^{1+2}c$, B^3, $B^{1+2}a + b$ are located at each apex of an equilateral triangle. The orifice of $B^{1+2}c$ is at right angles compared with those of B^3 and $B^{1+2}a + b$.

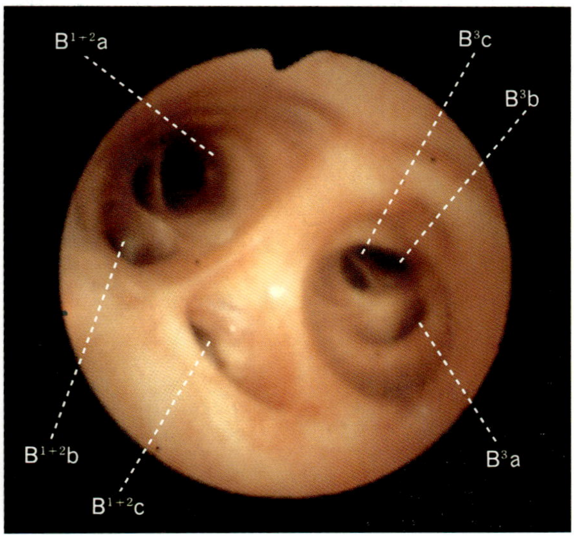

7.118 Upper division bronchus: trifurcation type (B^3, B^{1+2}). The orifice of $B^{1+2}c$ is at a right angle to the other bronchi.

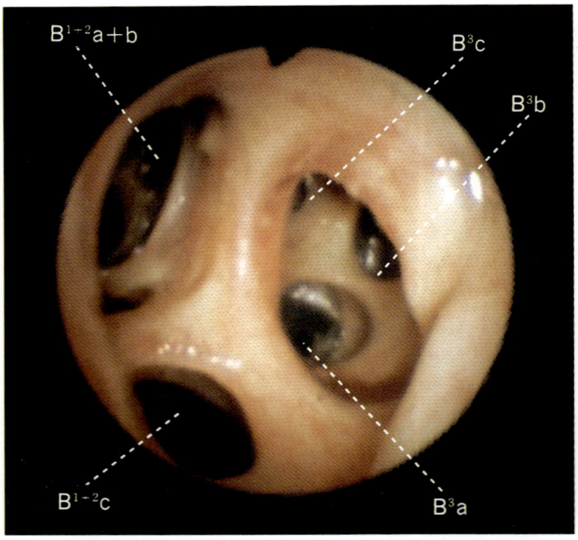

7.119 Upper division bronchus: trifurcation type (B^3, B^{1+2}). This case is a 69-year-old male who was a heavy smoker. Marked atrophy of the bronchial mucosa and anthracosis are observed.

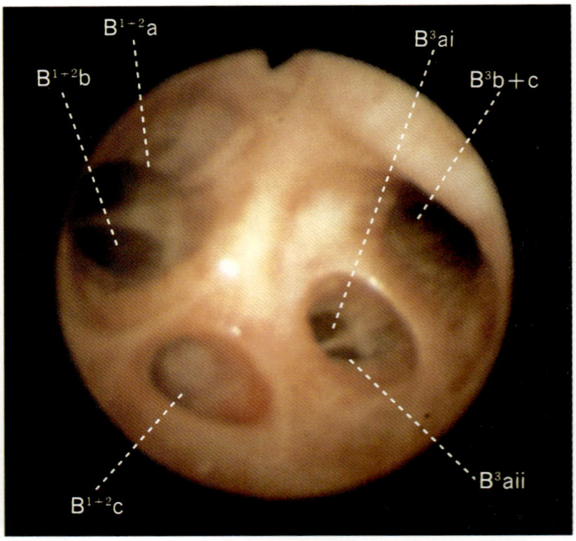

7.120 Upper division bronchus: quadrifurcation type (B^{1+2}, B^3). The diameters of the orifices of $B^{1+2}a + b$, $B^{1+2}c$, B^3a, and $B^3b + B^3c$ are similar. This type is extremely rare.

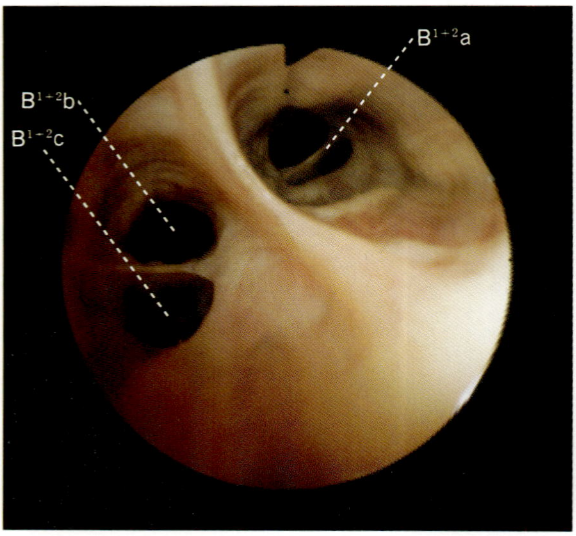

7.121 Left B^{1+2}. Three subsegmental bronchi of B^{1+2} are observed. $B^{1+2}a$ further bifurcates at its orifice.

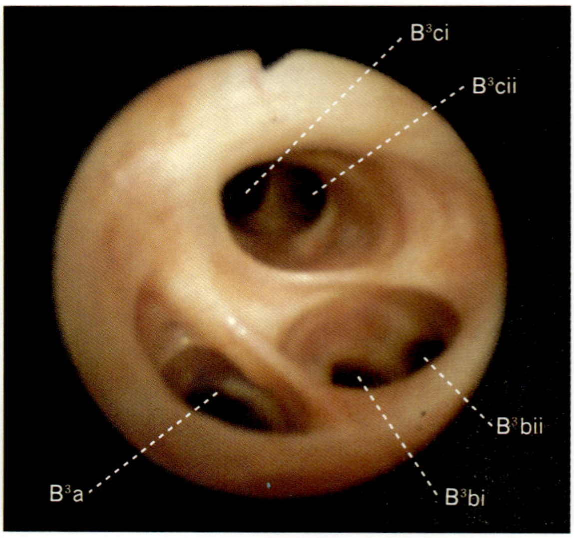

7.122 Left B^3. The subsegmental bronchi of left B^3 run anticlockwise. The orifices of the subsegmental bronchi are similar in diameter and present on the same level. Such a case is relatively rare.

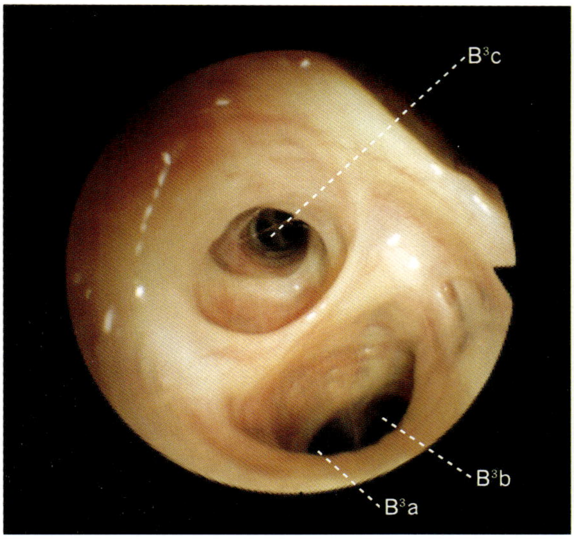

7.123 Left B^3. The most common type of division of left B^3. The subsegmental bronchi run anticlockwise.

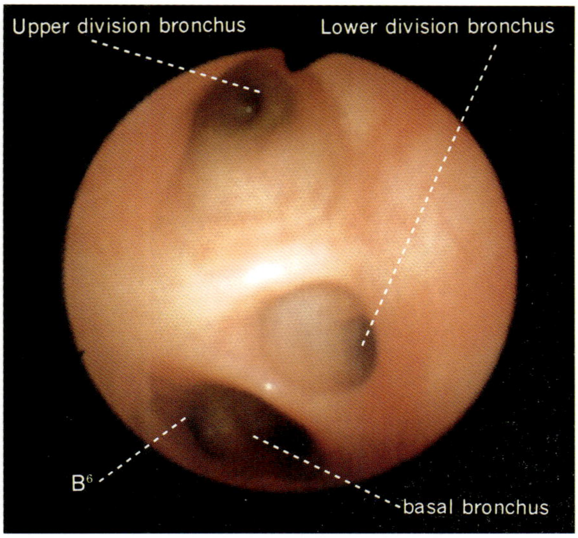

7.124 A variation of the bifurcation site into the left upper and lower lobe bronchi. The orifice of the lower division bronchus (B^4, B^5) is located not in the left upper lobe bronchus but in the centre of the bifurcation site into the upper and lower lobe bronchi. This type of case is extremely rare.

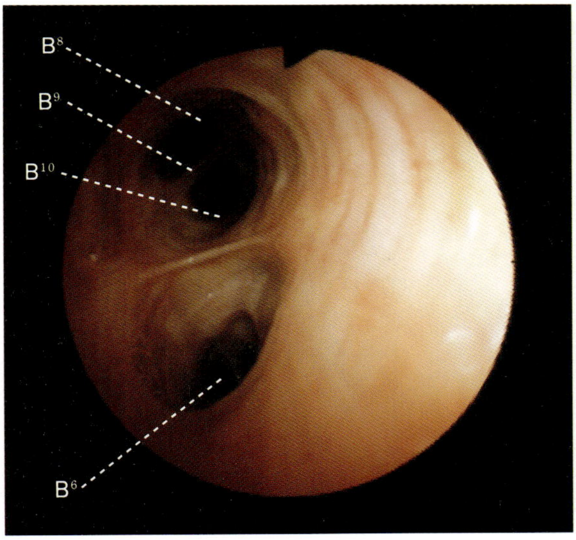

7.125 Left B^6 and left basal bronchus. This is a view from the orifice of the left lower lobe bronchus. The basal bronchi (B^8, B^9, B^{10}) are observed in the upper area and the orifice of B^6 in the lower area.

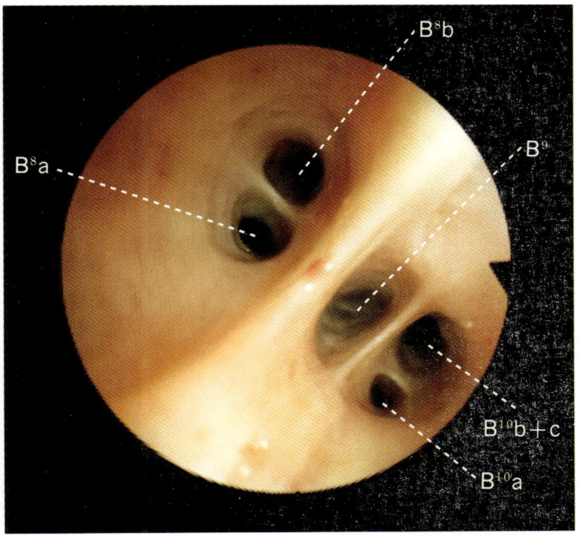

7.126 Left basal bronchus (B^8, $B^9 + B^{10}$). This is a standard type. B^8, B^9 and B^{10} are linear. There is a thick mucosal fold between B^8 and B^9.

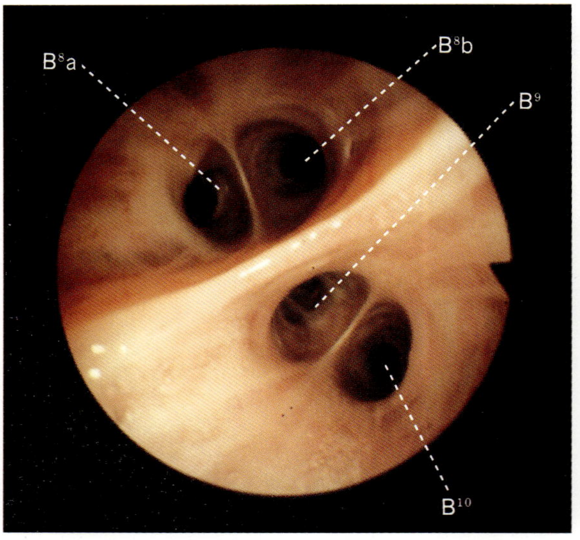

7.127 Left basal bronchus (B^8, B^9 + B^{10}). There is a thick mucosal fold between B^8 and B^9.

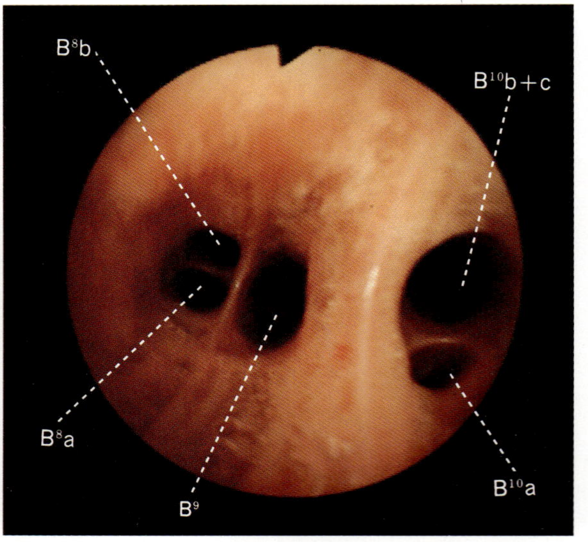

7.128 Left basal bronchus (B^8 + B^9, B^{10}). B^8, B^9 and B^{10} are linear. There is a thick mucosal fold between B^9 and B^{10}.

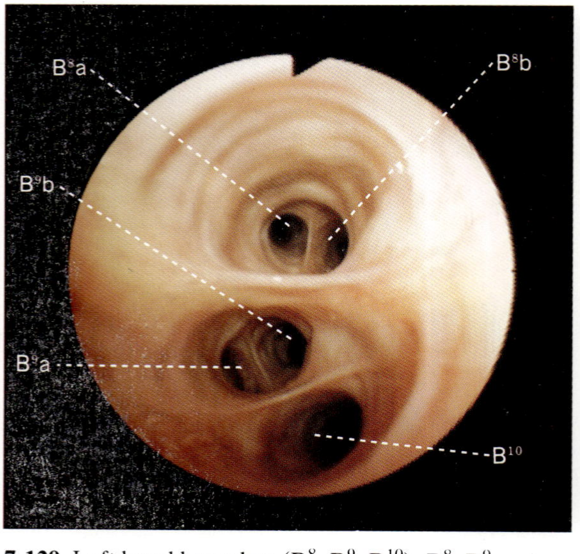

7.129 Left basal bronchus (B^8, B^9, B^{10}). B^8, B^9 and B^{10} are on a curve that is convex towards the left. There is a thick mucosal fold between B^8 and B^9.

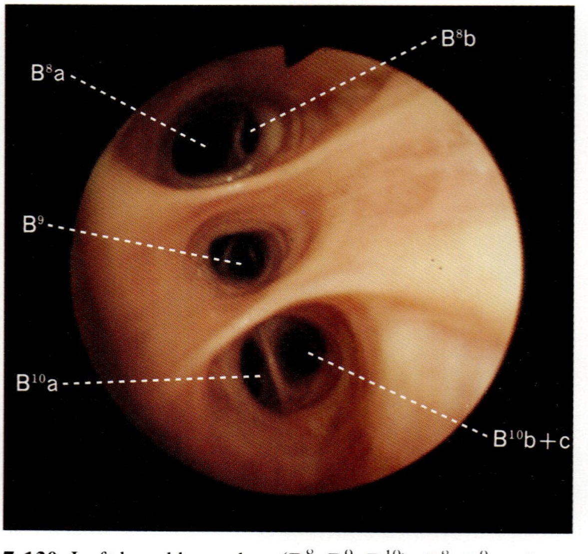

7.130 Left basal bronchus (B^8, B^9, B^{10}). B^8, B^9 and B^{10} are linear. The thickness of the mucosal fold between B^8 and B^9 is similar to that between B^9 and B^{10}.

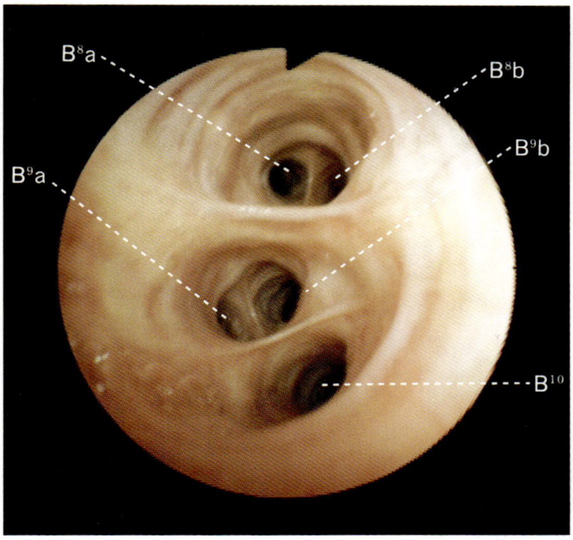

7.131 Left basal bronchus (B^8, B^9, B^{10}). B^8, B^9 and B^{10} are on a curve that is convex towards the left. The thickness of the mucosal fold between B^8 and B^9 is similar to that between B^9 and B^{10}.

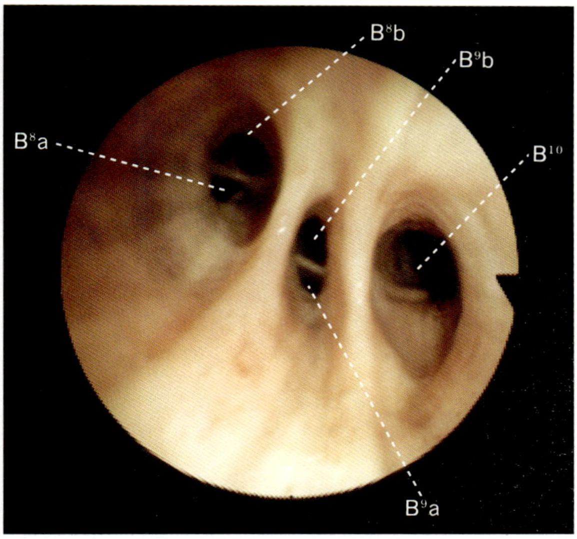

7.132 Left basal bronchus (B^8, B^9, B^{10}). B^8, B^9 and B^{10} are linear. The thickness of the mucosal fold between B^8 and B^9 is similar to that between B^9 and B^{10}. The orifice of B^9 is narrow and closed during expiration.

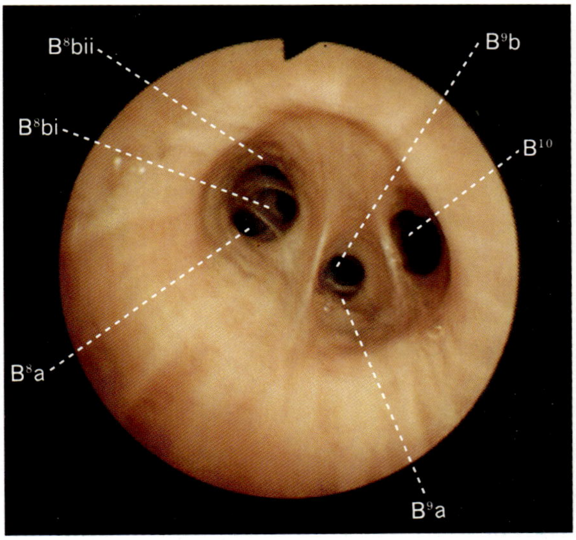

7.133 Left basal bronchus (B^8, B^9, B^{10}). B^8 and B^9 usually bifurcate. In this case B^8 trifurcates. Such a case is relatively rare.

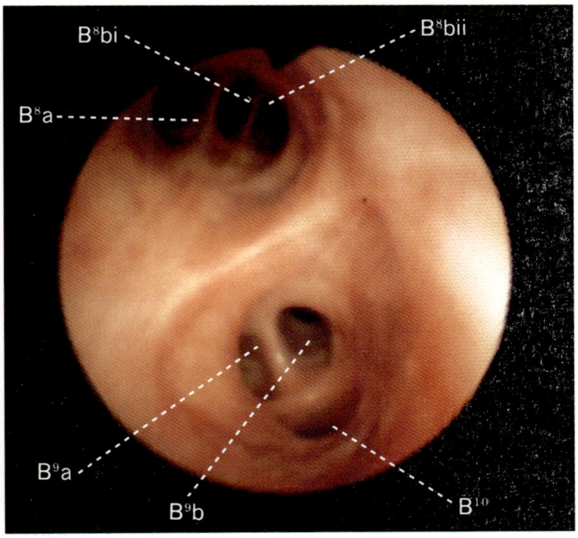

7.134 Left basal bronchus (B^8, B^9, B^{10}) B^8 trifurcates. The orifice of B^{10} is directed medioinferiorly (mediastinally).

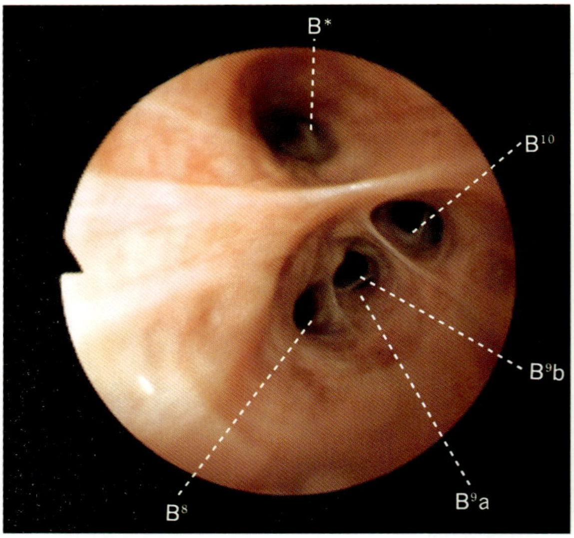

7.135 Left basal bronchus (B^8, B^9, B^{10}, B^*). B^* is sometimes observed in the left basal bronchus. In this case a large B^* is present anteriorly (ventrally) in the basal bronchus. B^8, B^9 and B^{10} in the basal bronchus are similar in size.

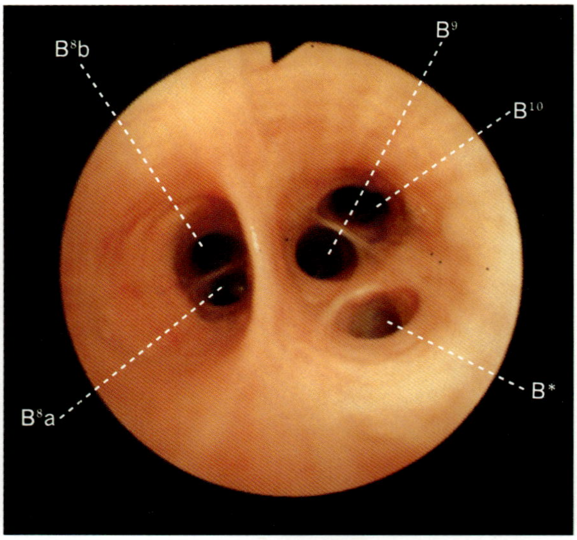

7.136 Left basal bronchus (B^8, B^9, B^{10}, B^*). This is the B^8 and $B^9 + B^{10}$ type. B^* is present dorsally in the orifice of $B^9 + B^{10}$.

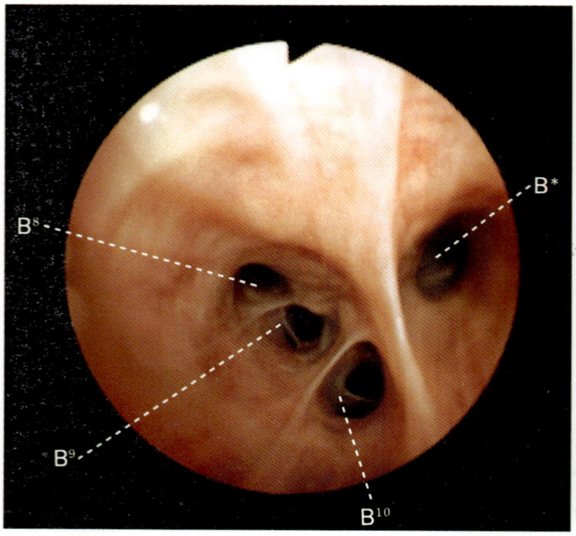

7.137 Left basal bronchus (B^8, B^9, B^{10}, B^*). B^8, B^9 and B^{10} are linear. B^* is located medially beyond a thick mucosal fold.

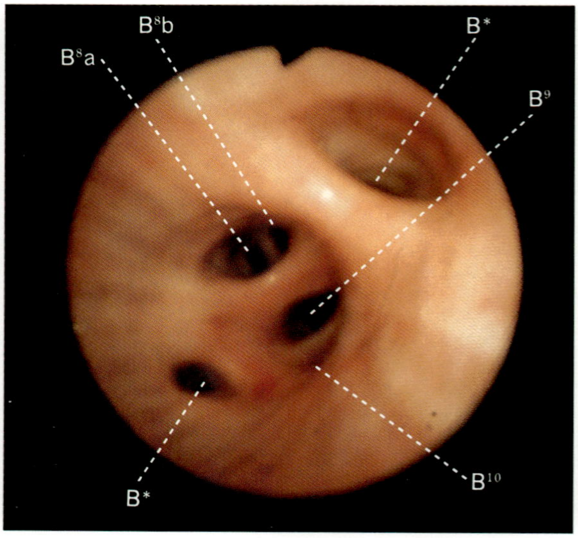

7.138 Left basal bronchus (B^8, B^9, B^{10}, B^*). B^* in the basal bronchus is not so rare. But B^* both anteriorly and posteriorly is rare.

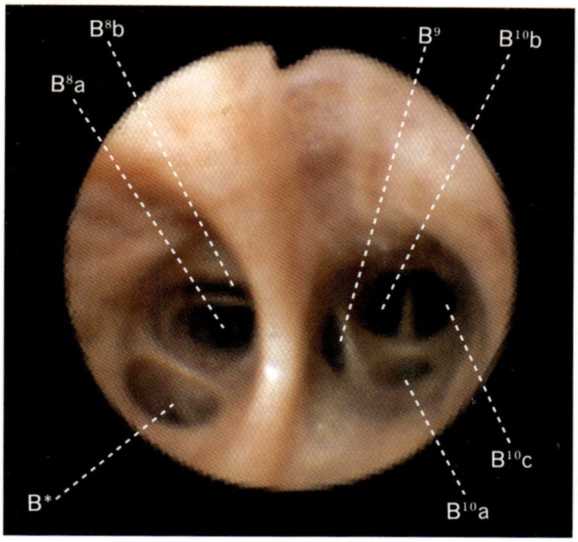

7.139 Left basal bronchus (B^8, B^9, B^{10}, B*). B* in all the above cases was located at the orifice of the basal bronchus or B^8 and B^9. In this case it is present at the orifice of B^8. B^9 is very small.

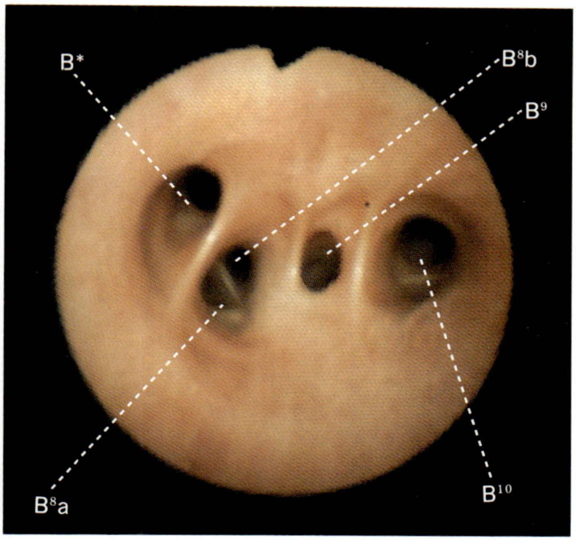

7.140 Left basal bronchus (B*, B^8, B^9, B^{10}). B^8, B^9 and B^{10} are linear. B* is present lateral to B^8.

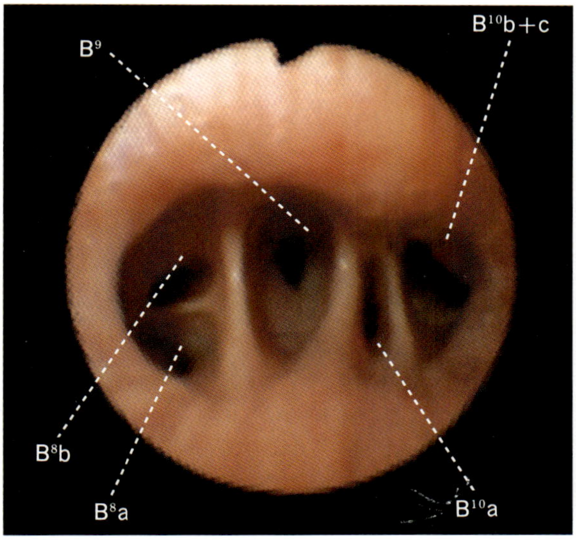

7.141 Left basal bronchus: quadrifurcation type. In this case, identification of segmental bronchi is very difficult. The possible nomenclature is, from the left, B*, B^8, B^9 and B^{10}; B^8, B^9a, B^9b, and B^{10}; B^8, B^9, B^{10}a, and B^{10}b + B^{10}c. The last seems to be appropriate.

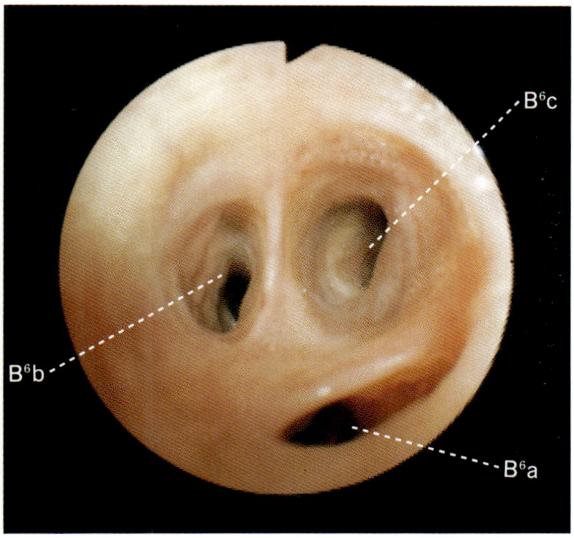

7.142 Left B^6: trifurcation type. B^6 arises first from the lower lobe bronchus posteriorly (dorsally). The incidence of trifurcation type (B^6a, B^6b, B^6c) was reported to be 14.5 per cent by Boyden[3], B^6a arises superiorly at right angles to the other bronchi.

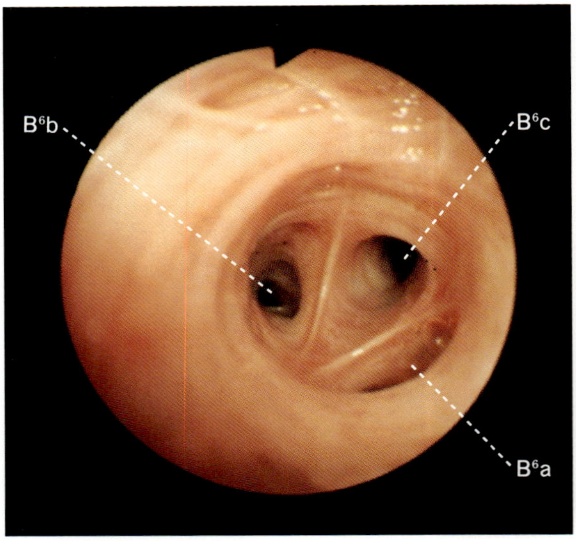

7.143 Left B^6: trifurcation type. Y-shaped trifurcation is observed.

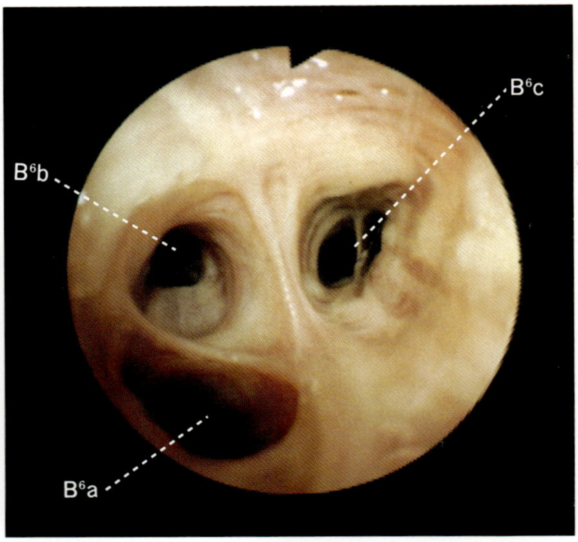

7.144 Left B^6: trifurcation type. The orifices of B^6a, B^6b and B^6c are located at an apex of an equilateral triangle. The branching angle at the orifices is also similar.

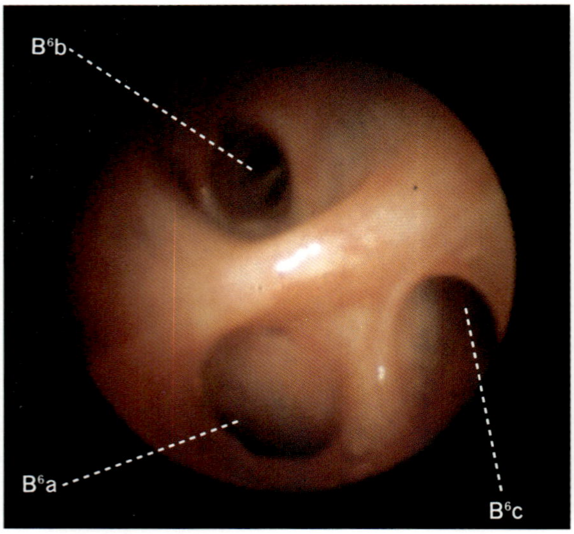

7.145 Left B^6: trifurcation type. The similar-sized orifices of B^6a, B^6b, and B^6c are located at each apex of an equilateral triangle. The branching angle is different.

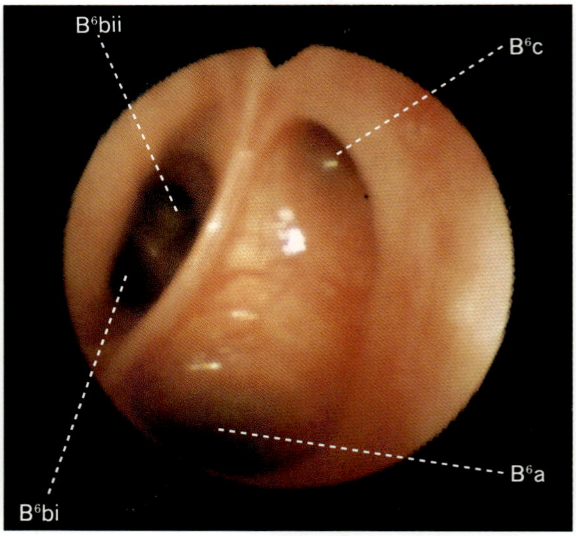

7.146 Left B^6: trifurcation type. B^6b is dependent, but B^6a and B^6c are in a common sulcus.

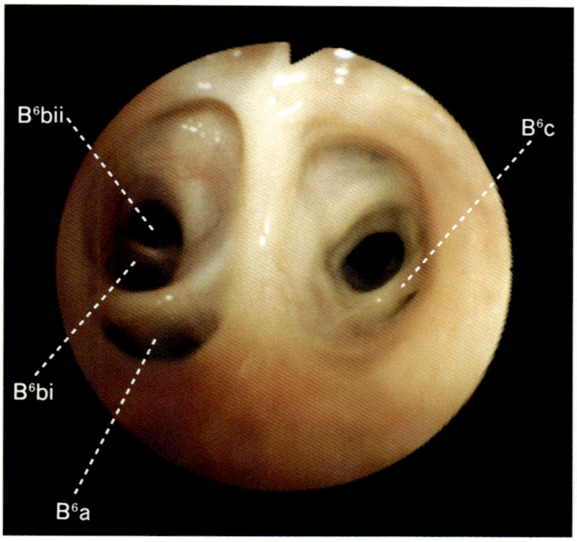

7.147 Left B^6: bifurcation type ($B^6a + B^6b$, B^6c). B^6a is adjacent to B^6b. B^6c is present at an opposite site beyond a thick mucosal fold. The incidence of this type is 42.7 per cent according to Boyden[3].

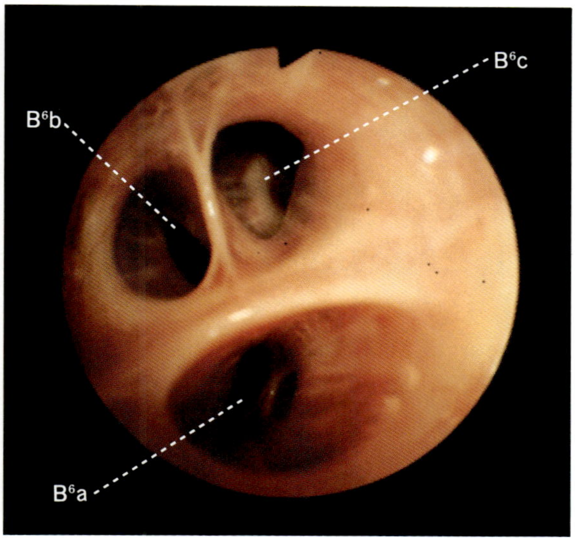

7.148 Left B^6: bifurcation type (B^6a, $B^6b + B^6c$). The incidence of bifurcation type (B^6a, $B^6b + B^6c$) was reported to be 29 per cent by Boyden[3].

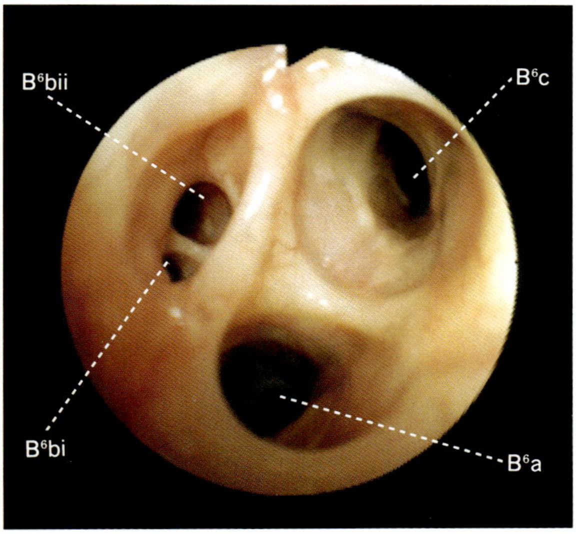

7.149 Left B^6: trifurcation type ($B^6a + B^6c$, B^6b). The origins of B^6a and B^6c are in a large common sulcus.

8 Classification of bronchoscopic findings

1 Endoscopic findings in the normal trachea and bronchi

It is very important to make precise and appropriate descriptions of bronchoscopic findings. Colour, shape and motility should be routinely observed. Today, endoscopic findings in the bronchi have been described not only in large-sized airways (trachea, lobar and segmental bronchi) but also in small-sized airways (subsegmental or even smaller bronchi). In particular, lesions in the bronchial lumen and wall have been described precisely. Categorisations for the classification of bronchoscopic findings were adopted by the Japan Lung Society in 1979 (Table 8.1).

Table 8.1 Categorisation of bronchoscopic findings

1 The bronchial wall
1) Redness or pallor
2) Absence of mucosal surface lustre
3) Swelling (oedema)
4) Vascular engorgement
5) Irregular mucosal surface
6) Indistinct cartilage ring
7) Protrusion of bronchial cartilage
8) Ulceration of the bronchial wall
9) Enlargement of the mucous glands
10) Transparent lymph nodes
11) Mucosal atrophy
12) Mucosal thickening
13) Tumour
14) Necrosis
15) Abnormalities in the mucosal folds

(irregularities, thickening, indistinctness, disappearance)

2 The bronchial lumen
1) Stenosis
2) Obstruction
3) Enlargement
4) Compression
5) Abnormal branching
—including diverticulum
6) Abnormal findings at bifurcation
(widening, compression, contriction)

3 Pathological substances
1) Abnormal secretions
2) Bleeding
3) Stones
4) Foreign bodies

4 Disturbance of movement
1) Abnormal movement during respiration
2) Abnormal movement on coughing

2 Endoscopic findings in patients with lung cancer

Squamous cell carcinoma usually grows in the hilar region (central type) and can be easily detected and diagnosed by fibreoptic bronchoscopy. Advanced lesions are seen most frequently in main or lobar bronchi and often in segmental or subsegmental bronchi. More peripheral lesions are rare. Usually tumours with an irregular surface and necrosis are seen as endoscopic findings of squamous cell carcinoma. Although about 10 per cent of squamous cell carcinomas proliferate in the peripheral parts of the lung, they will protrude within the lumen of the bronchi even in such cases.

Adenocarcinoma is a type of cancer which grows in the peripheral bronchi of the lung. Abnormal findings will be observed even in the segmental or subsegmental bronchi as tumours grow. They usually cannot be observed directly by routine fibreoptic bronchoscopy, because they grow in the 3rd or 4th divisions of peripheral bronchi. They often grow to invade regional lymph nodes and compress large bronchi.

Small cell carcinomas show unique findings at endoscopy. Especially in oat cell cancer, tumours usually invade submucosally and they do not appear in the bronchial lumen. The bronchial lumen often shows extreme redness and swelling. It is common to find indirect compression and loss of mucosal surface lustre[1]. In the past endoscopic findings in lung cancer were not described sufficiently, because we had few technical terms to describe these findings. For example, invasive findings were expressed only by the following terms—vascular engorgement, irregular mucosal surface, indistinct cartilage ring. After we accumulated new knowledge on these findings, in comparison with the pathological findings, we made up several new terms to express them. Table 8.2 illustrates bronchoscopic findings observed in patients with lung cancer by the Japan Lung Cancer Society.

Table 8.2 Findings in lung cancer cases

1 The bronchial wall
- 1) Tumour
  - a nodular
  - b multinodular
  - c smooth surface
  - d irregular surface
  - e granular surface
  - f necrosis
  - g vascular engorgement
- 2) Infiltration
  - a mucosal irregularity
  - b vascular engorgement
  - c loss of lustre
  - d necrosis
  - e pallor of mucosa
  - f swelling
  - g redness
  - h indistinct bronchial cartilage
  - i thickened mucosal folds
  - j indistinct mucosal folds

2 Changes in the bronchial lumen
- 1) Stenosis
  - a due to tumour
  - b due to infiltration
  - c due to external compression
- 2) Obstruction
  - a due to tumour
  - b due to infiltration
  - c due to external compression

3 Bronchoscopic findings in other diseases

Fibreoptic bronchoscopy has become a common investigative procedure. It has been used in many other respiratory diseases as well as in the diagnosis of lung cancer. Redness, swelling and indistinct cartilage rings are typical findings in patients with acute bronchitis, and sometimes purulent secretion is attached to the bronchial wall. Similar findings are observed in acute pneumonia patients; these findings are dominant in the lobar or segmental bronchus which leads to the inflammatory lesion.

In pulmonary tuberculosis, bronchoscopic findings differ according to the types of disease and the stage. In the acute phase, redness, swelling, indistinct cartilage rings and increase of secretion can be observed; these findings may suggest severe inflammatory change. Tracheal or bronchial tuberculosis is often complicated by pulmonary tuberculosis; in such cases granulomatous or white necrotic tissue can be observed on the bronchial wall[2].

In patients suffering from chronic bronchitis, redness, swelling and vascular engorgement will be present. Sometimes indistinct cartilage rings may be visible. The most characteristic change is the formation of a small diverticulum in the bronchial mucosa. It is formed by the dilatation of the mucous gland duct in the bronchial wall. At bronchography, the contrast medium shows a small protrusion in the bronchial wall, especially in the main, lobar or segmental bronchus.

In sarcoidosis, typical findings are frequently seen. Bronchial lesions are usually seen from the main up to the subsegmental bronchus. Epithelioid cell granulomas are seen in the submucosa of large bronchi. At bronchoscopy, diffuse small nodular lesions or networks caused by vascular engorgement can be observed. Irregularity and swelling of the bronchial wall can also be seen. The carina may be widened and the bronchial lumen may be narrowed[3].

Diffuse panbronchiolitis also shows characteristic findings at bronchoscopy. All bifurcations, from the carina to subsegmental bronchi, are widened. Bronchial mucosa may be red, swollen, thickened and irregular. Cartilage rings will be indistinct and purulent secretion may be increased[4].

Lymphangitis carcinomatosa shows a typical radiographic finding and can be diagnosed successfully by transbronchial lung biopsy (TBLB). Bronchoscopic findings will show widening of bifurcations from carina to subsegmental or further peripheral bronchi. Bronchial mucosa may be swollen and the cartilage rings may be indistinct, which may suggest the existence of a congested lymphatic circulation.

References

[1] Ikeda, S., Recent progress in fibreoptic bronchoscopy. *Jpn. J. Bronchoesophagology,* **30**, 63, 1979.

[2] Hayashi, R., Kitamura, S. *et al.,* A case of tracheobronchial tuberculosis observed serially by bronchofibrescopy. *Jpn. J. Thoracic Dis.,* **18**, 453, 1980.

[3] Kosuda, J. and Miyachi, J., Bronchofiberscopic findings in patients with sarcoidosis. *J. Jpn. Soc. Bronchology,* **2**, 7, 1980.

[4] Sugiyama, Y., Kitamura, S. *et al.,* Bronchofiberscopic findings and histological diagnosis by TBLB in patients with diffuse panbronchiolitis. *J. Jpn. Soc. Bronchology,* **3**(Suppl.) , 70, 1981.

9 Clinical application of fibreoptic bronchoscopy

A Diagnostic applications

The method of fibreoptic bronchoscopy has been improved; today it can be performed easily, safely and more comfortably. It is used in several clinical ways, especially as a procedure of diagnosis and treatment of various respiratory diseases. The following subsections describe the various practical applications of fibreoptic bronchoscopy.

1 Observation of intratracheal and intrabronchial lesions

This is one of the most popular applications of fibreoptic bronchoscopy. The inserted fibrescope visualises the pharynx, vocal cords, glottis, trachea, carina (bifurcation), lobar bronchus, segmental bronchus, and further peripheral bronchi. Not only direct viewing but also photographic observation is possible. It is also possible to observe conditions of the bronchial mucosa, and locate tumours or inflammatory lesions.

2 Collection of intrabronchial sputum for pathological and bacteriological examination

When inflammatory changes are present in the bronchial mucous membrane and malignant or infectious disease is suspected, a specimen of intrabronchial sputum should be collected for pathological and bacteriological examination. The examination should not only test for common bacteria but also for mycobacteria, fungi and parasites. To increase diagnostic yield lignocaine should not be used beyond the glottis, because it inhibits the growth of most micro-organisms. Pathological examinations should be carried out when inflammatory changes, white necrotic tissue and submucosal infiltration are seen in the bronchial mucous membrane.

3 Biopsy of tumours visible in the trachea or bronchi

Visible lesions, for example tumours or granulomas, can be biopsied by using various forceps. To prevent excessive bleeding, diluted epinephrine solution can be injected into the site before biopsy. If bleeding cannot be controlled, 2-3 ml of thrombin solution (1000u/ml) can be sprayed on to the biopsy site. Biopsied specimens stored in formaldehyde solution can be examined histologically.

4 Bronchial mucous membrane biopsy in cases of lymphangitis carcinomatosa and diffuse panbronchiolitis

Bronchial mucous membrane biopsy should be carried out when abnormal findings are present. Diffuse panbronchiolitis (DPB), sarcoidosis, Wegener's granulomatosis, lymphangitis carcinomatosa, or miliary tuberculosis can be diagnosed by bronchoscopy. The bifurcation of the right and left upper lobe bronchi, the bifurcation of the right middle lobe bronchus and the bifurcation of the bilateral B^6 bronchi are usual biopsy sites. Both main bronchi can sometimes be biopsied. Bleeding can be reduced usually by injecting a solution of epinephrine, but occasionally use of thrombin solution may be necessary to control excessive bleeding.

5 Collection of bronchoalveolar lavage fluid

Bronchoalveolar lavage is a method of collecting fluid through the channel of a wedged fibrescope after saline has been injected (**9.1A**). This method is used to collect and analyse liquid and cellular components from the bronchus and alveoli of specified lesions. Various diffuse lung diseases can be diagnosed by this method. Figure **9.1B** illustrates the collection of bronchoalveolar lavage fluid into an Argyll tube; this instrument is also suitable for collecting sputum from the bronchi.

As fibreoptic bronchoscopy becomes more popular today, not only 'the classical examinations', for example observation, tumour biopsy, transbronchial lung biopsy (TBLB), endobronchial brushing, and collection of sputum, but also 'the new analytic examinations' of cellular and liquid components in bronchoalveolar lavage fluid are carried out.

These methods are divided in two groups: 'bronchial lavage' (BL) and 'bronchoalveolar lavage' (BAL). The former instills saline into the proximal bronchi, and the latter instills saline into the peripheral airways which contain bronchioles and alveoli.

A practical common method of BAL has not been established yet. Usually, the patient is given a local anaesthetic using 4 per cent lignocaine spray; the fibreoptic bronchoscope is then inserted with the patient in the supine position. The fibreoptic bronchoscope is often wedged in the right middle lobe or left lingular segmental bronchi and 20-50 ml of warmed (36°C) saline is instilled and recovered by negative pressure three to six times. The author usually wedges the fibreoptic bronchoscope in the right B^3 bronchus and instills 50 ml of saline three times[1]. The recovered fluid is filtered through gauze, the number of cells are counted using a hemocytometer, and the cells are stained using the Wright–Giemsa stain. The cell fraction is examined from the sediment after low-speed centrifugation, and the liquid fraction is assessed from the supernatant. Of the liquid components, IgG, ACE, CEA, fibronectin, leukotriene, prostaglandin E_2, $F_2\alpha$, thromboxane B2, 6-keto-$PGF_1\alpha$, histamine, and serotonin are assayed; however, their pathophysiological roles have not been clarified yet.

The analysis of cellular components in bronchoalveolar lavage fluid (BALF) is important for the diagnosis of various lung diseases, especially idiopathic pulmonary fibrosis (IPF), sarcoidosis, and hypersensitivity pneumonitis[2]. It is also very useful to diagnose or judge the stages and activity of the disease. For example, in the cellular components of BALF, alveolar macrophages (AMs) are more than 95 per cent and lymphocytes are less than 5 per cent in healthy volunteers; on the other hand AMs are 50-60 per cent and lymphocytes are 30-80 per cent in sarcoidosis, hypersensitivity pneumonitis, and the active phase of IPF. By the analysis of T-cell subsets using the antibody of the OKT series, it has been clarified that the number of OKT4 positive cells (T4) increases and that of OKT8 positive cells (T8) decreases, thereby the T4/T8 ratio increases. In BALF of hypersensitivity pneumonitis, the number of T8 increases and the T4/T8 ratio decreases. T4 and T8 have been recognised as the helper/inducer cell and the suppressor/cytotoxic cell respectively. Izumi *et al*[3]. have showed that the number of activated T-lymphocytes increases significantly in the BALF of hypersensitivity pneumonitis and sarcoidosis, compared with the control group. On the other hand they have shown that the number of activated B-lymphocytes increases significantly in the BALF of idiopathic pulmonary fibrosis and collagen vascular diseases (see **9.2**). In addition, some specific findings are pointed out in the liquid component of BALF in several diseases (see **9.3**).

Many other substances in BALF liquid components will be analysed in the near future. These findings will be more important in diagnosing various lung diseases.

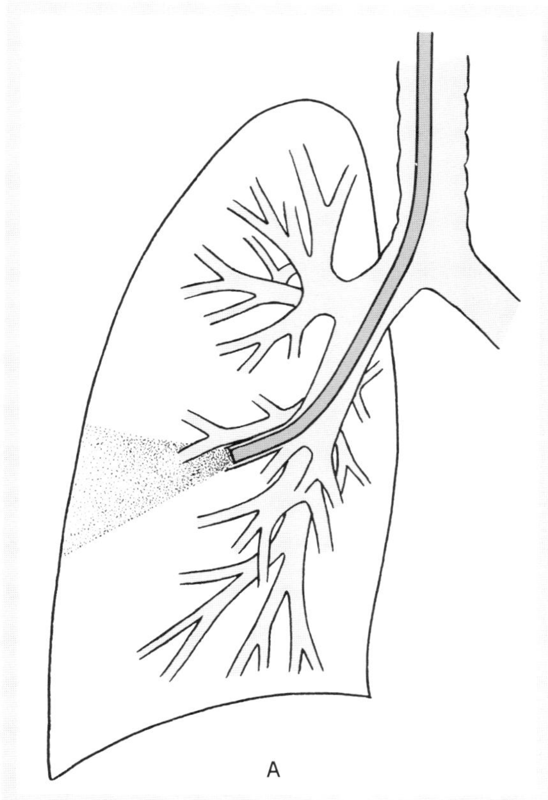

9.1A Technique for bronchoalveolar lavage (BAL).

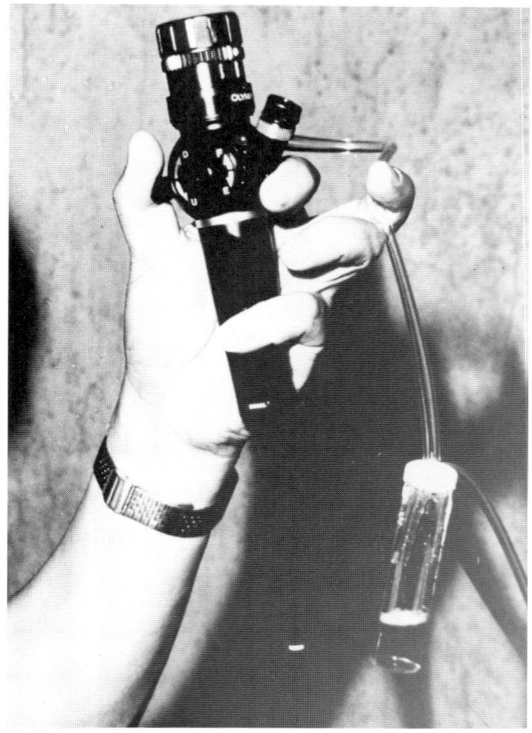

9.1B Collection of BAL fluid using an Argyll tube.

6 Biopsy of peripheral mass lesions

This procedure is used when mass lesions are not visible at bronchoscopy but apparent at fluorography. Essential instruments for this procedure, for example light source, aspirator, fibrescope and biopsy forceps, can be placed on a fibrescope trolley (**9.5**). The practical method is as follows: first locate the mass lesion by using chest radiographs, tomography and CT. The fibrescope is then inserted into the bronchus and routine photographs are taken (**9.6**). Guided by fluoroscopy, the forceps is eased forward with the utmost care through the channel of the fibrescope to reach the mass lesion. If the forceps overlaps the tumour shadow on fluoroscopy, the patient's body is rotated to ensure that the forceps is successfully attached to the mass lesion (**9.7**). The forceps are opened and closed within the tumour and biopsy specimens are extracted (**9.8**).

7 Brushing of peripheral lesions for pathological examination

To approach peripheral lesions, diffuse or solitary, the brushing method is used under fluoroscopy. The fibrescope is inserted in the bronchus of the patient and the brush instrument is inserted through the channel of the bronchoscope to reach the lesion, which is observed and recognised under

9.2 Changes in activated lymphocytes in BAL fluid in various lung diseases[3]. Grey columns indicate a significant increase compared with healthy controls.

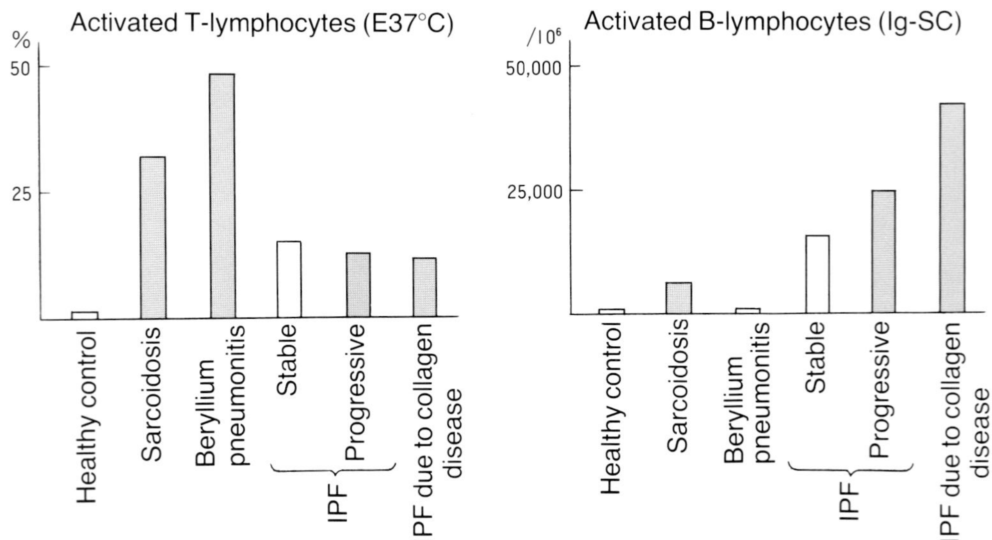

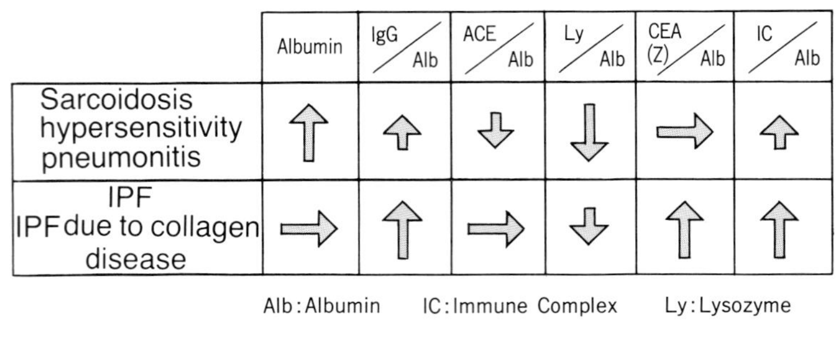

9.3 Change in humoral factors in BAL fluid in various lung diseases[3].

fluoroscopy. The brush is drawn to and fro several times, removed and run over glass plates for the material to be examined pathologically or bacteriologically. Next the brush from the brushed bronchus is washed in saline, and the solution can also be examined as above. The brushing procedure is shown in **9.9.**

8 Transbronchial lung biopsy (TBLB)

a) Clinical significance of TBLB

Various lung diseases show diffuse disseminated shadows on chest radiography. The main causes are miliary tuberculosis, pneumoconiosis, sarcoidosis, rheumatoid lung, diffuse panbronchiolitis, diffuse interstitial pulmonary fibrosis, pulmonary infiltration with eosinophilia, leukaemic infiltration, hypersensitivity pneumonitis, *Pneumocystis carinii,* lymphangitis carcinomatosa, eosinophilic granuloma, viral infection and alveolar proteinosis.

Diagnosing these diseases by using chest radiography alone is not easy. It is necessary to collect lung tissue specimens to make a pathological diagnosis. Open lung biopsy was commonly recommended in the past, but because it is an invasive procedure, few patients actually had to undergo this operation. However, today TBLB is an indispensable procedure in diagnosing diffuse lung diseases, because it is not so invasive and can be performed even at an out-patients clinic. The advent of HIV infection and AIDS has extended the use and value of the technique. The author performs TBLB on more than 200 patients a year and the pathological diagnoses have been established in 70 to 80 per cent of patients.

In lymphangitis carcinomatosa and miliary tuberculosis, the diagnosis was established in 100 per cent of patients. In diffuse panbronchiolitis and sarcoidosis, 64 per cent and 80 per cent were diagnosed respectively. These percentages may rise if we increase the number of biopsy procedures and/or of biopsy specimens.

b) Contraindications to TBLB

As a rule there are no contraindications to carrying out TBLB. However, patients with a tendency to bleed profusely, patients whose platelet count is less than 50,000/mm^3, patients with severe respiratory or heart failure, uraemia, cor pulmonale, or just after a heart attack may be exempted. Some patients have to be diagnosed as soon as possible, because they can be treated efficiently and successfully if diagnosed early. Typical diseases are drug-induced pneumonitis, leukaemic infiltration, intrapulmonary haemorrhage, and opportunistic infections such as virus, mycoplasma, or *Pneumocystis carinii.* If the number of platelets is less than 50,000/mm^3, platelet transfusion should be given 1-3 days before TBLB.

Patients with hypoxaemia whose P_aO_2 value is less than 50 Torr are not recommended for TBLB. If such patients must undergo this procedure, supplementary oxygen inhalation would be necessary during and for 12 hours after TBLB.

Patients prone to asthma or with a history of bronchial asthma are not always excluded; however, they sometimes suffer from a severe asthmatic attack or spasm of the glottis during local anaesthesia or immediately after insertion of the fibrescope. The author usually tells such patients to take a glucocorticoid agent (prednisolone 30-60 mg, P.O.) and a methylxanthine agent (aminophylline 250 mg, DIV) before TBLB. These prophylactic agents are usually very effective.

c) Practical considerations

i) Tools

The fibreoptic bronchoscope BF10 (Olympus) is most frequently used. BF-2T10 is useful because blood can be removed simultaneously from another channel during biopsy. Patients with a tendency to bleed heavily may have a BF-3C10 with small calibre used on them. BF-1T10 is useful to treat patients who tend to bleed because it has a large channel.

Fenestrated forceps with holes are used frequently because they prevent lung tissue specimens from being crushed. The author generally uses special forceps with crocodile teeth.

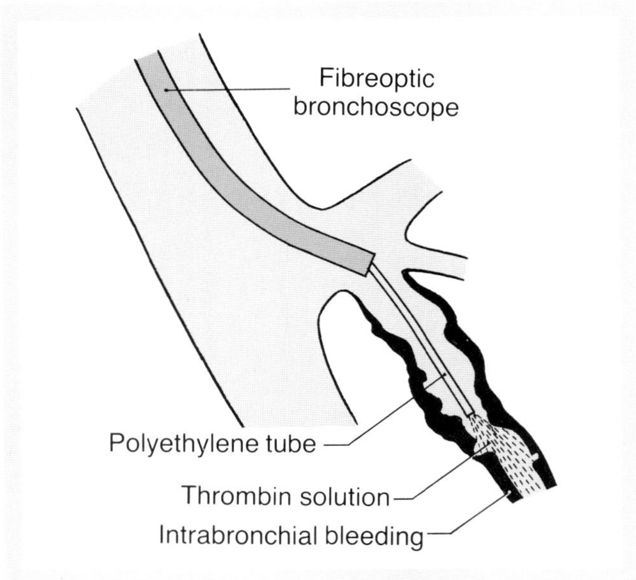

9.4 Thrombin instillation therapy for intrabronchial bleeding.

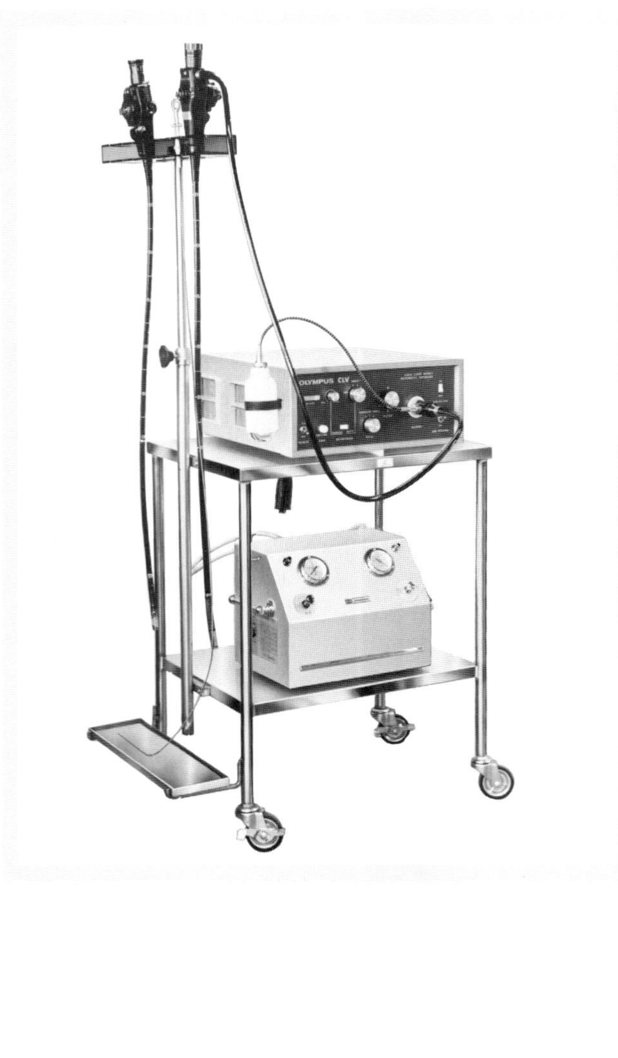

9.5 Trolley for fibreoptic bronchoscope.

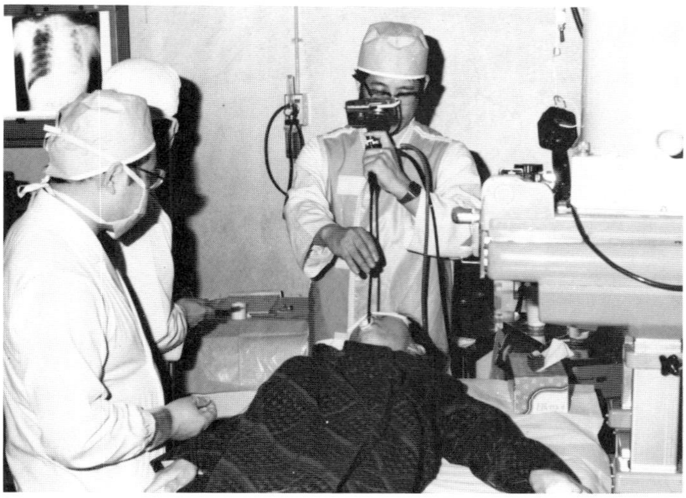

.6 Transbronchial tumour biopsy monitored by uoroscopy. At first, take a routine picture.

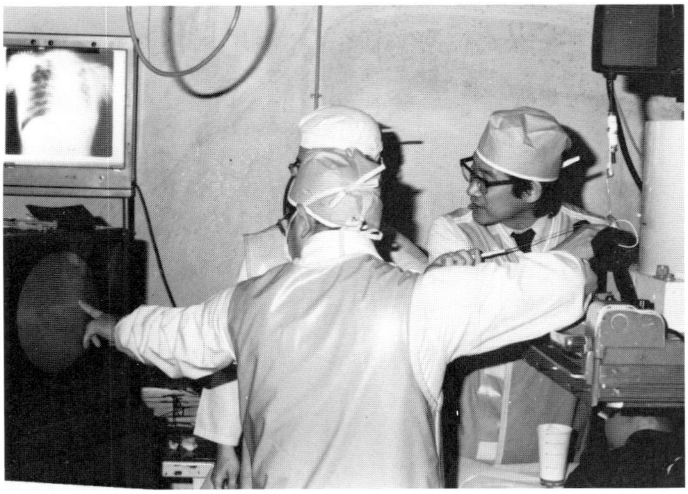

.7 Push the tip of the biopsy forceps up to the ımour monitoring the action by fluoroscopy.

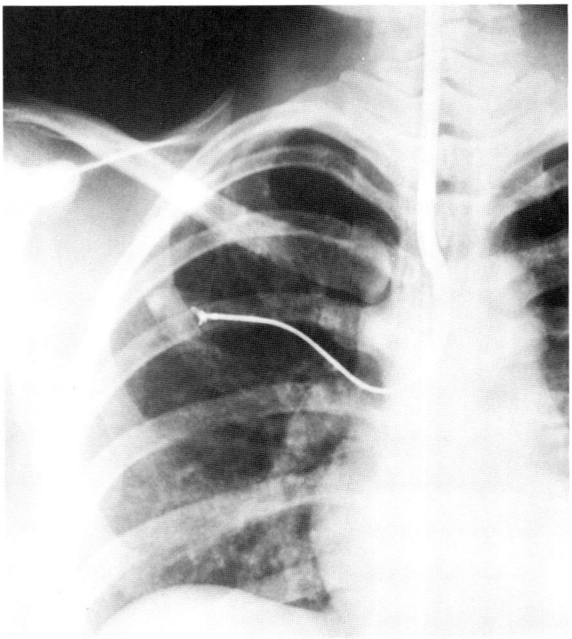

9.8 TBLB of a coin lesion. The forceps tip is pushed up to the coin lesion and the tissue sample is taken.

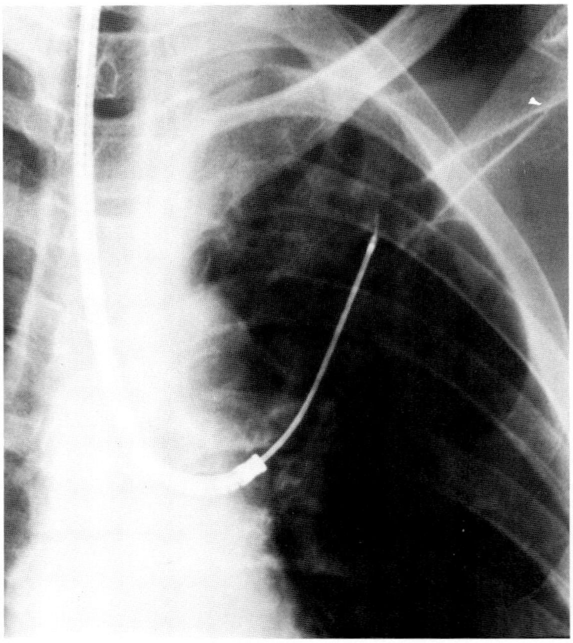

9.9 TBLB of infiltrative lesions. Under fluoroscopy the brush is pushed up to the lesion and the sample is taken.

ii) Selection of biopsy sites

It is very important to select the most suitable site for biopsy. If the lesion tends to be localised, the dominant site may be biopsied. In diffuse bilateral lesions, B^8a, B^8b, B^9a, B^9b, B^{10}a, B^{10}b, B^3ai and B^3aii of either side may be selected as biopsy sites. The author usually performs TBLB on the right side, because right lung fields are not hidden by the cardiac shadow. The frequency of unilateral pneumothorax is reported as 1-5 per cent. It should be emphasised that both lungs cannot be biopsied simultaneously in TBLB, because bilateral pneumothorax may occur and this can often be fatal.

It is not advisable to select right B^4 or B^5 for TBLB. The forceps may penetrate the lung or visceral pleura, because the middle lobe is located between the upper and lower lobes and the volume is very small. Do not perform TBLB on left B^6 or B^3b, because these bronchi lie vertically in the supine position and the localisation of the forceps cannot be recognised easily.

In bilateral diffuse lung diseases, we usually carry out TBLB from both right upper and lower lobes. In patients with collagen vascular diseases and hypersensitivity pneumonitis, fibrotic changes are dominant in the lower lung fields at chest radiography. Even in such cases, TBLB specimens taken from the upper lobes yield diagnostic information. In addition, it is reported that in cases of sarcoidosis, specimens taken from the upper lobe have more diagnostic significance than those from the lower lobe[4]. For the above reasons, lung tissue has to be collected from both upper and lower lobes.

Specimens should be taken from peripheral lung tissue adjacent to the visceral pleura. If we carry out TBLB on more proximal sites, only substances from the bronchial walls will be collected and bleeding will be frequent and profuse as a result of damaged bronchial artery walls.

Figure **9.10** illustrates a schema of TBLB procedure. The opened forceps can collect lung tissue which contains alveoli and bronchiolar walls.

iii) Methods of biopsy

The fibreoptic bronchoscope is inserted after local anaesthesia of the pharynx, trachea and bronchi. The top of the fibrescope is wedged and the forceps inserted into the target bronchus guided by fluoroscopy. We often instil diluted epinephrine solution into the bronchus before the forceps is inserted to prevent profuse bleeding. The forceps is carefully advanced until it reaches the visceral pleura and slight resistance is felt. Tell the patient before the procedure begins to raise his hand when he feels pain in his chest wall. If the patient raises his hand during forceps insertion, the operator must withdraw it 0.5-1 cm immediately.

Observe the position of the forceps in the most peripheral part of the lung on the monitor or request the co-operator to do so; the forceps should be withdrawn about 3 cm. Next, tell the co-operator to open the forceps and request the patient to inspire. After this the patient is told to expire slowly, and simultaneously the forceps is advanced towards the peripheral lung field, leaving 1 cm of lung beyond the forceps at the end of the expiratory phase. At the same time the forceps is pushed gently towards the peripheral lesion, and is closed to obtain a biopsy specimen and withdrawn. When profuse bleeding occurs, it will occur immediately after the forceps is withdrawn. If bleeding is light, it will occur several seconds after the forceps is withdrawn. Wedged fibrescopes have to keep to the initial position of insertion; the degree of bleeding should be observed for 1-2 minutes. Usually bleeding stops spontaneously; however, continuous bleeding should be treated by local injection of a thrombin solution (100μ/ml, 5 ml). The effects of giving a thrombin solution can be observed within 1-2 minutes in most patients.

Figures **9.11-9.14** show the practical methods of performing TBLB. The forceps is inserted into the bronchus to reach the peripheral lung field (**9.11**). The forceps is withdrawn 2-3 cm and opened (**9.12**). The opened forceps is advanced carefully according to the expiration rate of the patient to within 1 cm of the visceral pleura (**9.13**). Next, the forceps is closed (**9.14**).

iv) Complications

The most frequent complications of TBLB are pneumothorax and profuse bleeding. Other complications such as pneumomediastinum, septicaemia, heart attack, pneumonia, hypoxaemia, right heart failure, attack of bronchial asthma, and respiratory arrest have been reported[5]. However they are very rare. We experienced no pneumothorax in our patients; however, 3 patients lost 10-50 ml of blood and 2 patients lost 50-100 ml of blood.

The frequency of pneumothorax differs among operators and hospitals. Reported frequency is 1-5 per cent or 10 per cent[6]. Pneumothorax is easily diagnosed by fluoroscopy immediately after TBLB. Severe pneumothorax is rare and patients will recover completely by bed rest. Tube drainage is rarely necessary.

Profuse bleeding can be treated satisfactorily by the method described above. We usually supply oxygen (0.5-2l/minute) for 6-12 hours, depending on the state of the patient after TBLB. Antibiotics are also prescribed for preventing pneumonia or septicaemia.

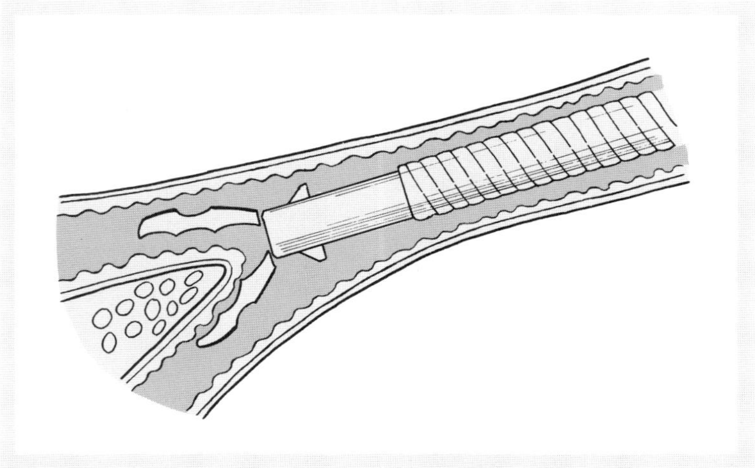

9.10 Schema of TBLB. The forceps tip is inserted into the peripheral part of the bronchus and sample tissue, which includes the wall of small bronchi and lung parenchymal tissue, is taken.

v) Preparation of biopsied material

Usually 4-6 specimens are collected by TBLB. If they are fixed immediately in formaldehyde solution (20 per cent), the alveolar structures could be crushed, making it difficult to examine the specimen pathologically. Dr Yamanaka[7] used a method of expanding lung tissues. The tissue is placed in 10 ml of saline in a 20 ml syringe, which is expanded by pulling on the plunger 2-3 times. After this step the specimens are fixed in formaldehyde solution. The method of expanding specimens directly by placing them in a formaldehyde solution turned out to be better. Figure **9.15** shows the method used for expanding lung tissue: A shows two tissue specimens in 6-8 ml of formaldehyde solution in a 20 ml syringe: B shows the expanded specimens, one of which expanded to twice its previous size.

9 Transbronchial needle aspiration biopsy
Fibreoptic bronchoscopy has made the diagnosis of bronchial carcinoma easier, but all primary lung cancers cannot be diagnosed by this procedure. Peripheral lesions which are located outside the wall of the 4th-5th division of the bronchus can be diagnosed by transcutaneous biopsy. But peripheral lesions which are located adjacent to the trachea, main bronchus, or lobar bronchus and in which no intrabronchial findings are observed, cannot be diagnosed easily.

In the latter cases transbronchial needle aspiration biopsy (TBAB) is used[8,9]. Primary lung cancer, metastatic lung cancer, sarcoidosis and malignant lymphoma can often be diagnosed by this method. The procedure is as follows: locate the appropriate position between the bronchus and the lesion by tomography, bronchography and CT. Having recognised the position of the large vessels, decide on a safe and effective biopsy site. A fibreoptic bronchoscope is inserted into the target bronchus and pressure is applied by pushing gently with the tip of the fibrescope. The point of the biopsy needle, which is inserted in the channel of the fibrescope, is pushed out of the instrument and the needle penetrates the wall of the bronchus. A 20 ml syringe is connected and checked for blood or air escaping by gently withdrawing the plunger while rotating the top end of the needle. The slight suction on the syringe is released and the top of the needle is withdrawn and removed from the channel of the fibrescope. Figure **9.16** illustrates the schema of TBAB. The collected sample is taken out of the syringe and placed on a glass slide, to be examined pathologically and bacteriologically. Bleeding from the biopsy sites should stop spontaneously or by applying pressure with the top of the fibrescope.

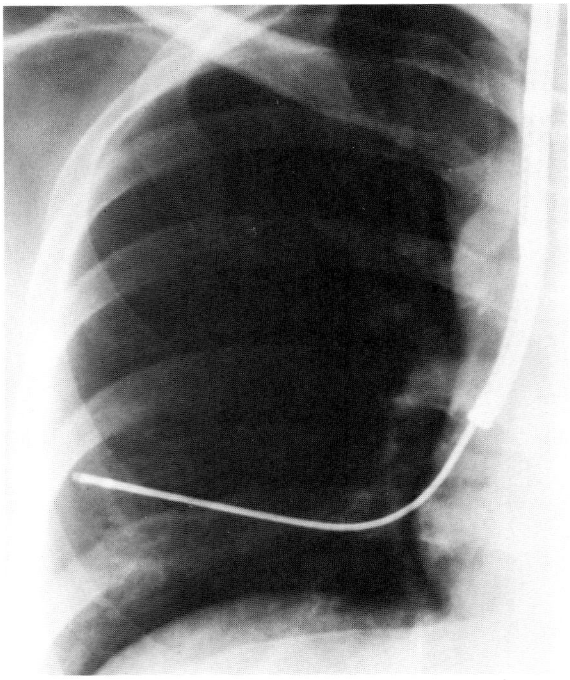

9.11 Fluoroscopic view during the TBLB procedure. The closed forceps tip is pushed through the fibreoptic bronchoscope in the peripheral part of right B^8a.

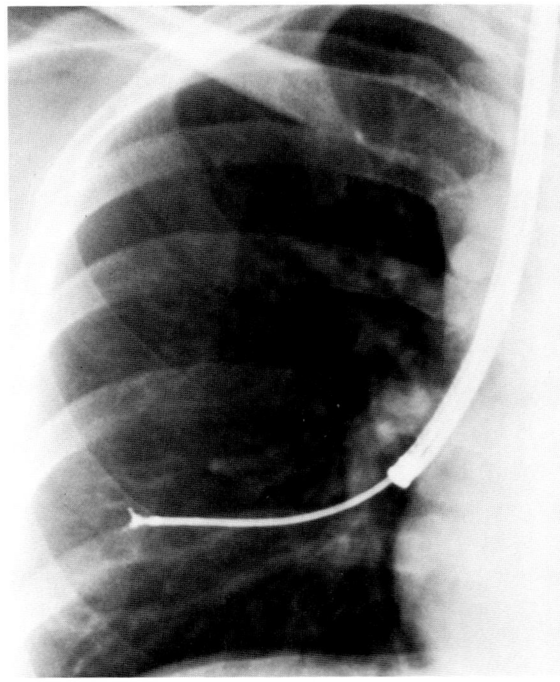

9.12 The forceps tip is pulled back about 3 cm and opened.

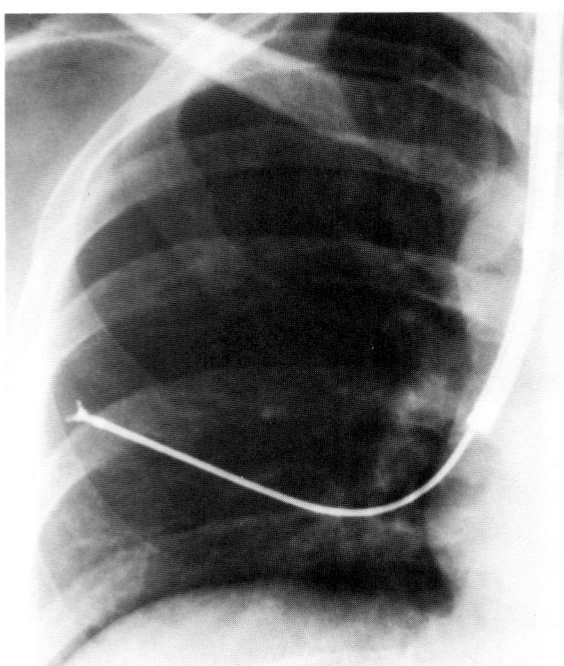

9.13 The open forceps tip is then positioned in the peripheral part of the bronchus, about 1 cm from the visceral pleura, and repositioned.

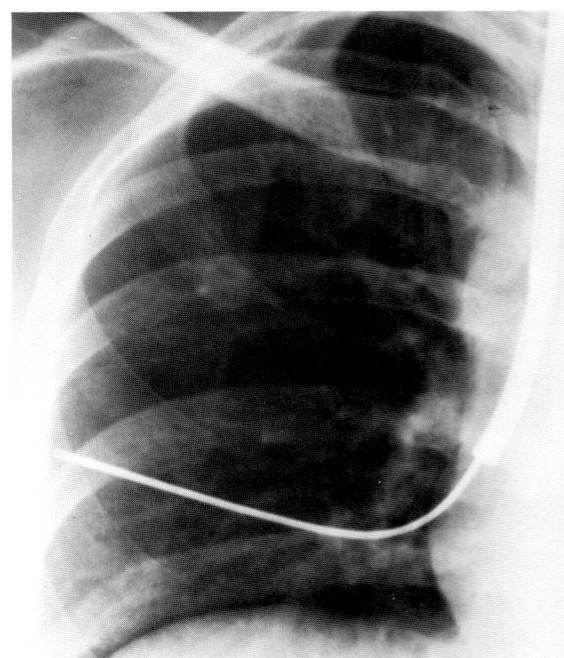

9.14 The forceps tip is closed and the procedure has been completed.

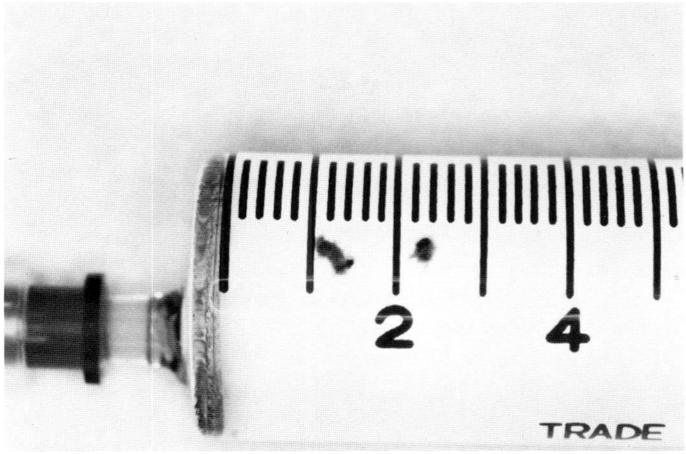

A

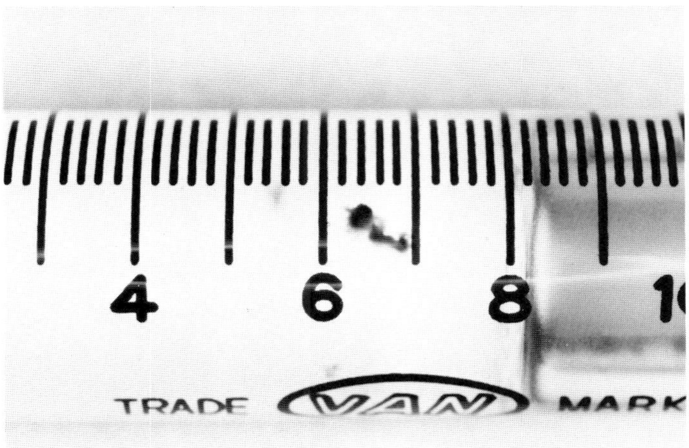

B

9.15 Preparation of biopsied lung tissue for pathological study. **A** Two lung tissue biopsy samples are placed in a syringe containing 20 per cent formalin solution; **B** Lung tissue samples are then expanded by negative pressure.

Figure **9.17** shows TBAB being performed in a sarcoidosis patient, whose bronchus has been penetrated at the inner side of the bifurcation between the right upper lobe bronchus and the intermediate bronchus. The tip of the biopsy needle is outside the bronchus. Figure **9.18** shows TBAB of the same patient. The inner side of the intermediate bronchus is punctured.

When using this method the operator must know the precise location of large vessels to prevent these being punctured. Generally, the inner side of the right upper lobe bronchus or the inner side of the intermediate bronchus can be biopsied safely at their bifurcations. In addition, TBAB can be carried out at the carina between the left upper and lower lobe bronchi, and at the bifurcation of the intermediate bronchus and the right middle lobe bronchus. Furthermore, the inner or dorsal side of either lower lobe bronchus seems a safe site for TBAB.

10 Bronchography

Nelaton and Metra catheters have been used for bronchography, but the authors exclusively use fibreoptic bronchoscopes. The following are the advantages of using the fibreoptic bronchoscope: i) Simultaneous observations of intratracheal lesions are possible; ii) Secretions which inhibit the procedure can be easily eliminated; iii) Instillation of the anaesthetic agent via the channel is possible and satisfactory local anaesthesia is obtained; iv) Reduced procedure time (the authors need only 15 minutes for routine pictures using a fibrescope for bilateral bronchography); v) Target bronchus can be examined selectively; vi) Cleaning of the bronchus after the procedure and removal of the contrast medium is easy; this reduces the patient's effort to expectorate and prevents side-effects, such as fever, after bronchography. Figure **9.22** shows bronchography of the left lung. Almost all of the segmental or subsegmental bronchi are visualised. Figure **9.23** shows the state of the bronchus after the contrast medium has dispersed by forced coughing after the examination.

B Therapeutic applications

1 Bronchial toilet

Bronchial toilet can be carried out by fibreoptic bronchoscopy in patients with primary lung cancer, lung abscess and bronchiectasis. More effective toilet can be performed by using a fibrescope with a large channel, for example BF-1T10 (Olympus). This method is used especially when the patient cannot expectorate sputum because of general weakness or pain resulting from a chest or abdominal operation. This procedure can be easily carried out at the patient's bedside.

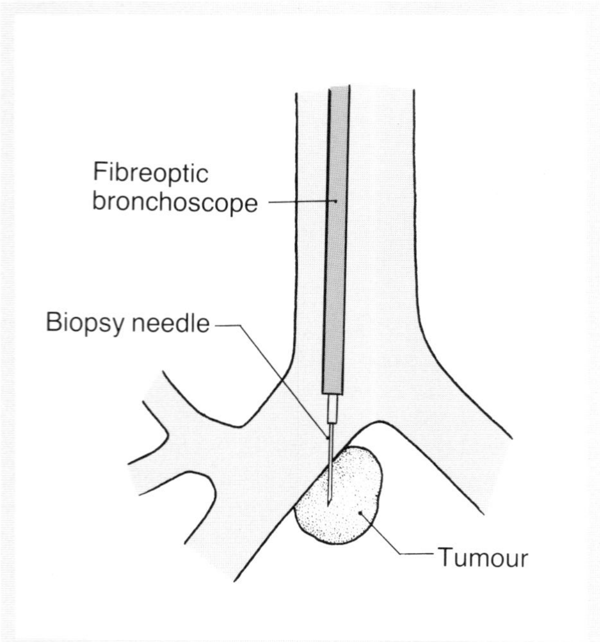

9.16 Schema of a TBAB procedure.

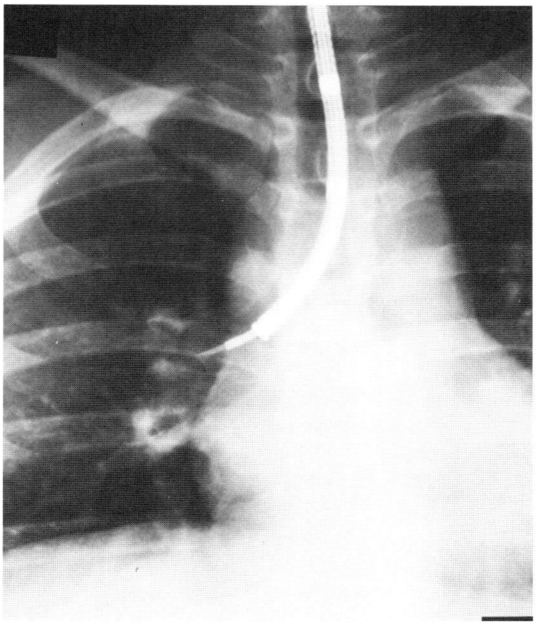

9.17 TBAB procedure. This radiograph shows the needle in the right upper lobe bronchus which was punctured at the bifurcation of right upper lobe bronchus and truncus intermedius.

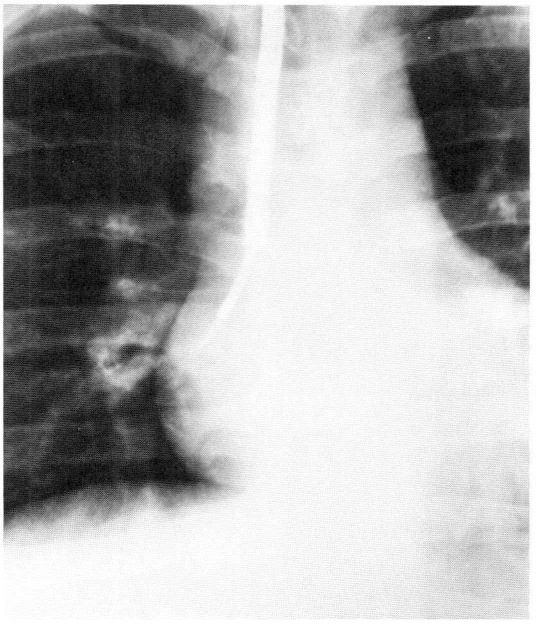

9.18 TBAB procedure. In the same case the inner wall the truncus intermedius was punctured. A biopsy needle penetrates the wall of the bronchus.

2 Removal of foreign body from the trachea or bronchi

A fibreoptic bronchoscope as well as a rigid bronchoscope is available for the removal of foreign bodies. Any type of inhaled foreign body can be removed by means of a fibreoptic bronchoscope, using various grasping instruments. The most common foreign bodies are prosthetic teeth, beans, peanuts and metal clips.

3 Local administration of thrombin solution into the bronchus or onto the tumour where bleeding occurs

This method[10] to stop bleeding by using a thrombin solution was established by the author. A fibrescope is inserted into the bronchus of the patient suffering from haemoptysis; the bronchus which contains fresh blood or a clot is recognised, either visually or by washing with saline. Next, a thrombin solution (5 ml of 100 μ/ml) is instilled to stop haemorrhage. If bleeding is from a visible tumour in the bronchus, the thrombin solution is directly applied to it (**9.4**).

4 Local administration of anticancer drugs

Drugs such as BCG, BCG-CWS, and bleomycin have been tried on endotracheal and endobronchial tumours. These drugs are infiltrated by using a special needle which is inserted in the channel of the fibrescope. Local applications of anticancer drugs were successful in many patients, whose tumours were visible during fibreoptic bronchoscopy. This method of treatment is very effective; for example, atelectasis caused by intraluminal narrowing usually disappears after local application of drugs once or twice[11]. Figure **9.19** illustrates the schema of local application of anticancer drugs. Figure **9.20** shows the injection of anticancer drugs into an endobronchia tumour.

Figure **9.21** shows a special set for local application of oil-suspended bleomycin; this instrument was designed by Dr Arakawa.

This method seems to be more effective when combined with radiation therapy, systemic chemotherapy or biological response modifier (BRM).

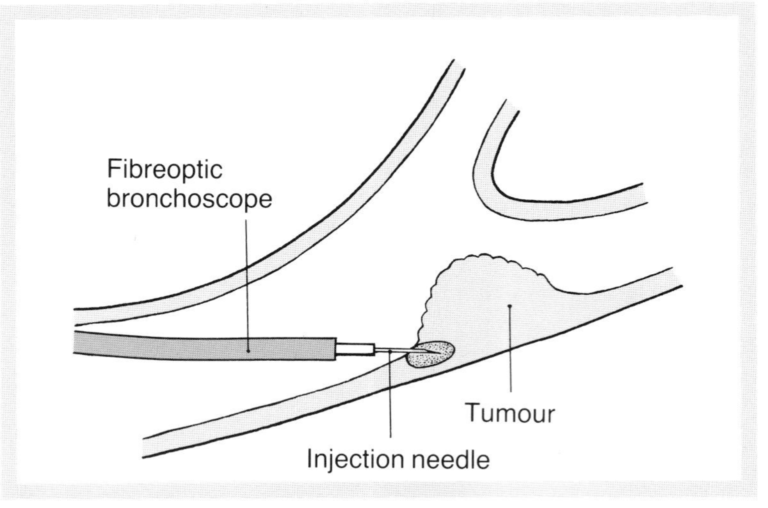

9.19 Method of local injection of anticancer drugs.

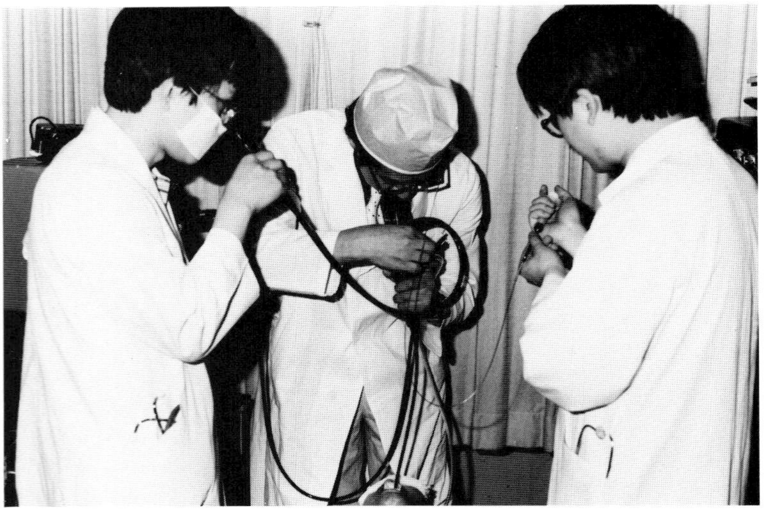

9.20 Local injection of anticancer drugs.

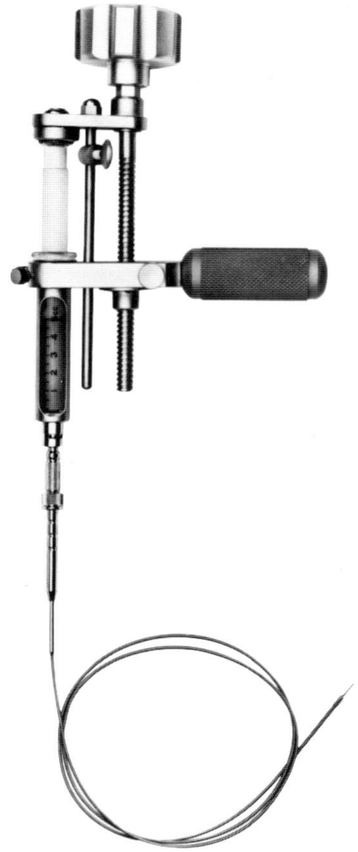

9.21 Transbronchial injection apparatus for oil-suspended bleomycin.

5 Bronchoalveolar lavage for patients with alveolar proteinosis or aspiration pneumonia (Mendelson's syndrome)

Bronchoalveolar lavage is used to treat alveolar proteinosis and aspiration pneumonia. Patients with alveolar proteinosis can be treated by wedging the bronchoscope in each segmental or subsegmental bronchus and washing repeatedly with large amounts of saline. In some cases this method of treatment is successful for several years and no supplementary therapy is necessary. In patients with aspiration pneumonia, bronchial toilet and drug administration are carried out through the channel of a fibrescope. Aspirates which contain food and gastric juice can be removed and washed repeatedly with saline. Drugs such as corticosteroids and antibiotics should also be instilled via the bronchoscope. These therapeutic procedures have markedly improved the prognosis of cases of aspiration pneumonia; in the past prognosis had been very poor[3].

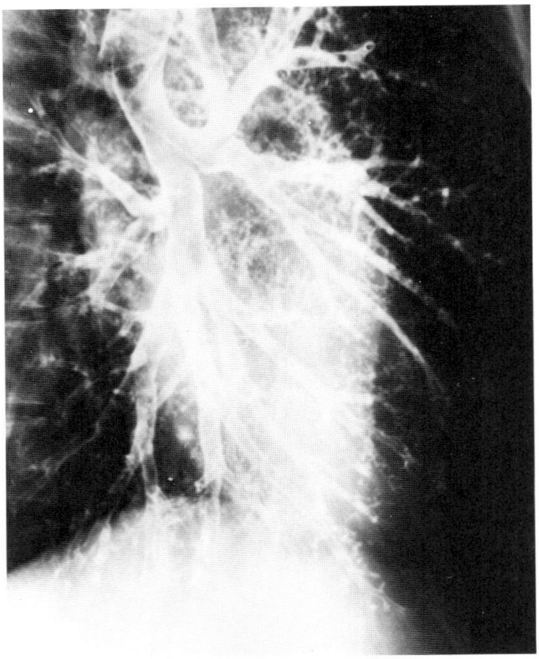

9.22 Bronchography of the left lung.

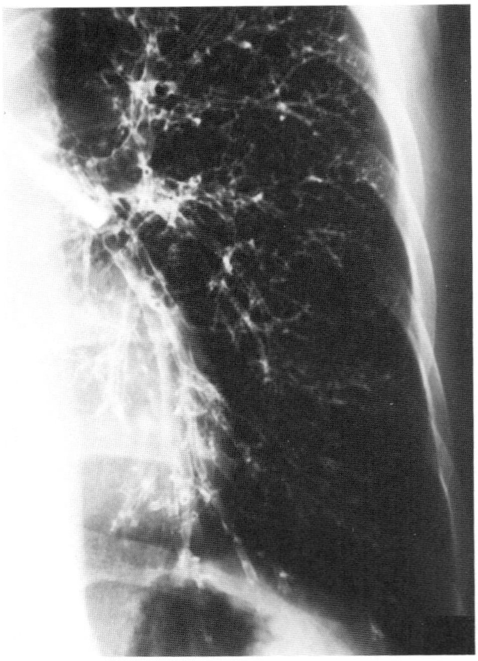

9.23 After the bronchography, contrast medium was aspirated by using a fibreoptic bronchoscope.

6 Insertion of tracheal tube

The insertion of an endotracheal tube is not always an easy procedure, especially in an emergency. However, fibrescope guided intubation is used in many instances. The fibrescope is passed through the endotracheal tube before it is inserted in the trachea (**9.24**). After the fibrescope is inserted in the trachea, the endotracheal tube is slid easily along the fibrescope. This method is useful in an emergency, because it takes less than 30 seconds.

7 Endoscopic surgery

Endoscopic surgery is performed in the proximal airway rather than in the distal one. Patients with squamous cell carcinoma, whose tumour grows from the carina towards the lower part of the trachea, are in danger of becoming victims of asphyxia by airways obstruction. In such cases emergency endoscopic surgery is necessary to keep the airway open.

According to Dr Oho *et al.*[12], these operations are classified into three groups: i) Electric surgery by microwaves; ii) Laser surgery (chiefly by Yag laser); iii) Forceps reduction using biopsy forceps.

Endoscopic surgery is necessary for patients with stenosis caused by tuberculosis or trauma, with granulomatous lesions caused by tracheobronchoplastic surgery, and with benign or low-grade malignant tumours of the trachea and bronchi. Further on we shall present a patient who was treated with laser therapy (Case 113).

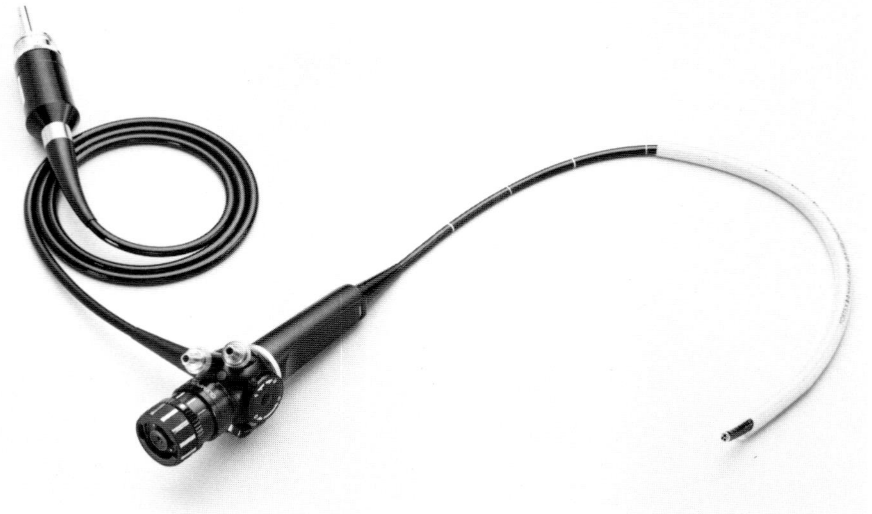

9.24 The fibreoptic bronchoscope inserted into a tracheal tube. The tracheal tube is then passed into the trachea.

References

[1] Shiraki, R., Kitamura, S. *et al.*, Biochemical and immunological studies on BAL fluid in patients with primary lung cancer. *Lung Cancer,* **21**: 335, 1981 (in Japanese).
[3] Izumi, T., Kitamura, S. *et al.,* Diagnosis and therapy for patients with aspiration pneumonia by fibreoptic bronchoscopy. *J. Jpn. Soc. Bronchology,* **3** (suppl.), 68, 1981 (in Japanese).
[2] Kado, M., Izumi, T., *et al.*, Applicability and limitations of BAL and TBLB in diagnosing diffuse interstitial pulmonary diseases. *J. Jpn. Soc. Bronchology,* **8**: 501, 1986 (in Japanese).
[10] Kinoshita, M., Kitamura, S. *et al.*, Thrombin instillation therapy through the fibreoptic bronchoscope in patients with hemoptysis. *Jpn. J. Thoracic Dis.,* **20**: 251, 1982 (in Japanese).
[4] Takagi, H., Matsuoka, R. *et al.*, Diagnostic usefulness of TBLB in patients with sarcoidosis. *J. Jpn. Soc. Bronchology,* **3**(suppl.), 91, 1981 (in Japanese).
[5] Zavala, D.C., Transbronchial biopsy in diffuse lung disease. *Chest,* **73**: 727, 1978.
[6] Andersen, H.A., Transbronchoscopic lung biopsy for diffuse pulmonary diseases. Results in 939 patients. *Chest,* **73**: 734, 1978.
[7] Yamanaka, A., Usefulness of lung biopsy judged by a pathologist. *Jpn. J. Chest Dis.,* **39**: 259, 1980 (in Japanese).
[9] Oho, K., Kato, H., Ogawa, I. *et al.*, A new needle for transfibreoptic bronchoscopic use. *Chest,* **76**: 497, 1979.
[10] Wang, K.P., Marsh, B.R., Summer, W.K. *et al.*, Transbronchial needle aspiration for diagnosis of lung cancer. *Chest,* **80**: 48, 1981.
[11] Wagai, F., Kitamura, S. *et al.*, Direct injection of several anticancer drugs into the primary lung cancer lesion through a fibreoptic bronchoscope. *Jpn. J. Thoracic Dis.* **20**: 170, 1982 (in Japanese).
[12] Oho, K. and Amemiya, R., *Practical Fibreoptic Bronchoscopy*. Igaku-Shoin, Tokyo, 1981.

10 Complications of fibreoptic bronchoscopy procedures

Fibreoptic bronchoscopy has become very popular recently, mainly as a result of the improvements made on the appliance itself and its accessories. No physician specialising in respiratory medicine today is considered adequately trained unless he is competent with a fibreoptic bronchoscope. With the rapid increase of fibreoptic bronchoscopy procedures, there are an increasing number of reports where complications have arisen. Therefore, in order to classify the complications associated with fibreoptic bronchoscopy, we made a study based on a nationwide questionnaire. This study was conducted in Japan from July 1984 to February 1985.

1 Questionnaire study

We sent questionnaires to 1,028 major hospitals in Japan and received 495 answers. The contents of the questionnaire are shown in Table 10.1. The specialities of 495 medical departments were 321 (64.8 per cent) of internal medicine, 119 (24 per cent) of surgery, 24 (4.9 per cent) of radiology and 7 (1.4 per cent) of otolaryngology.

There were 47,744 fibreoptic bronchoscopies (FBS) per year with a grand total of 279,280 cases. Complications were reported in 1,381 cases (0.49 per cent). Intrabronchial tumour biopsy (IBTB) or transbronchial lung biopsy (TBLB) was carried out in 32 per cent of all procedures.

Table 10.2 shows the major complications of FBS procedures. There were 611 cases (0.219 per cent) of pneumothorax, 169 cases (0.061 per cent) of lignocaine intoxication, 137 cases (0.049 per cent) of haemorrhage estimated as greater than 300 ml, 125 cases (0.045 per cent) of high fever, 57 cases (0.020 per cent) of respiratory arrest, 53 cases (0.019 per cent) of extrasystole, 41 cases (0.015 per cent) of lignocaine shock, 39 cases (0.014 per cent) of a decrease in blood pressure, 20 cases (0.007 per cent) of pneumonia and 34 cases (0.012 per cent) deaths. Table 10.3 shows rare complications of FBS procedures, such as asthmatic attacks, hoarseness and dislocation of the jaw.

Table 10.4 shows causes of death in FBS procedures. They are 13 cases (38.2 per cent) of intrabronchial tumour biopsy, 9 cases (26.4 per cent) of transbronchial lung biopsy, 4 cases (11.8 per cent) of endoscopic laser surgery and so on. Table 10.5 shows direct causes of death in FBS procedures. They are 20 cases (58.8 per cent) of profuse bleeding, 4 cases (11.8 per cent) of pneumothorax, 3 cases (8.8 per cent) of respiratory insufficiency, 2 cases of circulatory insufficiency and 2 cases of lignocaine shock.

Table 10.6 shows intervals between FBS procedures and death. Of 34 cases, 20 (58.8 per cent) died during or immediately after the procedure, 5 cases (14.7 per cent) within 24 hours and 4 cases (11.8 per cent) within a week.

Table 10.1 Contents of the questionnaire

1. Name of hospitals
2. Cumulative cases of FBS procedures
3. Annual cases of FBS procedures
4. Cumulative and annual cases of bronchial biopsies and lung biopsies
5. Complications: fatalities, haemorrhage (more than 300 ml of blood), pneumothorax, cardiac arrest, respiratory arrest, xylocaine overdose shock, other complications

Table 10.2 Major complications of FBS procedures

Complication	Number of cases	%
1 Pneumothorax	611	0.219
2 Lignocaine intoxication	169	0.061
3 Haemorrhage (more than 300 ml)	137	0.049
4 High fever (38°C~)	125	0.045
5 Respiratory arrest	57	0.020
6 Extrasystole	53	0.019
7 Lignocaine shock	41	0.015
8 Fall in blood pressure	39	0.014
9 Death	34	0.012
10 Pneumonia	20	0.007
11 Cardiac arrest	16	0.006
12 Laryngospasm	12	0.004
13 Exacerbation of pulmonary tuberculosis	8	0.003
14 Myocardial infarction	7	0.003

Table 10.3 Rare complications of FBS procedures

Complication	Number of cases	Complication	Number of cases
Asthmatic attack	5	Pulmonary abscess	2
Hoarseness	5	Tachycardia	2
Dislocation of jaw	5	CO_2 narcosis	2
Dyspnoea	4	Injury to trachea	2
Tracheal stenosis	3	Cerebral apoplexy	2
Vomiting	3	Cyanosis	2
Disturbance of consciousness	3	Rupture of aortic aneurysm	1
Hyperventilation	3	Dysuria	1
Pulmonary haemorrhage	2	Atrial flutter	1
Subcutaneous emphysema	2	Coma	1
		Primary infiltration with eosinophilia*	1

* drug-induced, probably propyliodone

Table 10.4 Causes of death in fibreoptic bronchoscopy

Cause	No of patients	(%)
Intrabronchial tumour biopsy	13	(38.2)
Transbronchial lung biopsy	9	(26.4)
Endoscopic laser surgery	4	(11.8)
Observation by FBS	2	(5.9)
Lignocaine overdose shock	2	(5.9)
Intubation by FBS	1	(2.9)
Bronchial toilet	1	(2.9)
Unknown	2	(5.9)
Total	34 cases	

Table 10.5 Direct causes of death in fibreoptic bronchoscopy

Direct cause	No. of patients (%)	Procedure	
Massive bleeding	20 (58.8)	IBTB	11
		TBLB	3
		Laser surgery	3
		Observation by FBS	2*
		Bronchial toilet	1
Pneumothorax	4 (11.8)	TBLB	3
		IBTB	1
Respiratory insufficiency	3 (8.8)	TBLB	1
		IBTB	1
		Laser surgery	1
Circulatory insufficiency	2 (5.9)	TBLB	2
Lignocaine overdose shock	2 (5.9)		
Unknown	5 (14.7)		
Total	34 cases		

* includes a case of rupture of aortic aneurysm
IBTB: intrabronchial tumour biopsy

Table 10.6 Time lapse between FBS procedures and death

Interval	No. of cases (%)
During or immediately after the procedures	20 (58.8)
Within 24 hours	5 (14.7)
Within a week	4 (11.8)
More than 2 weeks	3 (8.8)
Unknown	2 (5.9)
Total:	34 cases

2 Precautions and treatment of complications

Pneumothorax, the most frequent complication after transbronchial lung biopsy, is easily detectable by fluoroscopy. Usually, if pneumothorax is not so severe, it is sufficient to monitor it. Sometimes, needle aspiration or aspiration via a small lumen catheter is carried out. It is also possible to insert a chest tube to drain fluid.

Lignocaine intoxication is the next most frequent complication. Exercise a great deal of care to avoid an overdose. About 4-8 ml of 4 per cent lignocaine is a safe dose. Intoxication due to excessive use of lignocaine is manifested by marked weakness or loss of consciousness and at times convulsions. Treatment is by maintaining an open airway and supplying sufficient oxygen.

Haemorrhage of more than 300 ml of blood, induced by transbronchial lung or tumour biopsy, is the third most frequent complication. Usually, it is sufficient just to insert the tip of the fibreoptic bronchoscope into the affected bronchus to start the bleeding. However, if there is still more bleeding, instill the cooled saline into the bronchus, clamp the bronchus with the tip of fibreoptic bronchoscope and wait for 30-60 seconds[1]. However, if these procedures are not effective, then instill 5 ml of thrombin solution (5,000 U of thrombin dissolved in saline) into the affected bronchus through a polyethylene tube via a fibreoptic bronchoscope and wait for 1-2 minutes. This method, which was invented by the author, is very effective for treating patients with profuse bleeding which has been induced by TBLB[2].

Fibreoptic bronchoscopy and TBLB are very useful and safe procedures for diagnosing various pulmonary diseases. However, at times severe complications, including death, could occur. Before carrying out this procedure, prepare a tracheal tube, an ambu bag, an oxygen supply and an infusion set in case an emergency arises.

References

[1] Kitamura, S. *et al.*, Local administration of cold saline for the treatment of bleeding induced by transbronchial lung biopsy. *J. Jpn. Soc. Bronchology,* **6**: 309, 1984.

[2] Kitamura, S., Local administration of thrombin solution for the treatment of intrabronchial bleeding. *Internal. Med.,* **53**: 747, 1984.

11 Analysis of bronchoscopic findings in various lung diseases

So far the sources of information relating to various lung diseases have been limited to chest radiographs, clinical manifestations, physical examination, cytological and bacteriological examination of sputum, pulmonary function tests and arterial blood gases. Although such data may be adequate for diagnosing some diseases, it is frequently not possible to diagnose diseases such as bronchial adenoma, carcinoid of the bronchi, tuberculosis of the trachea or bronchi, haemangioma of the bronchi, early-stage epidermoid carcinoma and tracheobronchopathia osteochondroplastica.

On the other hand, in some diseases where bronchoscopy was not thought to supply useful diagnostic information, specific diagnostic findings have been revealed: for example in sarcoidosis, lymphangitis carcinomatosa, interstitial pneumonia, mitral stenosis and diffuse panbronchiolitis. Recently the author observed and took photographs of dilated bronchial walls in bronchiectatic patients, using fibreoptic bronchoscopes. It was interesting to note that in some cases of heart disease, particularly where right heart overload or right heart failure is present, engorgement of the submucosal vessels was clearly visible. Lymphangitis carcinomatosa supplies specific bronchoscopic data—the bronchial mucosa appears oedematous because of lymphatic stagnation.

This section comprises 15 chapters: congenital and healed tracheobronchial lesions, inflammatory tracheobronchial lesions, sarcoidosis, other bronchial lesions, tuberculosis of lungs and lymph nodes, primary lung cancer (small cell carcinoma), primary lung cancer (epidermoid carcinoma), primary lung cancer (large cell carcinoma), primary lung cancer (adenocarcinoma), metastatic lung cancer, bronchial lesions of malignant tumours adjacent to lungs, benign bronchial tumours and foreign bodies in the airway, cardiovascular diseases, mucoepidermoid carcinoma, other lesions of the lungs and bronchi. One hundred and thirteen cases of bronchoscopic findings are presented and analysed; these are compared with chest radiographs, CT scans and pathology investigations.

Case 1: Anomaly of bronchial tree (tracheal bronchus) in a 39-year-old male.

A previously healthy male, who smoked more than 3,000 cigarettes per year, presented with a recent productive cough.

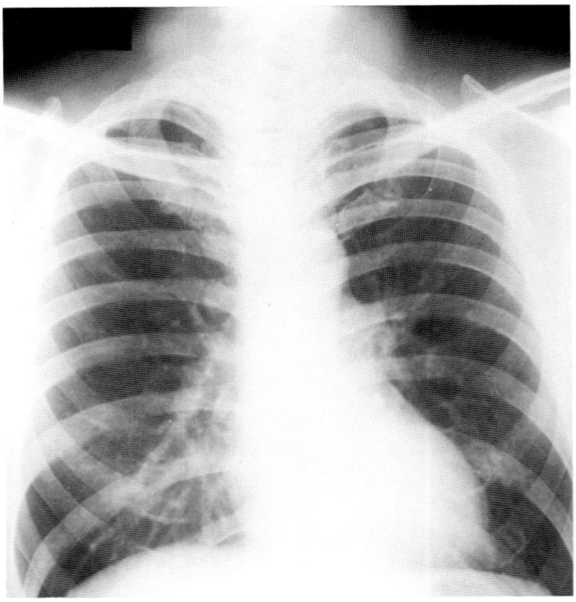

1.1 Posteroanterior chest radiograph. No abnormal shadows are visible in the lungs, except for considerable lower branching of the RUL bronchus.

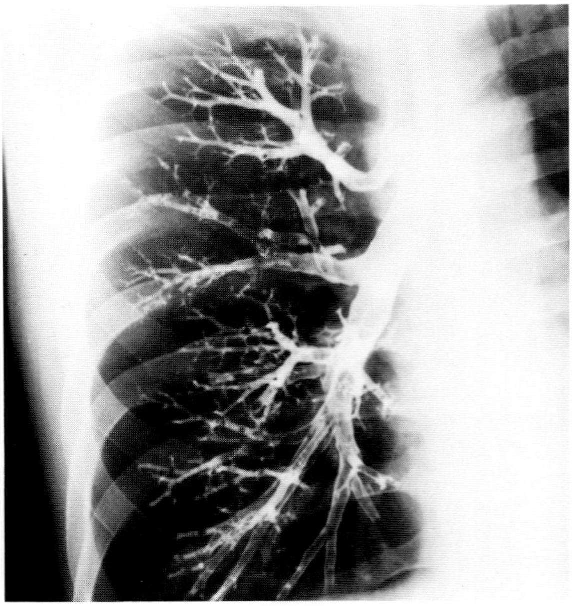

1.2 Posteroanterior bronchogram of the right lung. B^1 directly stems from the lower portion of the trachea, despite B^2 and B^3 taking off from the main bronchus.

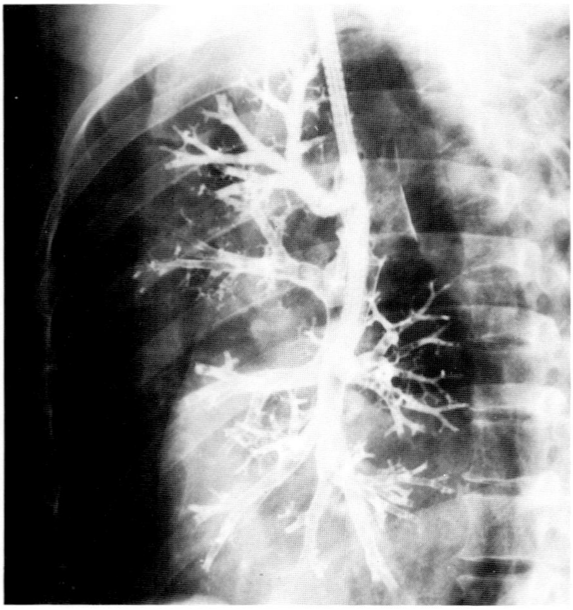

1.3 Left oblique bronchogram of the right lung. B^1 comes directly off the trachea, while B^2 and B^3 are located as usual.

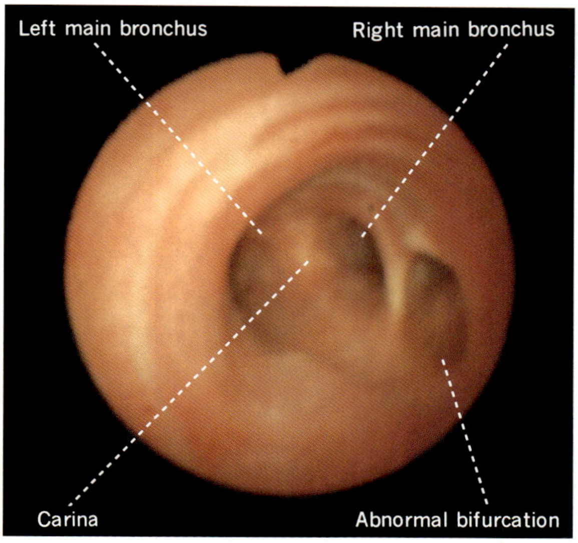

1.4 Bronchoscopic findings of the lower portion of the trachea. The orifice of B^1 (tracheal bronchus) is seen on the right wall of the trachea, just above the carina.

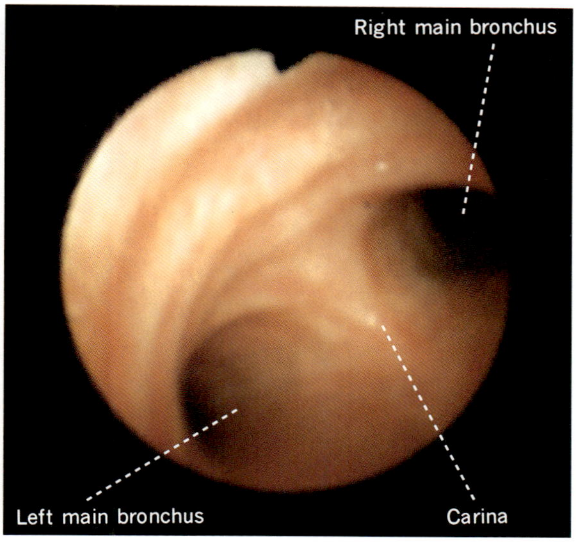

1.5 Bronchoscopic findings of the carina. No abnormalities can be seen.

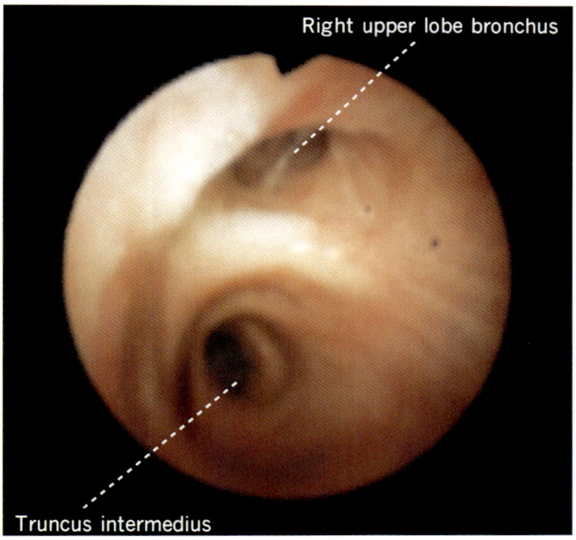

1.6 Bronchoscopic findings of the RUL bronchus (B^2, B^3).

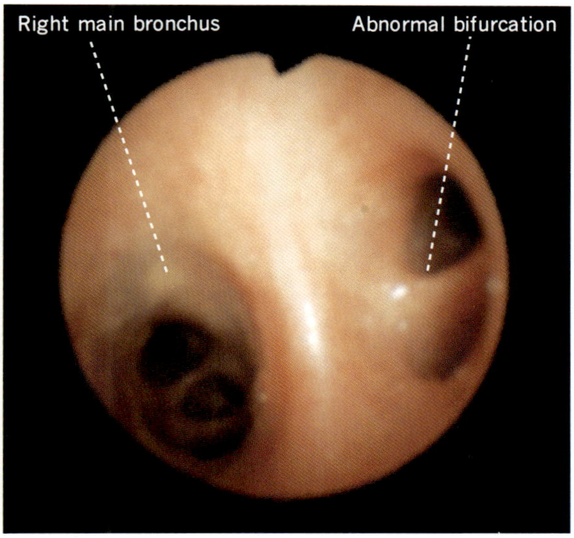

1.7 Close-up of abnormal branching. The bifurcating orifice of B^1 is visible.

Case 2: Bronchial stenosis in a 30-year-old male.

The patient had a history of pneumonia while he was at junior high school; this was followed by frequent bouts of common colds, usually presenting with a cough. His chest radiograph showed relatively homogeneous tumour-like shadows in the right lower lung zone, which had gradually increased in size since he first visited us six years ago.

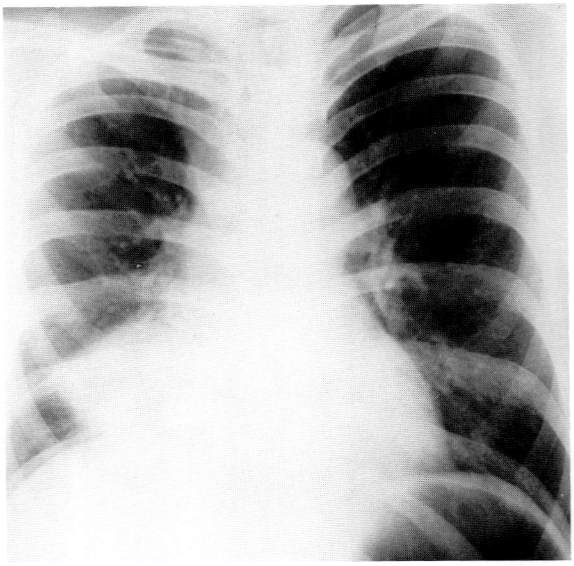

2.1 Posteroanterior chest radiograph. Obliteration of the right heart border (silhouette sign) indicates atelectasis of the right middle lobe.

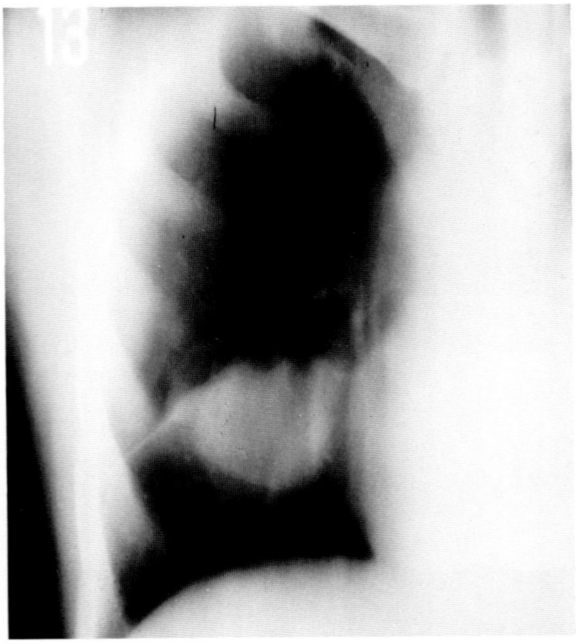

2.2 Anteroposterior tomogram (13 cm from the back). A well-demarcated shadow (6 × 5 cm in size) is seen in the right middle lobe.

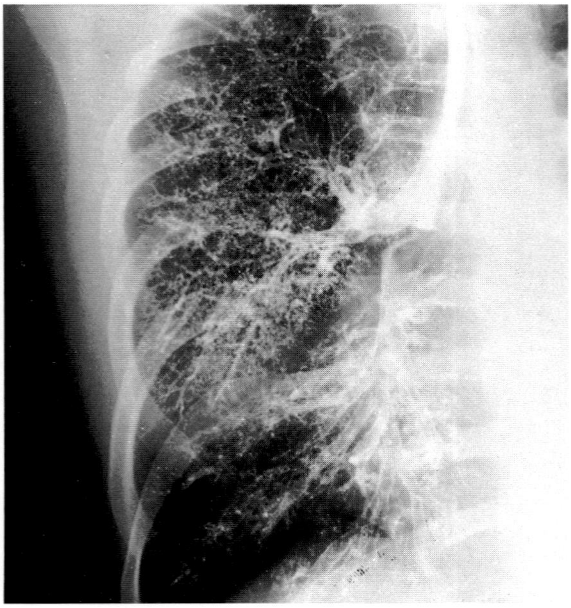

2.3 Right bronchogram. Truncus intermedius shows prominent stenosis beneath the RUL bronchus with deviating B^3a and B^3b underneath. None of B^4a, B^4b, B^5a or B^5b is demonstrated. B^6b, B^6c, B^9a, and B^9b reveal mild cylindrical dilatation. B^{10} shows marked cylindrical dilatation.

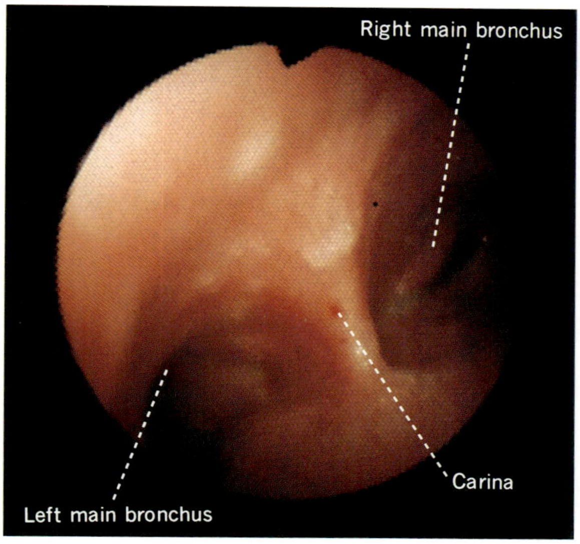

2.4 Bronchoscopic findings of the carina. Right main bronchus branches into the RUL bronchus and the stenotic truncus intermedius.

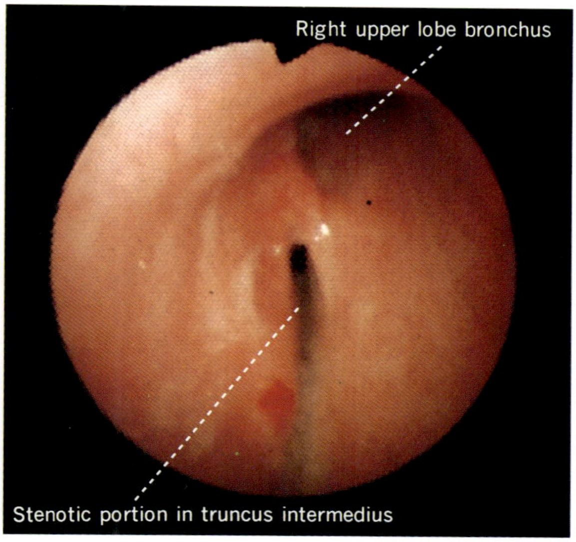

2.5 Close-up of **2.4**. The stenotic truncus intermedius is visible.

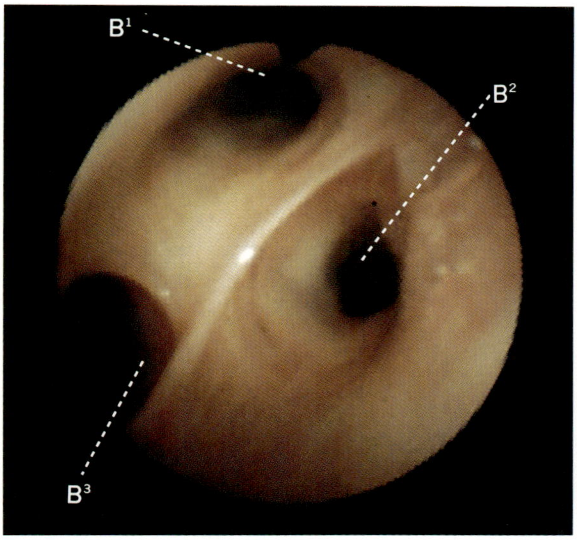

2.6 Bronchoscopic findings of the RUL bronchus. No abnormal findings are observed at the orifice of B^1, B^2 or B^3.

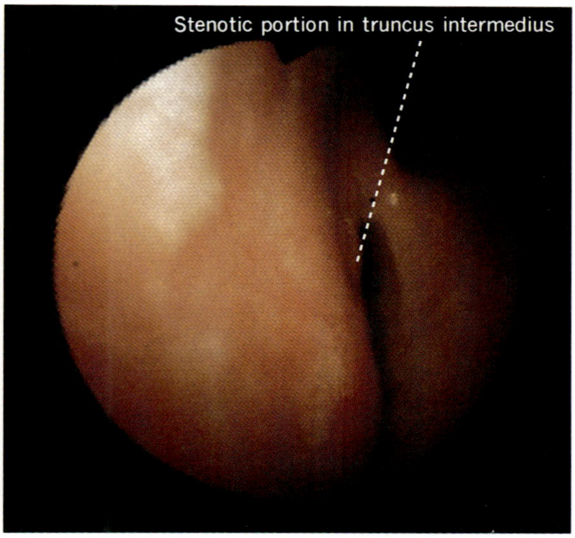

2.7 Close-up of the stenotic truncus intermedius. It is not possible to insert a fibreoptic bronchoscope through this portion, which is 2 mm wide. Note the slight reddening on the bronchial mucosa, which is likely to be caused by an inflammation such as tuberculosis.

Case 3: Bronchial stenosis in a 40-year-old male.

The patient suffered from pulmonary tuberculosis several years ago and complained of frequent upper respiratory infections, with cough, during the last 2 years. He did not have dyspnoea. This is a case of stenosis of the left main bronchus caused by bronchial tuberculosis.

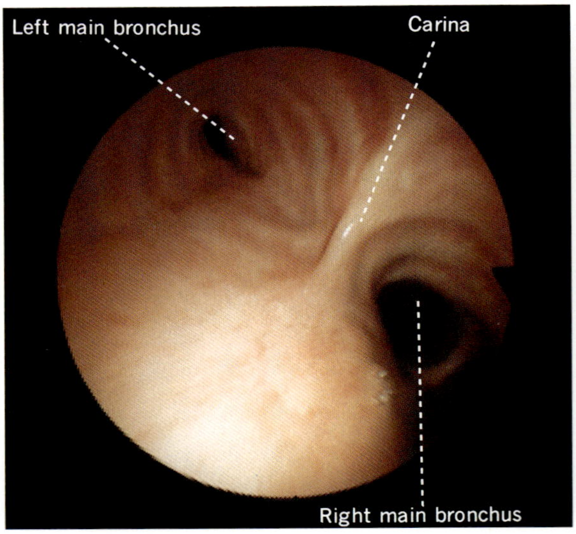

3.1 Bronchoscopic findings at the carina. The left main bronchus appears stenotic at the fourth cartilage ring, although the carinal spur remains sharp.

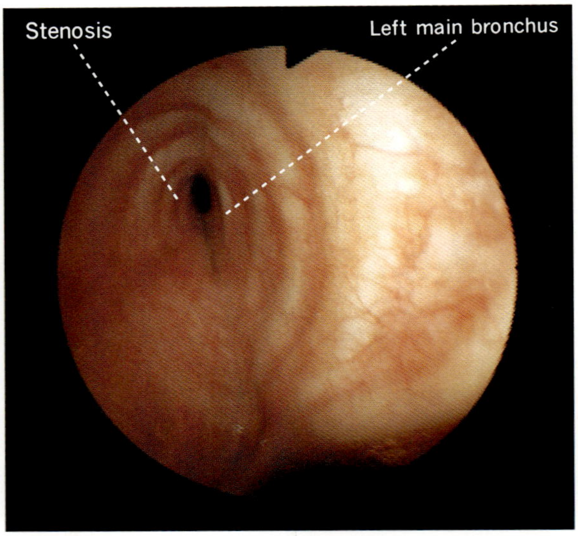

3.2 Bronchoscopic findings in the left main bronchus. Engorgement of the small vasculature of the bronchial mucosa is visible.

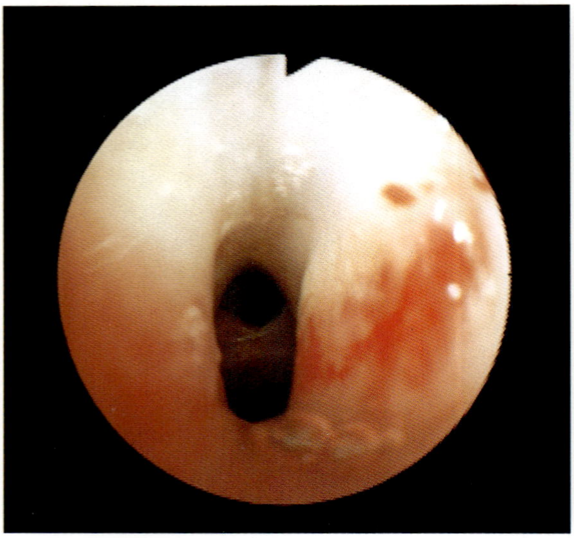

3.3 Close-up of the stenotic portion. A fibreoptic bronchoscope is barely able to get through the stenosis, which is approximately 5 mm in width.

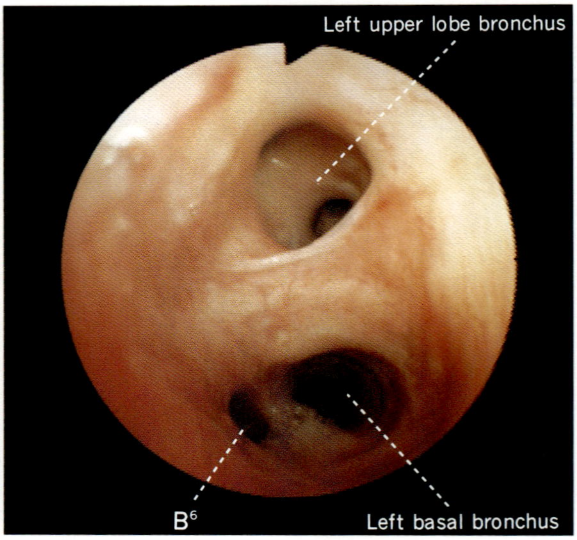

3.4 Distal to the stenosis of the left main bronchus, approximately 1 cm in length, bronchoscopic examination reveals almost normal mucosa including the bifurcation between the LUL and the LLL bronchi.

Case 4: Abnormal vasculature of the bronchi in a 61-year-old female.

The patient complained of fever without any respiratory symptoms. Chest radiograph revealed obliteration of the right heart border which suggested the presence of the silhouette sign.

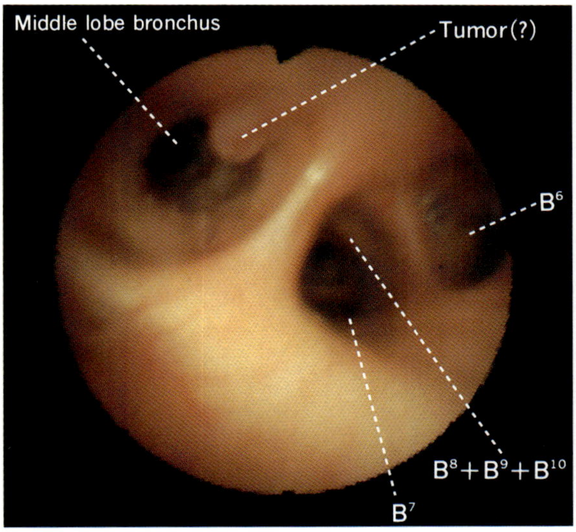

4.1 Bronchoscopic findings in the lower portion of the truncus intermedius. The basal bronchus and B^6 are seen. A spherical 'tumour', with a smooth surface, is located at the orifice of the RML bronchus.

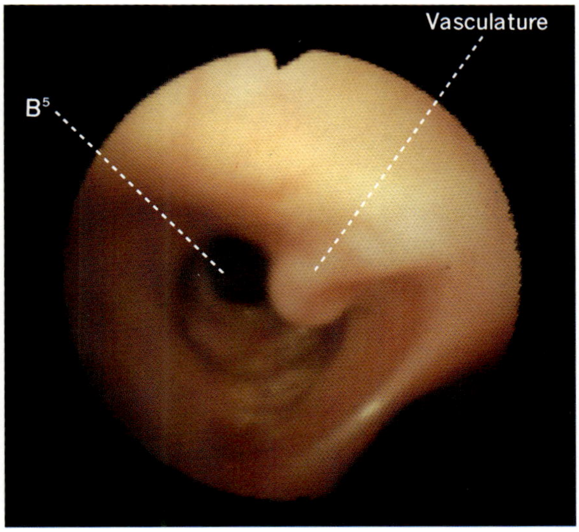

4.2 Close-up of the RML bronchus. The 'tumour' is located from the orifice of the RML bronchus to the distal side.

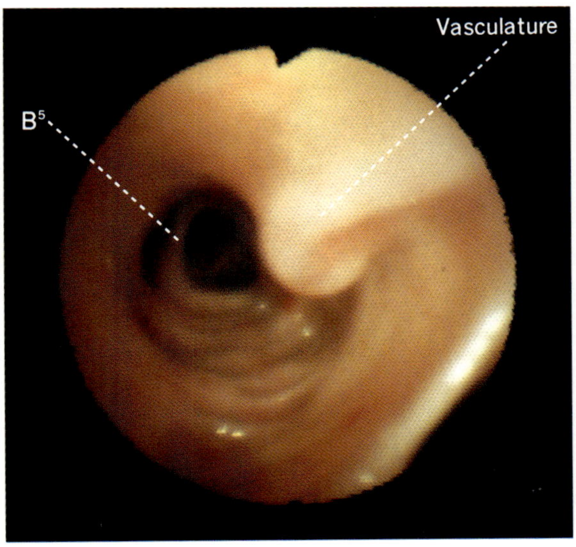

4.3 Close-up of the 'tumour'. It appears trabecular or looks like a 'worm', beyond which the segmental bronchus is visible.

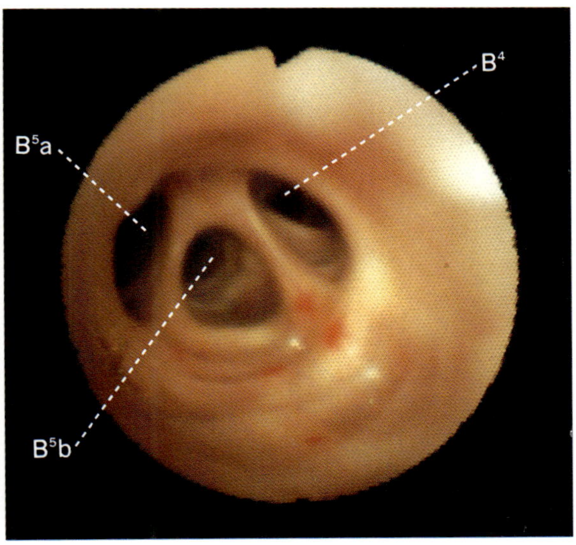

4.4 The trifurcated RML bronchus beyond the trabecular 'tumour'. Biopsy of the 'tumour' induced pulsatile bleeding in volume of some 300 ml, which was controlled with an intrabronchial injection of thrombin. It revealed an abnormal blood vessel beneath the bronchial mucosa. Before carrying out a biopsy on a 'worm'-like 'tumour', think about it with utmost care.

Case 5: Anthracosis in a 69-year-old male.

This patient had been a coal miner for 30 years. He presented with a productive cough during winter, which suggested he suffered from chronic bronchitis.

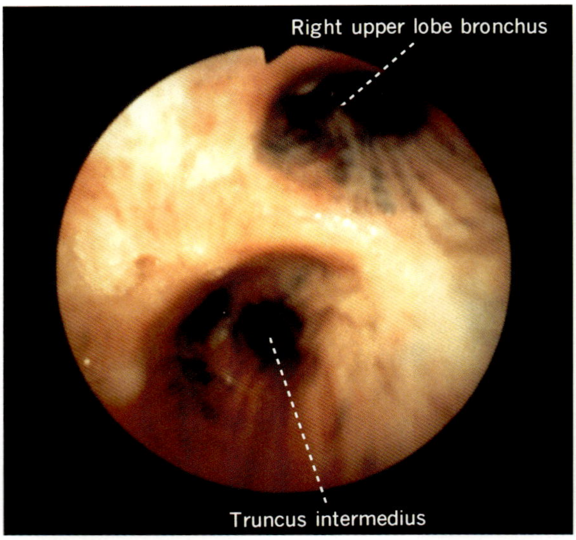

5.1 Bronchoscopic findings at the bifurcation between the RUL bronchus and the truncus intermedius. The bifurcation is a little widened and there is irregularity of the bronchial mucosa, which is associated with anthracosis of the mucosal folds.

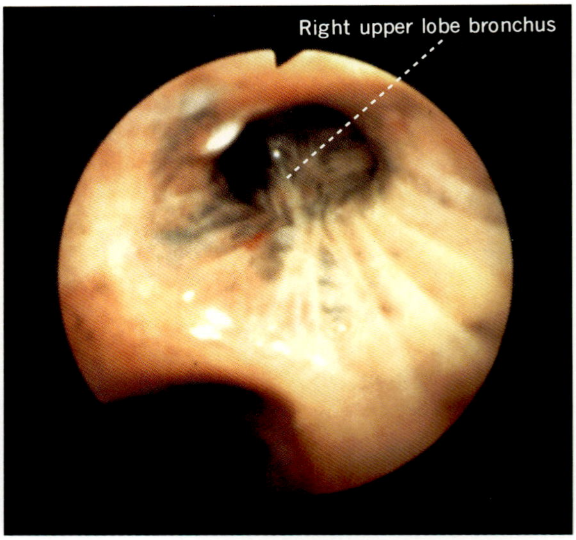

5.2 Bronchoscopic findings at the orifice of the RUL bronchus. Anthracosis is present along the mucosal folds and a white nodule is visible on the bronchial wall around the orifice, which suggests an inflammatory granuloma.

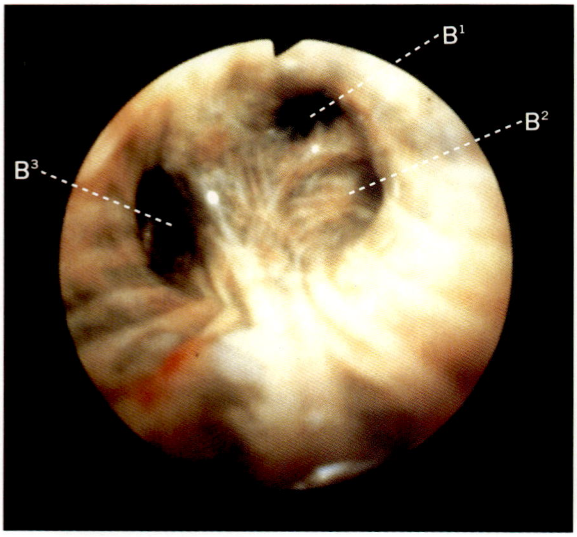

5.3 Close-up of the RUL bronchus. Marked anthracosis and widening of the bifurcation is present. The mucosa is in part reddened probably as a result of inflammation.

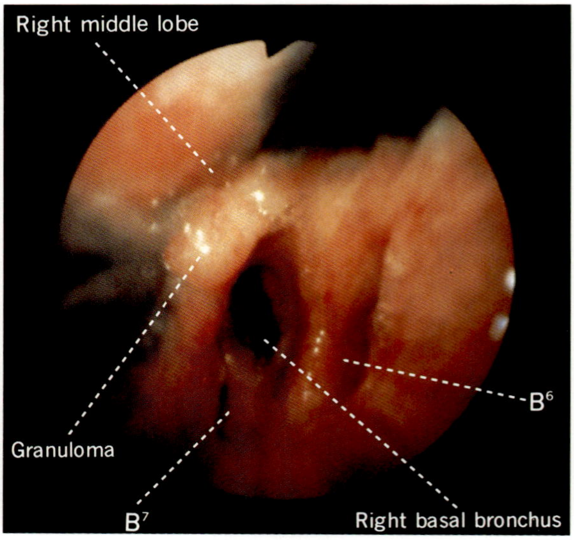

5.4 Bronchoscopic findings in the RML bronchus and the RLL bronchus in another case (77-year-old male). The RML bronchus is obstructed and a granulomatous nodule overlies the widened bifurcation with accompanying prominent anthracosis on each side. Biopsy of the granuloma revealed a tuberculous lesion (bronchial tuberculosis).

Case 6: Stenosis of the trachea in a 44-year-old female.

The patient, who had suffered from Wegener's granulomatosis a few years earlier, had been almost free of the disease until she presented with severe exertional dyspnoea with wheeze, both on expiration and inspiration, 6 months previously. Chest radiograph revealed no abnormalities and anti-asthmatic therapy failed to improve the symptom. This is a case of cicatricial stenosis of the trachea just beneath the vocal cords, caused by Wegener's granulomatosis.

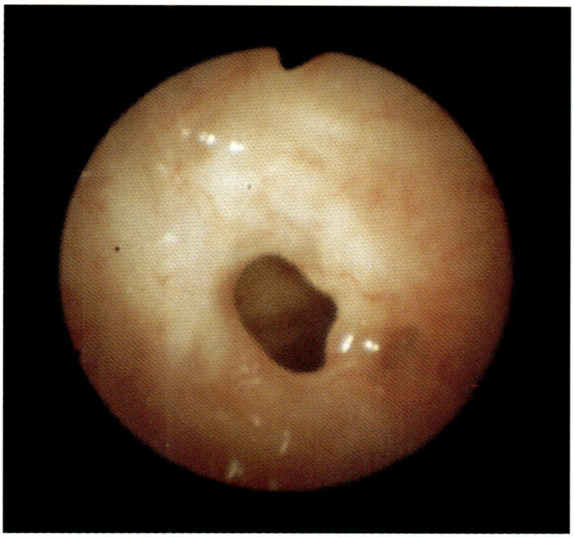

6.1 Bronchoscopic findings in the area of the vocal cords. There is generalised, irregularly oval narrowing of the trachea. The shorter diameter is approximately 4.5 mm, which makes it impossible for a fibreoptic bronchoscope to pass through the orifice.

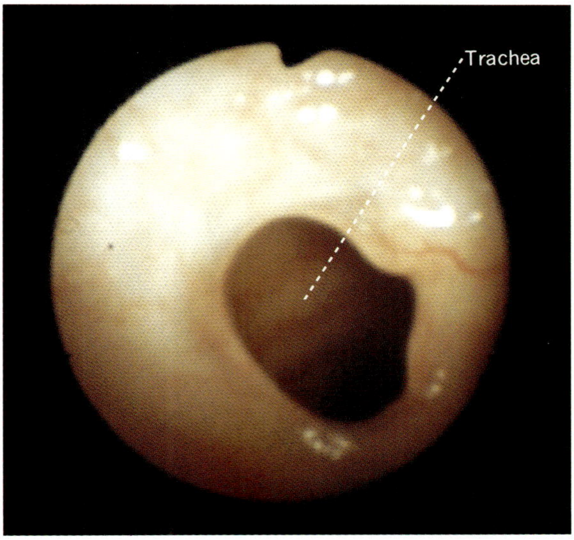

6.2 Close-up beyond the stenosis. The trachea appears normal. Because biopsy of this portion revealed fibrosis without any active lesion, it was removed by electrocautery.

Case 7: Cicatricial obstruction of a bronchus in a 32-year-old male.

This patient was noted to have an enlargement of the hilar lymph nodes on a chest film, while he was at junior high school. An abnormal shadow had been noted in the right upper zone for more than 10 years; this shadow had remained unchanged. The patient is in good condition, and has no cough or sputum production.

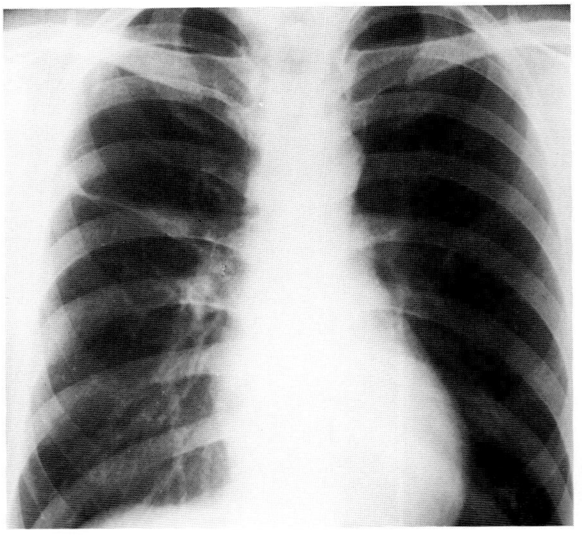

7.1 Posteroanterior chest radiograph. A tumour-like shadow, about 3-4 cm, is visible just above the thickened minor fissure.

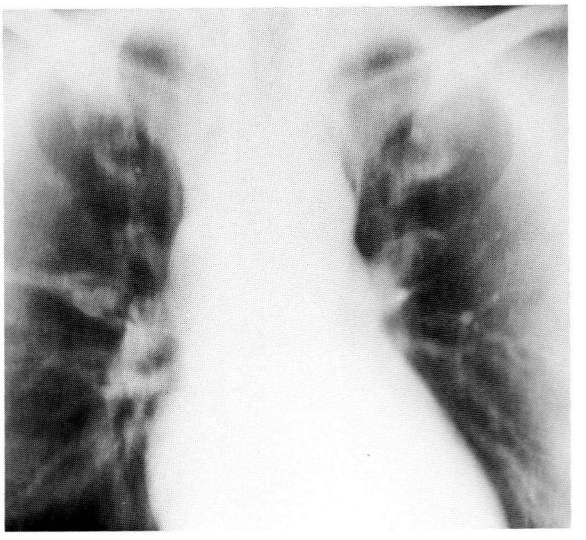

7.2 Chest tomogram (12 cm from the back). The thickened minor fissure and a tumour-like shadow are visible.

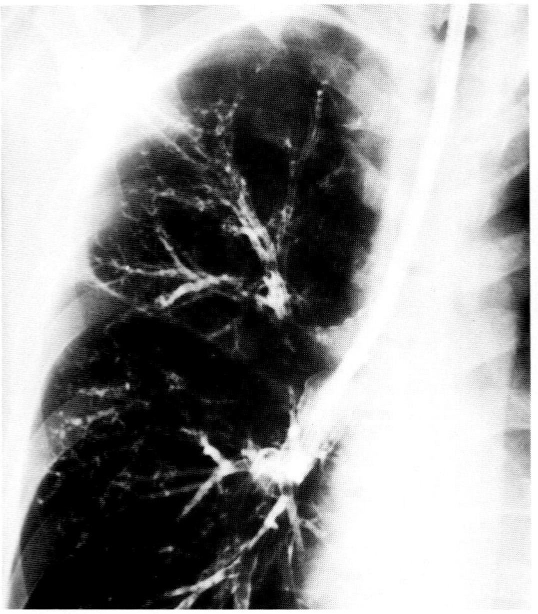

7.3 Posteroanterior right bronchogram. B^3 is completely missing.

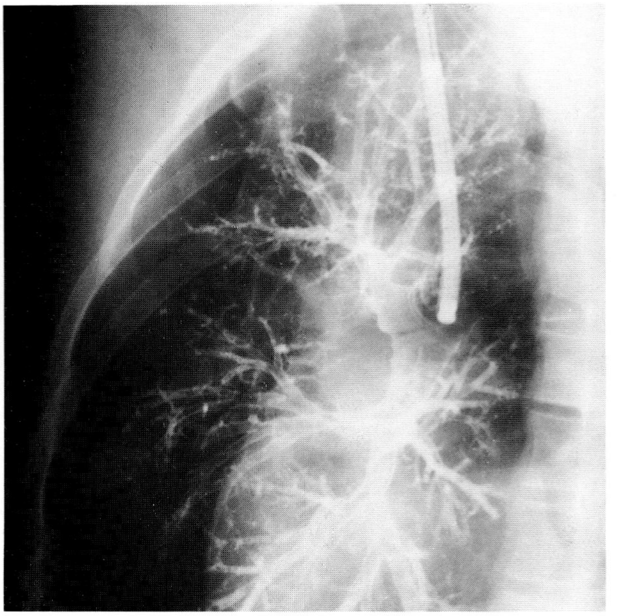

7.4 Lateral right bronchogram. B^3 is not visible.

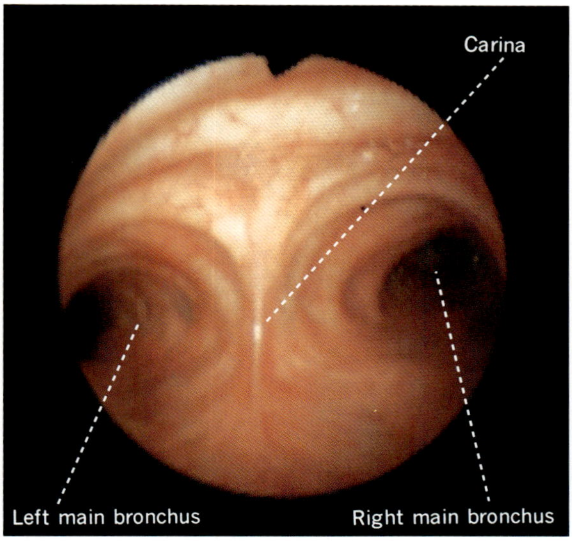

7.5 Bronchoscopic findings at the carina. No abnormalities are visible.

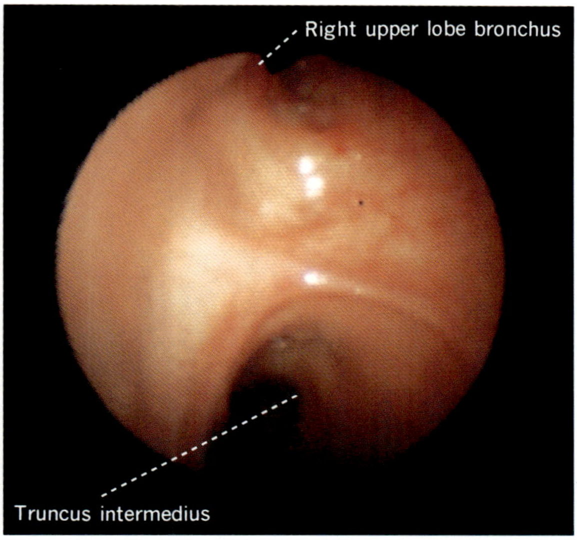

7.6 Bronchoscopic findings at the bifurcation between the RUL bronchus and the truncus intermedius.

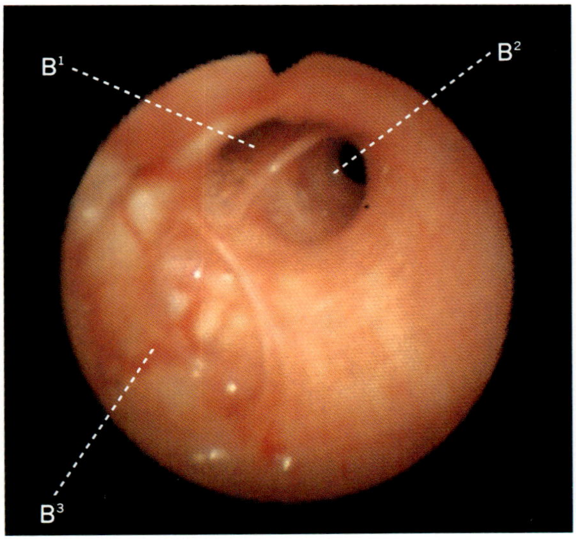

7.7 Bronchoscopic findings in the RUL bronchus. While B^1 and B^2 are recognised, the orifice of B^3 is completely occluded by the vascular dilatation and the scar caused by previous inflammation.

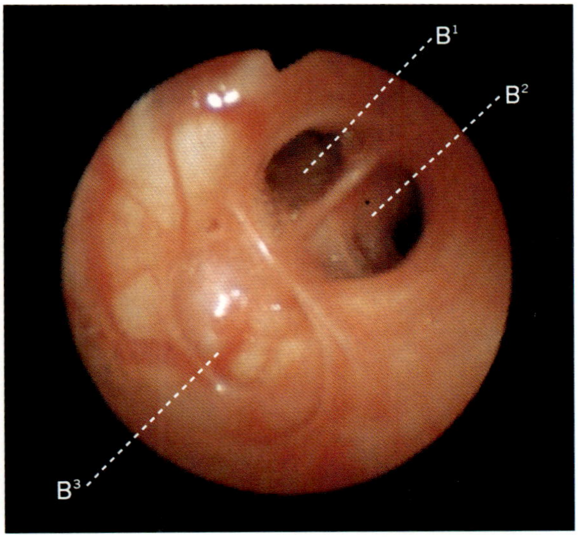

7.8 Close-up of the RUL bronchus. In spite of intact B^1 and B^2 the orifice of B^3 is completely occluded by a previous inflammation (probably tuberculosis).

Case 8: Acute bronchitis in a 36-year-old male.

This patient presented with flu-like symptoms. He had fever and a persistent cough, and produced sticky white sputum in small quantities. Although no pathological bacteria were detected on sputum cytology, acute bronchitis was suspected. His symptoms resolved 1 week after an antibiotic and a non-steroidal anti-inflammatory agent had been prescribed.

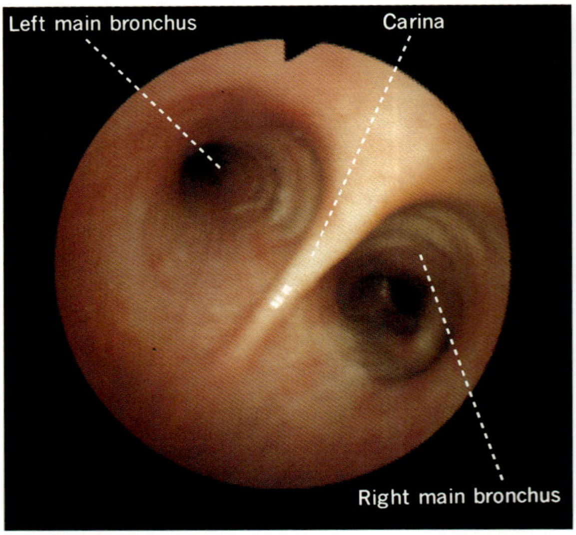

8.1 Bronchoscopic findings at the carina. The carina is moderately widened and the bronchial mucosa of the proximal main bronchi, on each side, is markedly reddened.

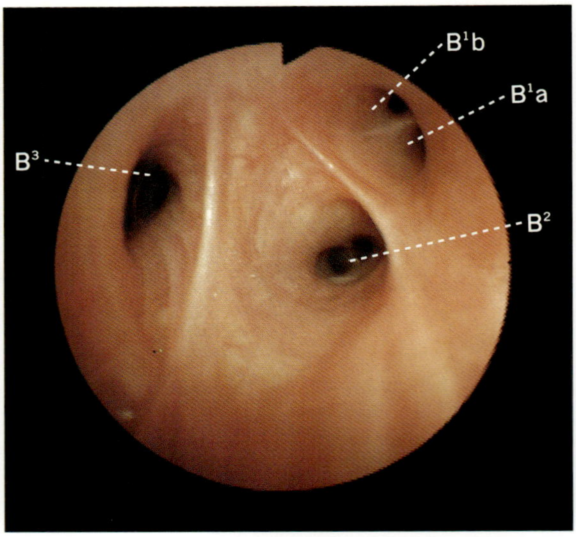

8.2 Bronchoscopic findings at the RUL bronchus. While the bifurcation remains sharp, the bronchial mucosa is reddened with marked dilatation of the small vessels.

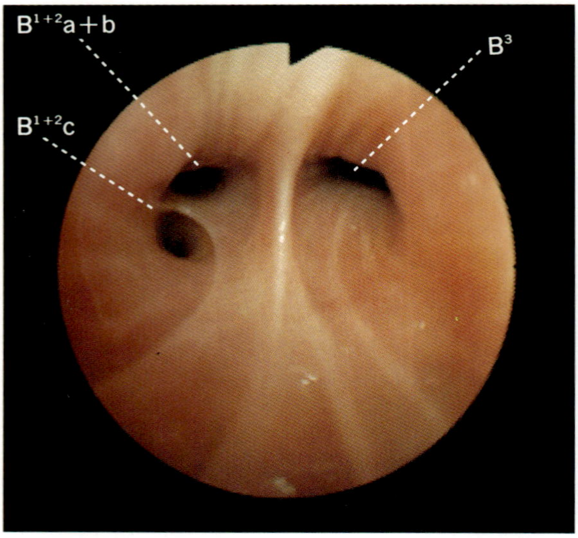

8.3 Bronchoscopic findings at the left upper-division bronchus. While the mucosal folds of the membranous portion are well shown here, mucosa around the orifice is much reddened with narrowing of B^3.

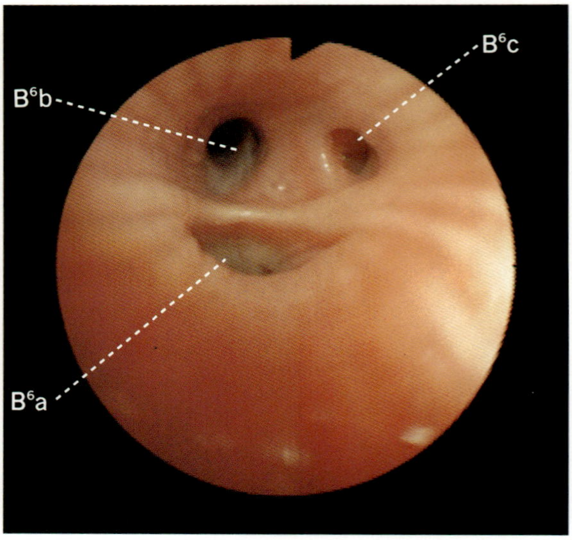

8.4 Bronchoscopic findings in left B^6. The bifurcation is somewhat widened and swollen with a narrowed orifice.

Case 9: Chronic bronchitis in a 58-year-old male.

This patient who smoked more than 12,000 cigarettes per year presented with a productive cough. The sputum was usually white and mucoid but at times purulent.

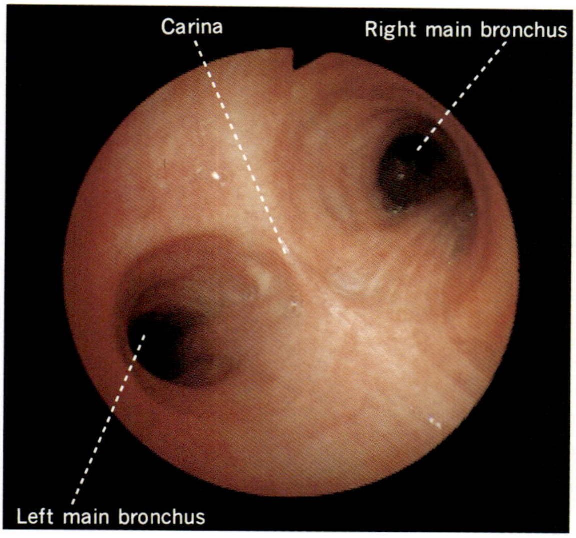

9.1 Bronchoscopic findings at the carina. While the carina remains sharp, the mucosa is diffusely reddened with dilated vessels.

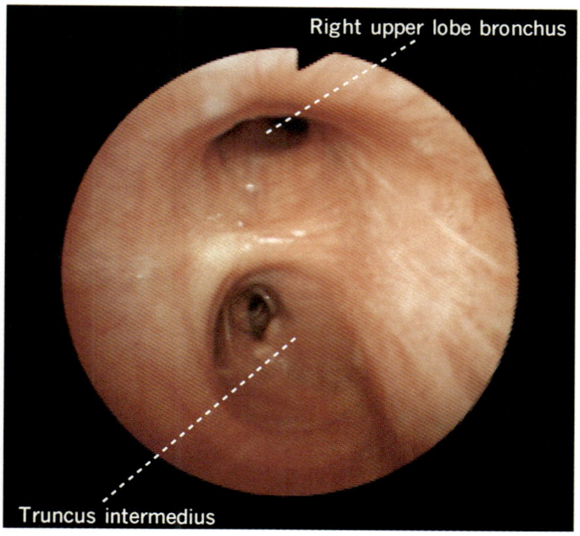

9.2 Bronchoscopic findings in the RUL bronchus and truncus intermedius. The bifurcation is moderately widened with reddening and engorgement of vessels on the mucosa.

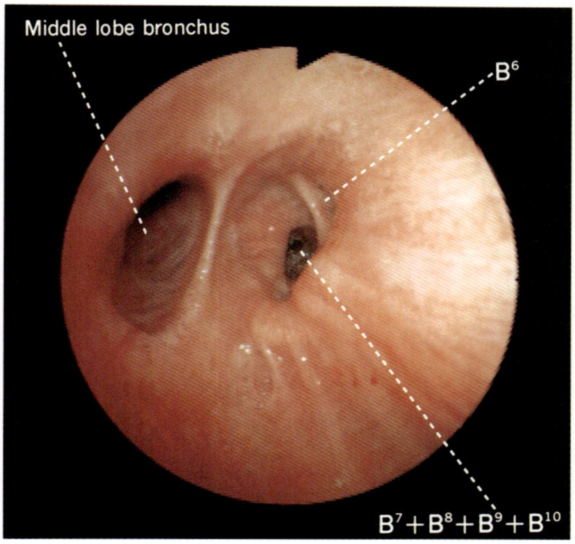

9.3 Bronchoscopic findings in the RML bronchus and the RLL bronchus. While the sharp-edged bifurcation remains intact, diffuse reddening and engorgement of small vessels are seen on the bronchial mucosa. Longitudinal folds run deep. An elevated lesion is seen at the orifice of the RLL bronchus.

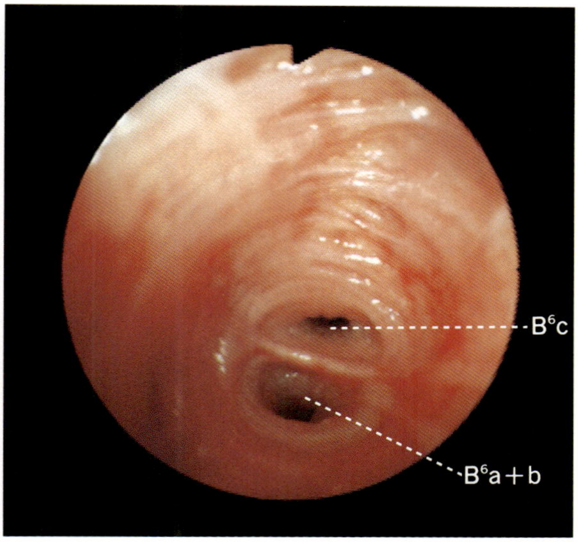

9.4 Bronchoscopic findings in left B^6. The circular mucosal folds are well defined with some pits, suggesting mucosal atrophy. The mucosa is prominently reddened.

Case 10: Bronchiectasis in a 55-year-old male.

The patient complained of a non-productive cough for 2½ years. He had produced purulent sputum, sometimes bloodstained, for six months. Laboratory data revealed the following: erythrocyte sedimentation rate 7 mm/h, C-reactive protein negative, cold agglutinin test 4+. No pathological bacteria were detected on sputum examination. Pulmonary function was normal.

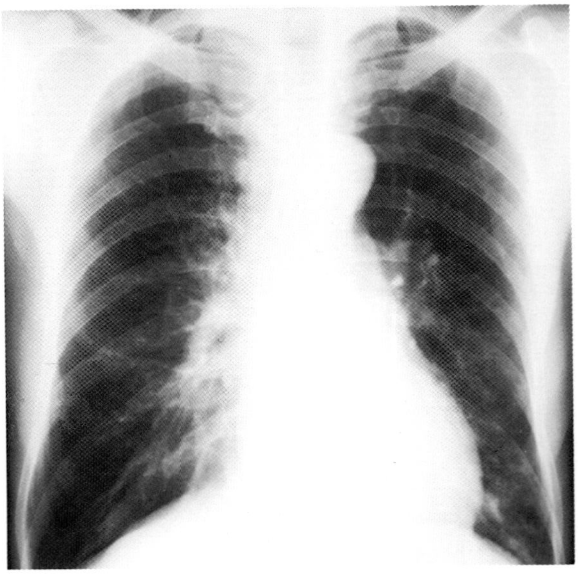

10.1 Posteroanterior chest radiograph. Nodular as well as ring shadows are visible in the left lower lung zone.

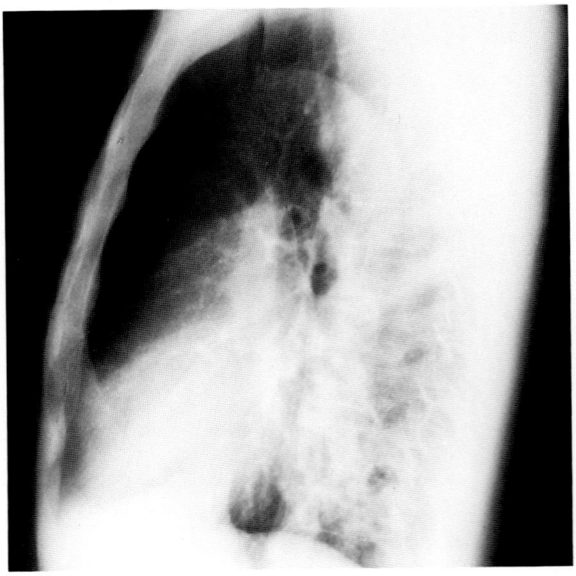

10.2 Lateral chest radiograph (R-L). An irregular-shaped shadow exists along the bronchial tree in the area of B^8, B^9, and B^{10}.

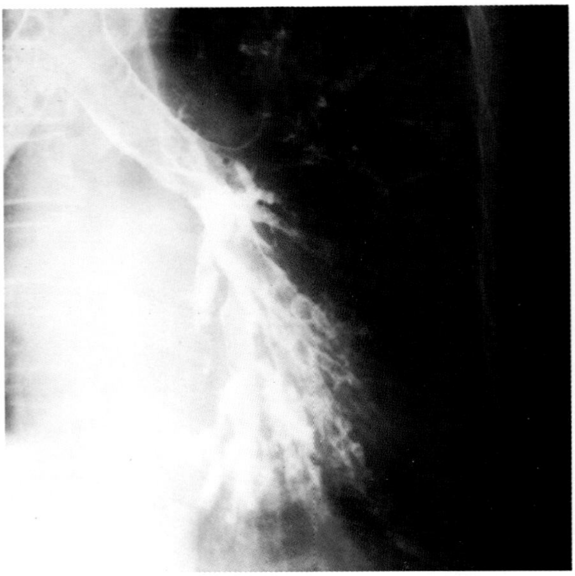

10.3 Left bronchogram: posteroanterior view. Prominent tubular dilatation of B^6, B^8, B^9, and B^{10} is visible.

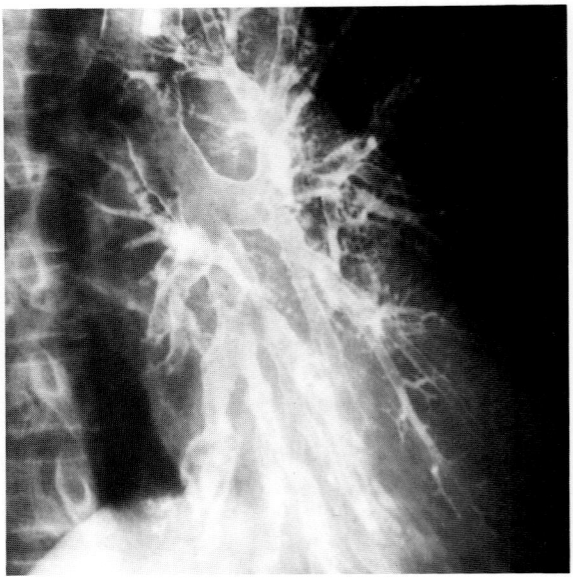

10.4 Left bronchogram: oblique view. Tubular or cystic dilatation as well as irregularity of the wall are seen in B^5, B^6, B^8, B^9, and B^{10}.

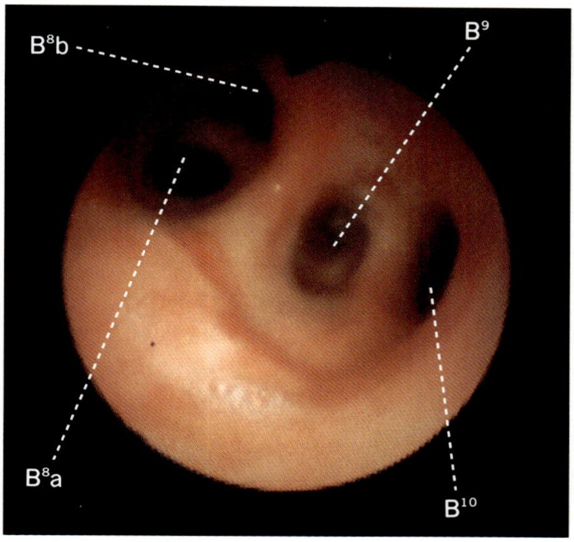

10.5 Bronchoscopic findings in the left basal bronchus. The bronchial mucosa is reddened and swollen. Bifurcations into segmental and subsegmental bronchi are widened, with purulent secretion partly attached to the wall.

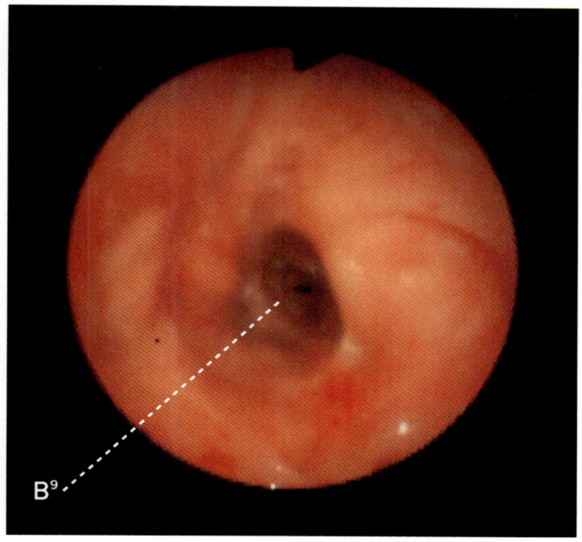

10.6 Bronchoscopic findings of left B^9. The mucosa is strikingly reddened, swollen and irregular, with obliteration of longitudinal corrugations.

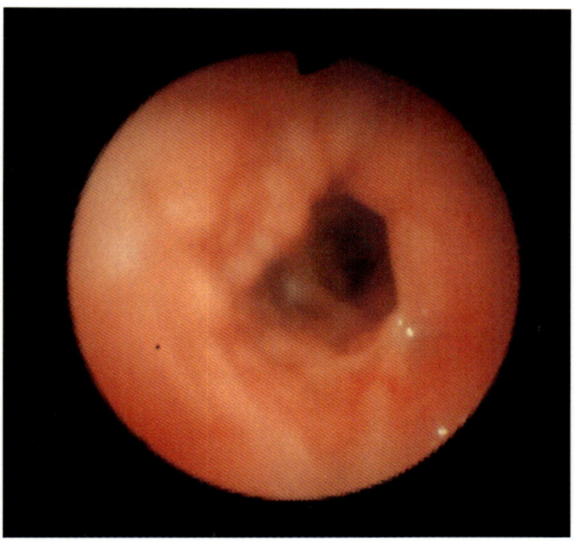

10.7 Close-up of left B^9. The reddened and irregular surface is associated with loss of tapering of the lumen.

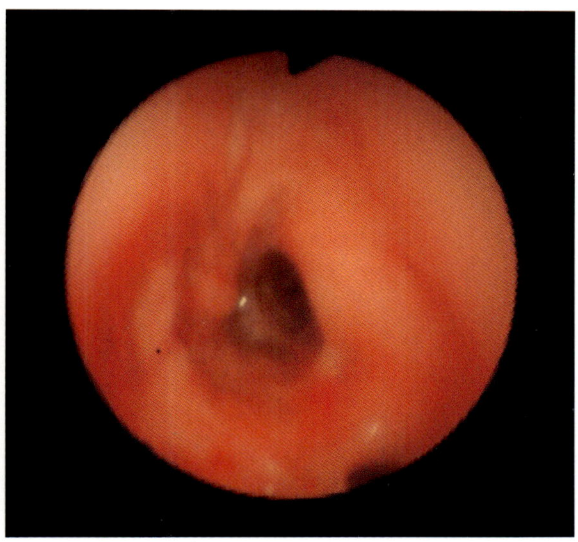

10.8 Close-up beyond the orifice of B^9. The mucosa is markedly nodular, with loss of tapering of the lumen.

Case 11: Haemoptysis (bronchiectasis) in a 55-year-old male.

The patient had a history of pulmonary tuberculosis and had undergone right thoracoplasty 30 years earlier. Although he had been well since this operation, he presented with haemoptysis of 50–100 ml daily.

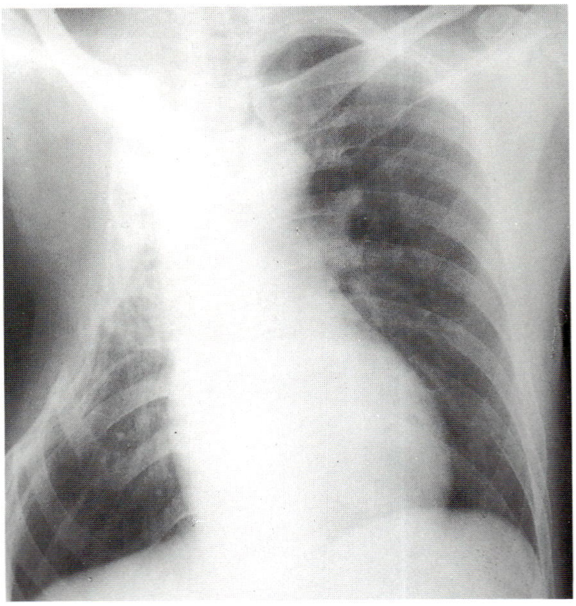

11.1 Posteroanterior chest radiograph. Prominent distortion of the right thorax caused by thoracoplasty. Bronchoscopy was performed because of persistent haemoptysis.

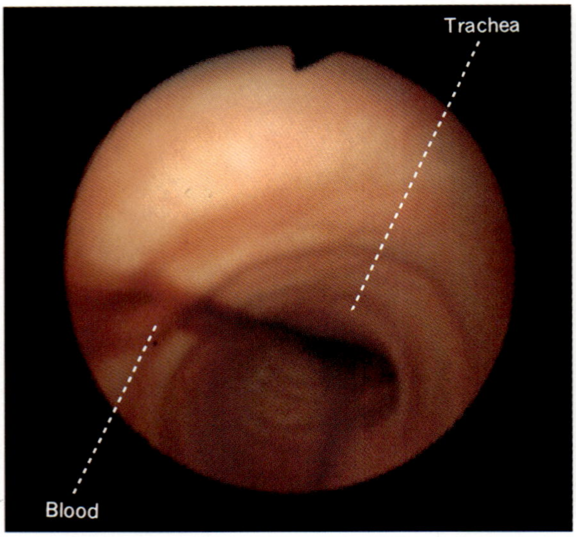

11.2 Bronchoscopic findings in the trachea. The blood is welling up into the upper portion of the trachea.

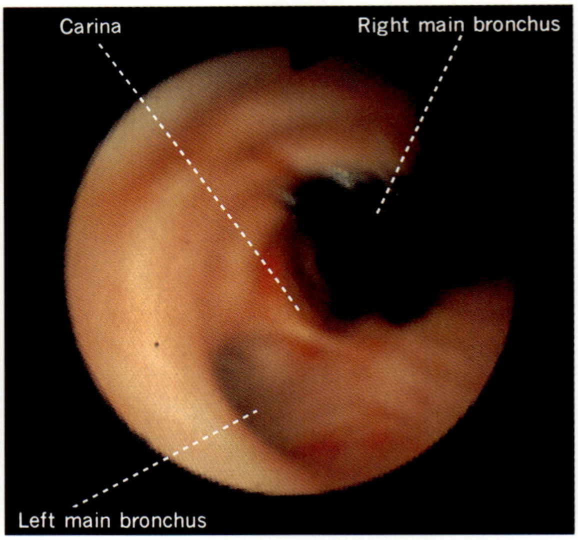

11.3 Bronchoscopic findings of the R main bronchus. A black coagulum completely overlies the orifice.

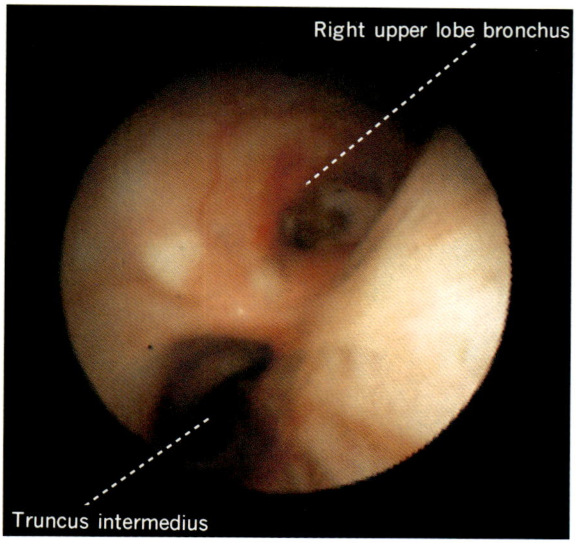

11.4 After lavaging the bronchus with physiological saline, removal of the coagulum uncovered the RUL bronchus and truncus intermedius.

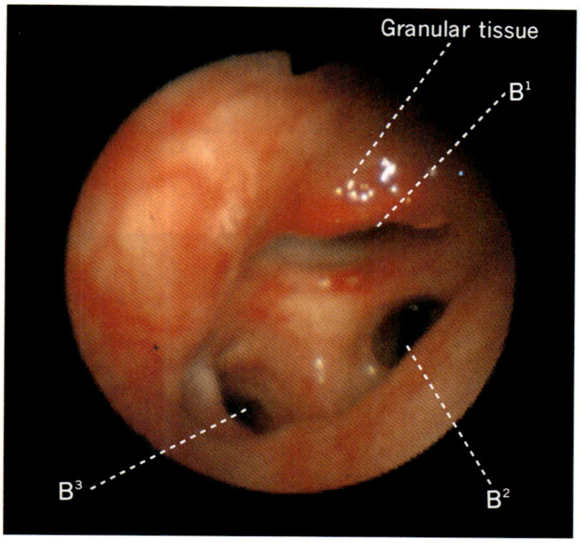

11.5 Bronchoscopic findings in the RUL bronchus. The bronchial mucosa is strikingly reddened with accompanying vascular dilatation. There is a granulomatous lesion at the orifice of B^1.

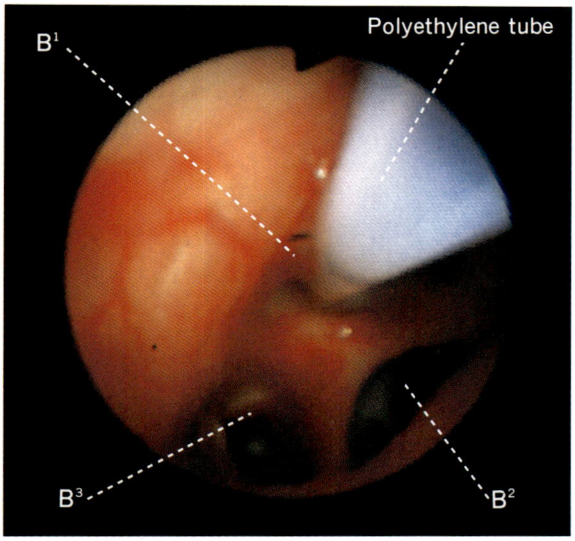

11.6 After confirming that the bleeding was arising from B^1, thrombin solution was instilled into B^1 via a polyethylene tube.

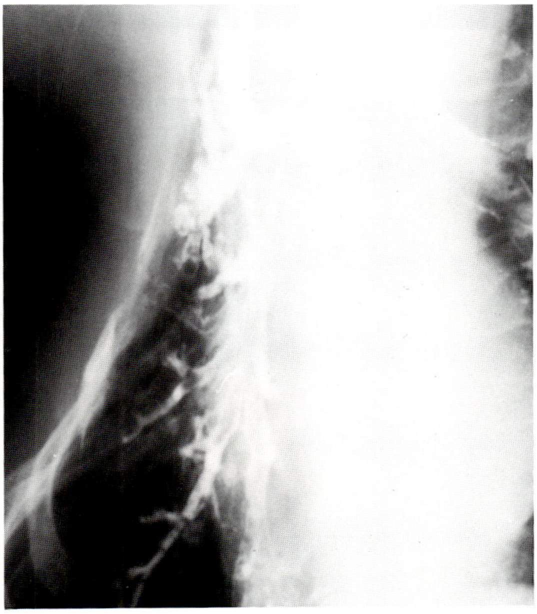

11.7 A right bronchogram was carried out 2 weeks later. Haemoptysis subsided completely after the injection of thrombin solution. The bronchiogram revealed a prominent dilatation of the RUL bronchus, suggesting that bleeding originated from the dilated B^1.

Case 14: Pulmonary aspergillosis in a 26-year-old male.

Because of massive haemoptysis caused by pulmonary aspergillosis, the patient underwent right pneumonectomy, including removal of a fungus ball. Nevertheless, he again attended hospital with a cough.

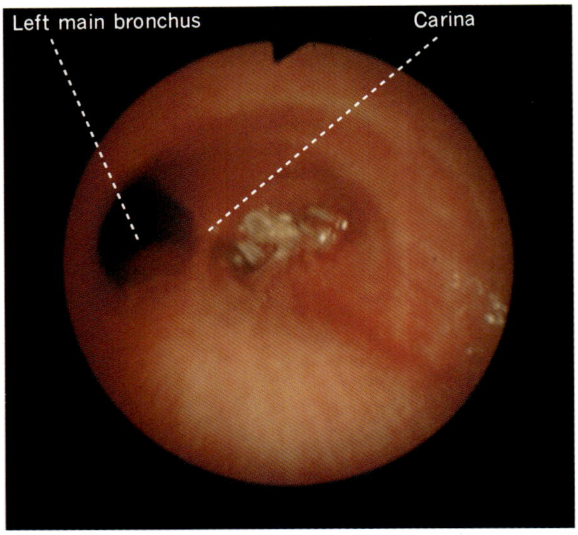

14.1 Bronchoscopic findings at the stump of the right main bronchus. Note the white material attached around the suture. The mucosa is generally reddened and swollen around these changes, including the lower portion of the trachea.

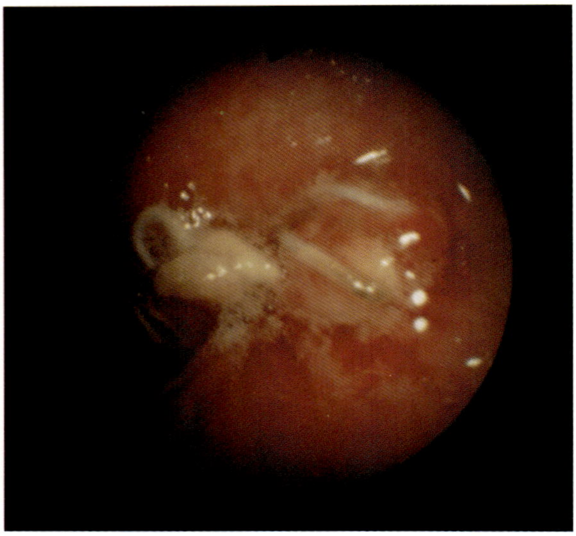

14.2 Close-up of the suture. On the suture and the mucosa surrounding these changes, a white layer of *Aspergillus fumigatus* is present. The bronchial mucosa is so reddened and swollen that it bleeds very readily.

Case 15: Pulmonary aspergillosis in a 67-year-old male.

The patient underwent left upper lobectomy for primary lung cancer (epidermoid carcinoma). Several months later he complained of a cough.

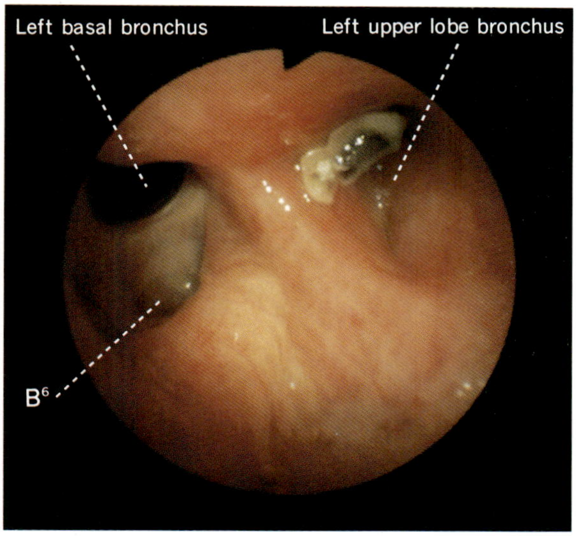

15.1 Bronchoscopic findings at the bifurcation between the LUL and LLL bronchi. B^6 as well as the basal bronchus are distorted. The suture in the stump of the LUL bronchus is covered with white material, with reddening on the surrounding mucosa.

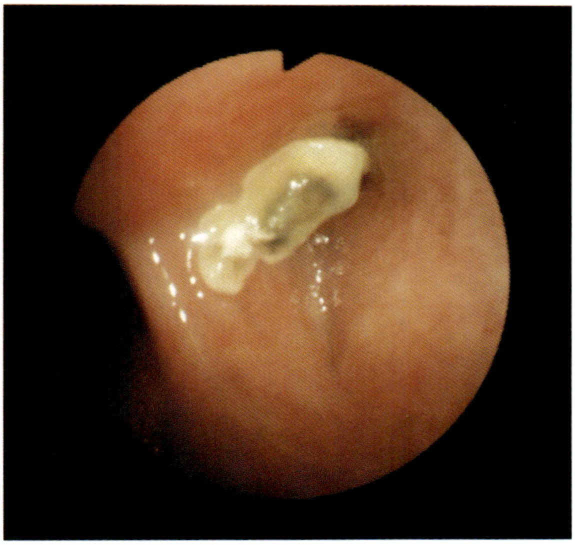

15.2 Bronchoscopic findings in the stump of the LUL bronchus. A yellow-white deposit of *Aspergillus fumigatus* overlies the suture.

Case 16: Burn of the airway in a 45-year-old male.

During a fire at the patient's home, he collapsed at the entrance. He was brought to hospital with burns on his face and had a wheeze.

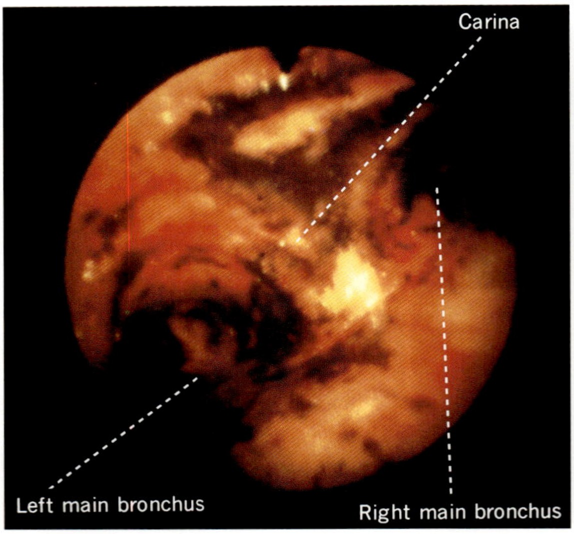

16.1 Bronchoscopic findings at the carina on the patient's fifth day in hospital. A black crust of soot is attached to the mucosa, which is strikingly reddened and swollen.

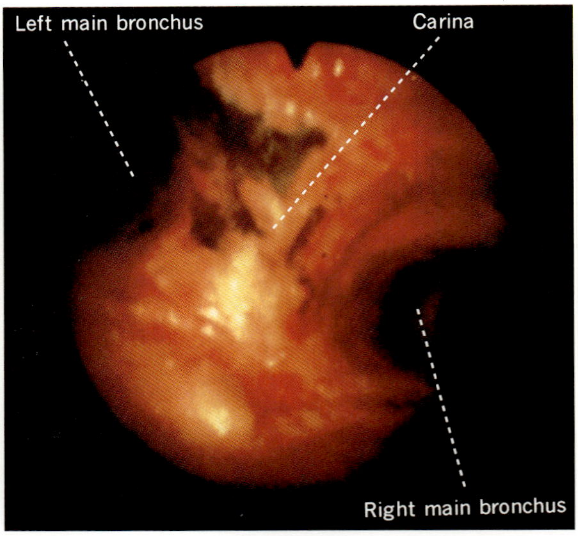

16.2 Bronchoscopic findings at the carina on the patient's eighth day in hospital. On the bronchial mucosa there is a black crust which is associated with necrosis and yellow-white granulomatous tissue. The mucosa is so reddened and swollen that it bleeds readily.

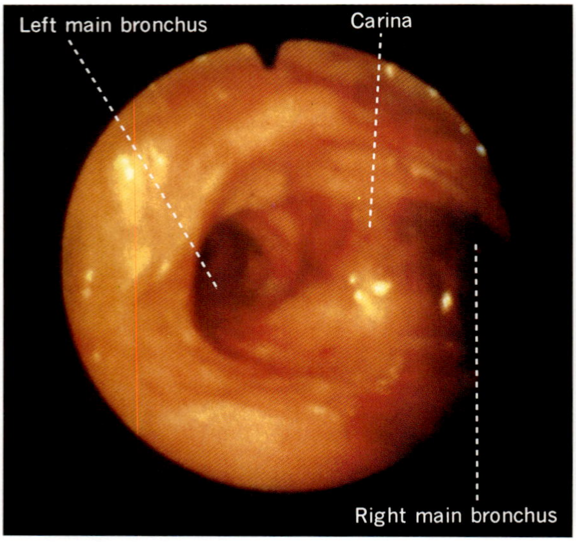

16.3 Bronchoscopic findings at the carina on the patient's fifteenth day in hospital. Inflammation of the mucosa decreased gradually and the cartilage rings are well defined. Yellow-white granulomatous tissue which bleeds readily is present.

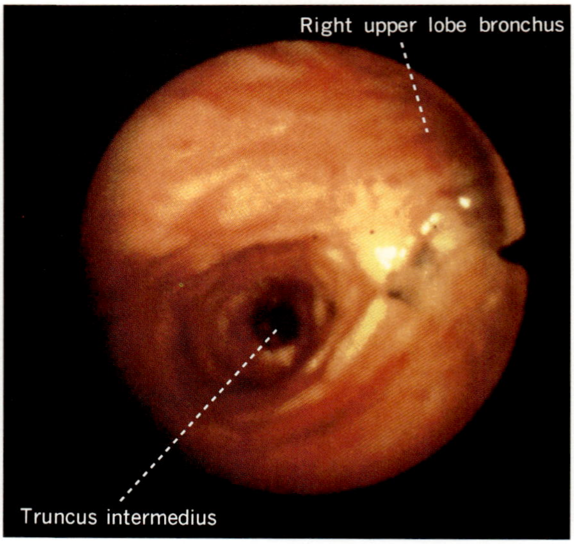

16.4 Bronchoscopic findings at the bifurcation into the RUL bronchus and truncus intermedius. Apart from the black necrotic tissue in one area, inflammation of the mucosa has improved.

Case 17: Tuberculosis of trachea and bronchi in a 64-year-old female.

The patient had been treated for rheumatoid arthritis with steroids for several years. She presented with a non-productive cough that had lasted a few months, which persisted despite therapy for bronchitis. Her erythrocyte sedimentation rate was 24 mm/h.

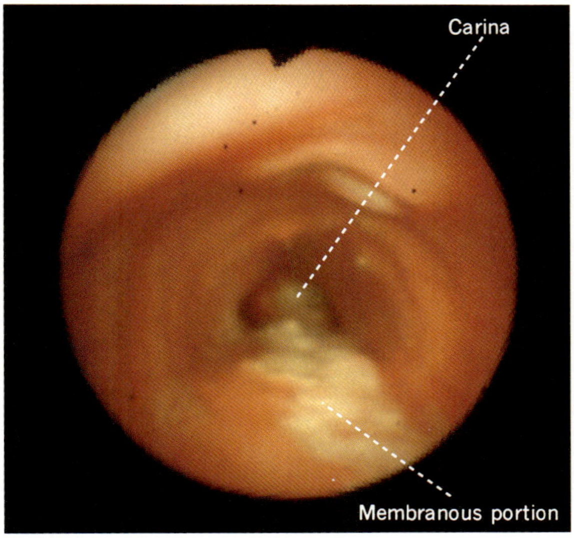

17.1 Bronchoscopic findings in the subglottis and trachea. A diffuse white coating is seen on the membranous portion of the trachea. Irregularly elevated lesions exist on the cartilage, where the white coating is present.

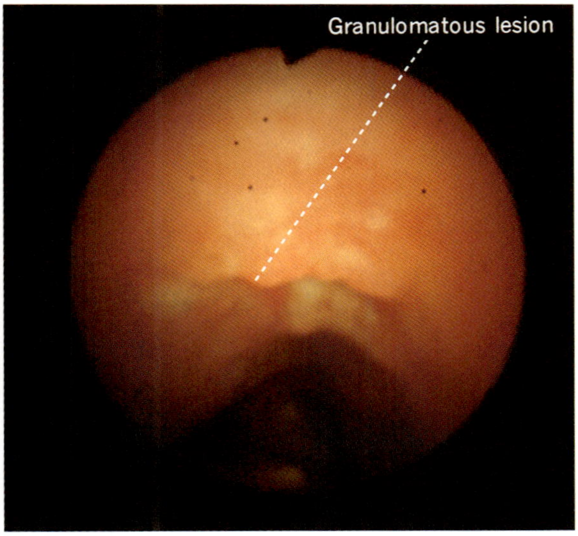

17.2 Close-up of **17.1**. Several granulomatous lesions, with irregular surfaces, are visible on the cartilage of the trachea, surrounded by a white coating.

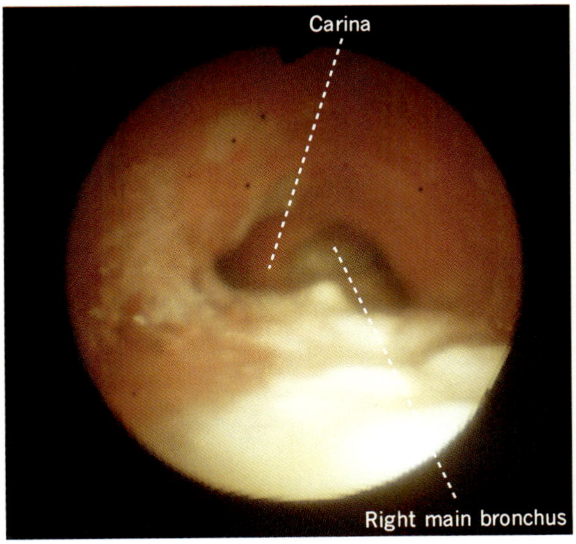

17.3 Close-up of the carina. The membranous portion, covered with a thick white coating, shows a markedly irregular surface. A sticky secretion is visible on the left.

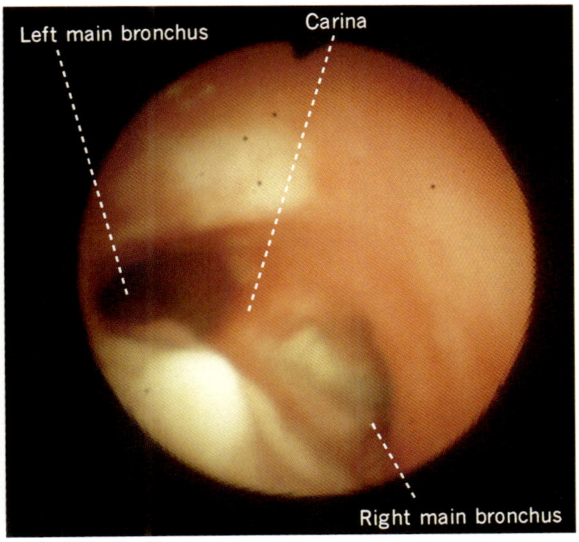

17.4 Another close-up of the carina. The membranous portion is elevated and covered with a white coating. The carina is widened and reddened. The white coating continues up to the right main bronchus.

Case 18: Tuberculosis of the bronchi in a 21-year-old male.

The patient had been well until 6 months earlier, when he developed a cough. His chest radiograph revealed an abnormality and sputum examination proved the presence of mycobacterial infection (Gaffky 2 on sputum smear). He was hospitalised at once for further investigations. His erythrocyte sedimentation rate was 36 mm/h, C-reactive protein double positive.

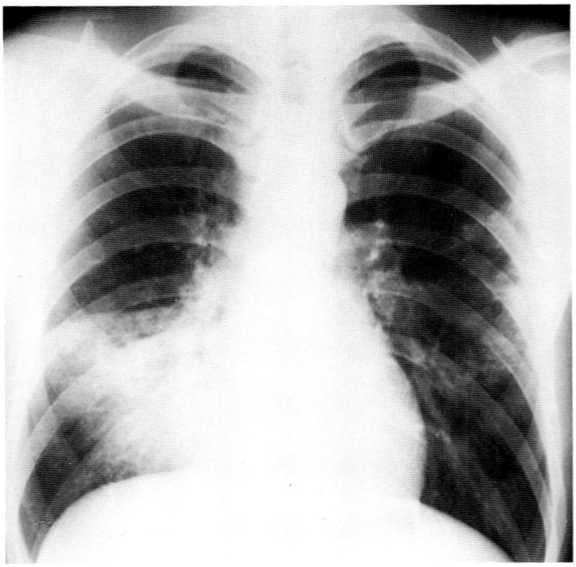

18.1 Posteroanterior chest radiograph. There is atelectasis of the RML, scattered shadows in right S^8 and S^9, and an infiltrative shadow in left S^{3a} and S^4.

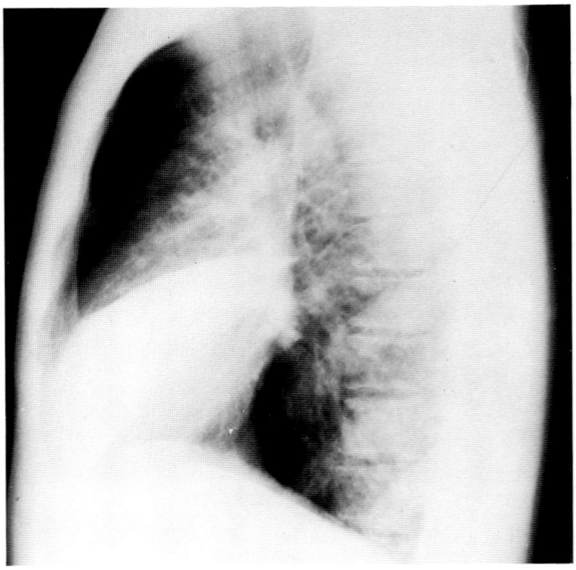

18.2 Lateral chest radiograph (R-L). Atelectasis of the RML (mainly S^4b) and a micronodular shadow in the RLL are visible.

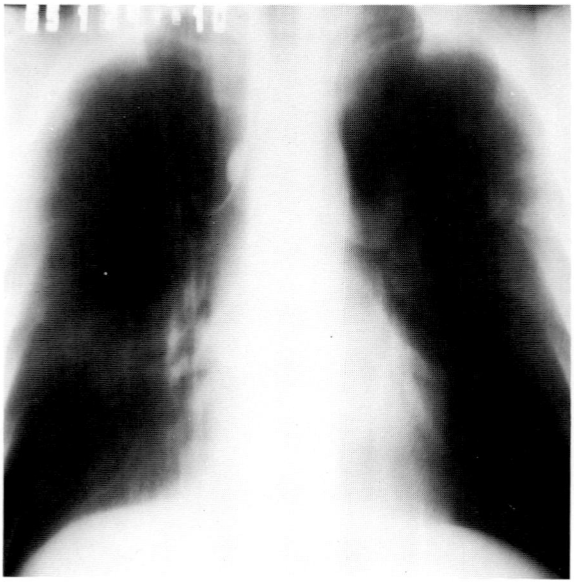

18.3 Chest tomogram (10 cm from the back). Right main bronchus, truncus intermedius, and left main bronchus are clearly seen, in addition to an infiltrative shadow in left S^3a.

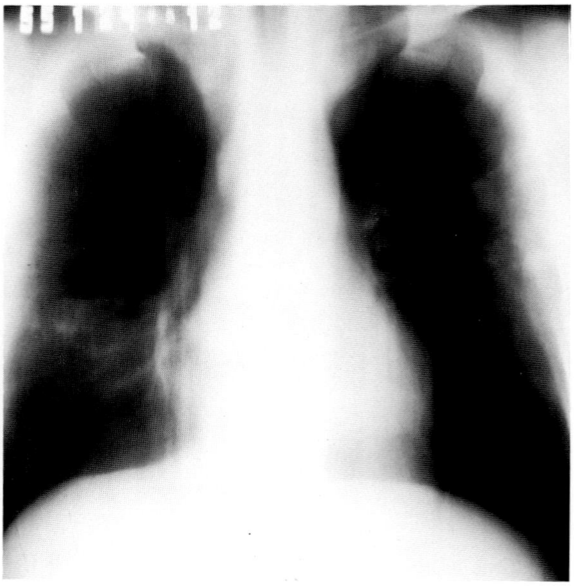

18.4 Chest tomogram (12 cm from the back). Note loss of volume of right S^4a and infiltrates in left S^3a and S^4a.

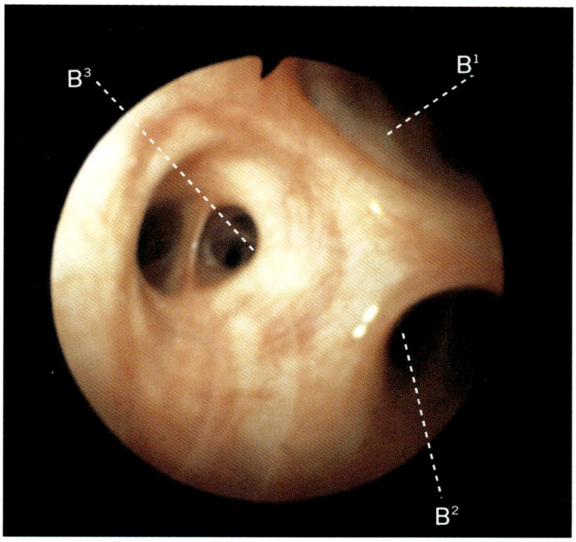

18.5 Bronchoscopic findings in the RUL bronchus. The reddened and swollen mucosa accompanies vascular engorgement and minimal widened bifurcation.

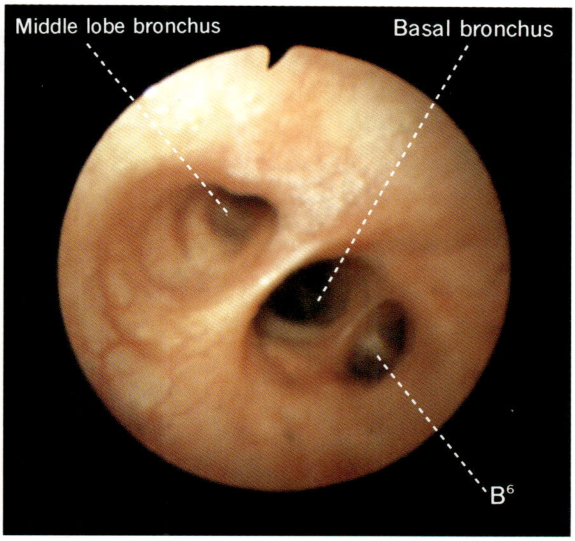

18.6 Bronchoscopic findings in the RML and RLL bronchi. The mucosa is mildly reddened and is associated with vascular dilatation.

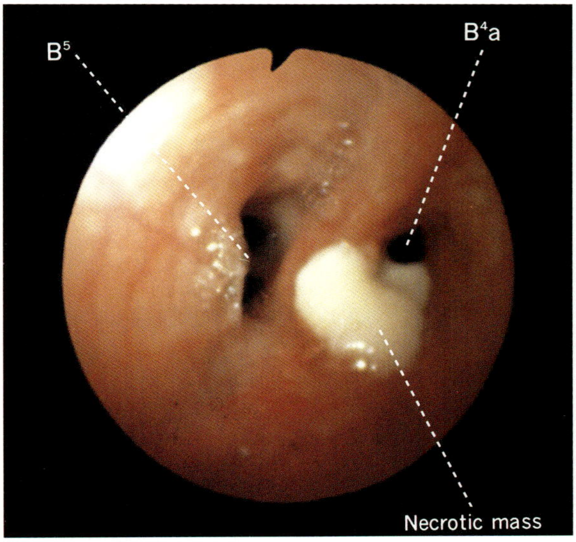

18.7 Bronchoscopic findings at the RML bronchus. There is a striking mucosal reddening, irregularity, and vascular dilatation on it, associated with obliteration of circular folds. Note the white coating from the bifurcation between B^4 and B^5, to the orifice of B^4.

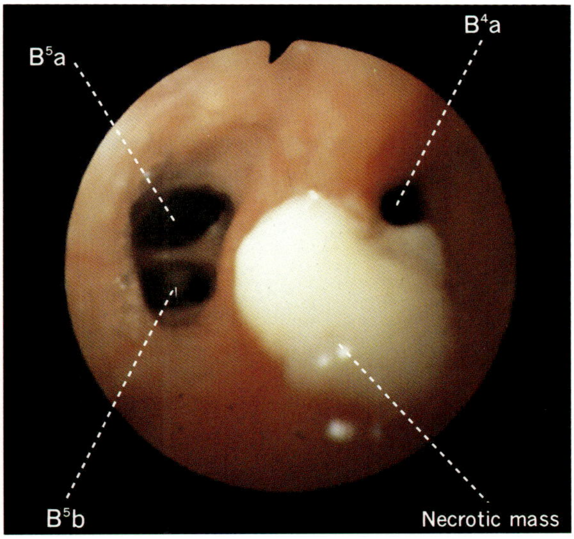

18.8 Close-up of **18.7**. The white coat spreads from the bifurcation between B^4 and B^5 to the orifice of B^4, leaving the orifice of B^4 barely patent.

Case 20: Tuberculosis of the bronchi in an 82-year-old male.

The patient, who suffered repeatedly from pneumonia for 10 months, complained mainly of a non-productive cough.

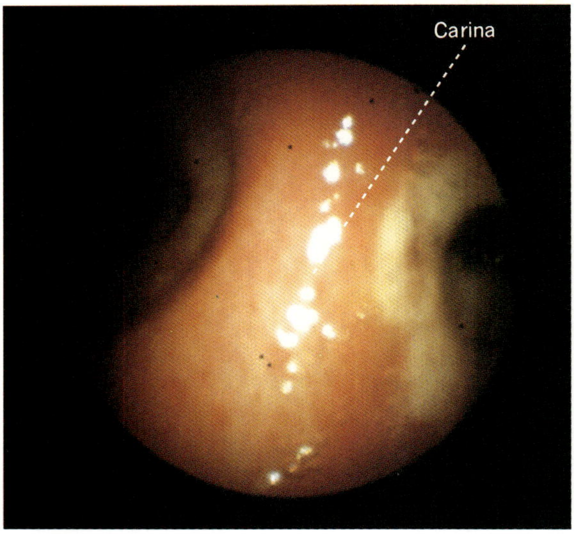

20.1 Bronchoscopic findings at the carina. The bifurcation is swollen and widened; note the white coating at the orifice of the right main bronchus.

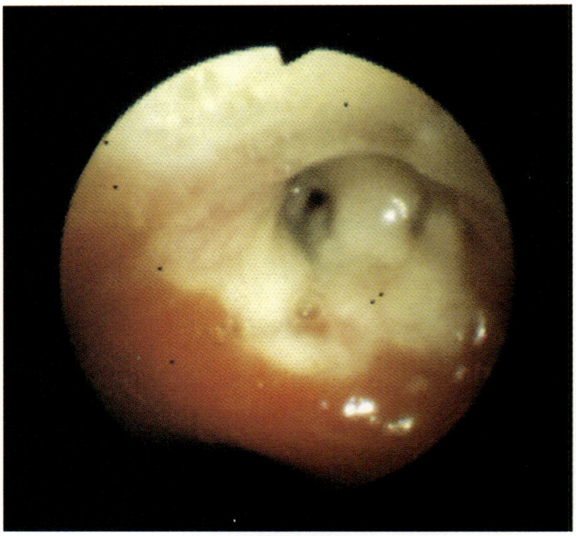

20.2 Bronchoscopic findings at the RUL bronchus. The bifurcation is widened and reddened, and there is a white coat around the orifice of the RUL bronchus.

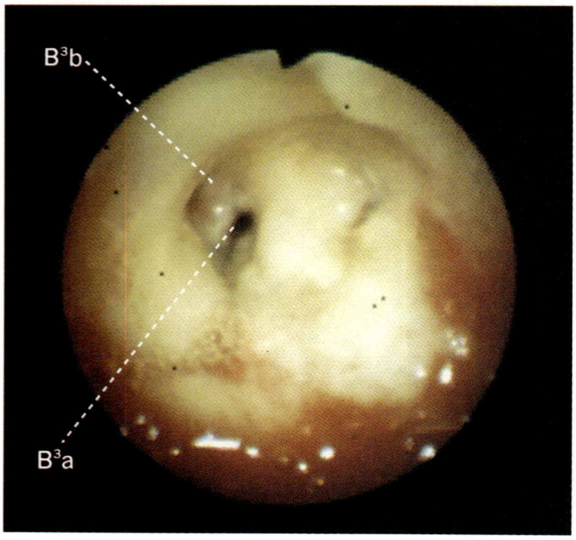

20.3 Close-up of the RUL bronchus. The bifurcation into the truncus intermedius is covered with a thick white coating and shows an irregular surface.

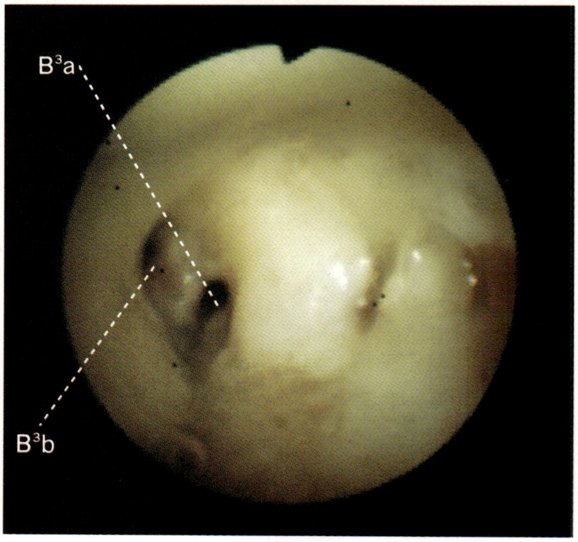

20.4 Close-up of **20.3**. The orifices of B^1 and B^2 are completely occluded with the white coating, which barely spares B^3. Mycobacterium was detected in this white coating.

Case 21: Tuberculosis of the trachea in a 62-year-old female.

The patient presented with cough and low-grade fever. However, her chest radiograph showed no abnormality. At bronchoscopy a tumour was detected in the trachea. Biopsy confirmed it to be a tuberculous granuloma.

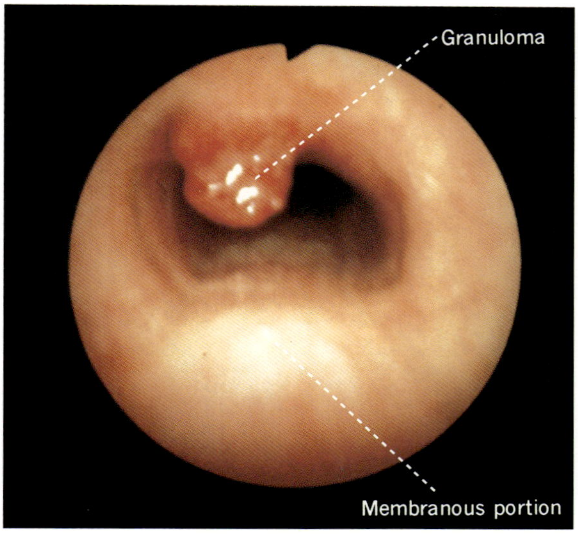

21.1 Bronchoscopic findings in the trachea. On the anterior wall of the upper trachea, a tumour with an irregular surface and vascular dilatation, partly covered with white necrotic lesions, is visible. The mucosa around it is reddened.

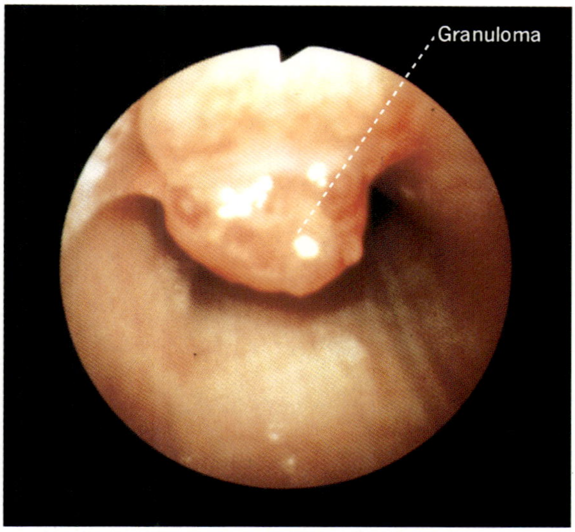

21.2 Close-up of the tumour. It showed an irregular surface with vascular dilatation and revealed a soft-tissue mass during biopsy, which enabled the histological diagnosis to be obtained. The surrounding mucosa is oedematous.

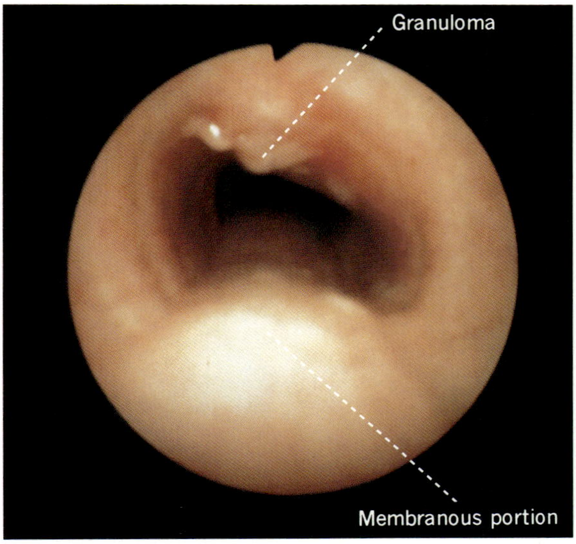

21.3 Bronchoscopic findings in the trachea 4 weeks after anti-tuberculosis therapy, which included isoniazid, ethambutol and rifampicin. The tumour, covered with necrotic tissue, decreased in size, reducing the posteroanterior diameter of the trachea.

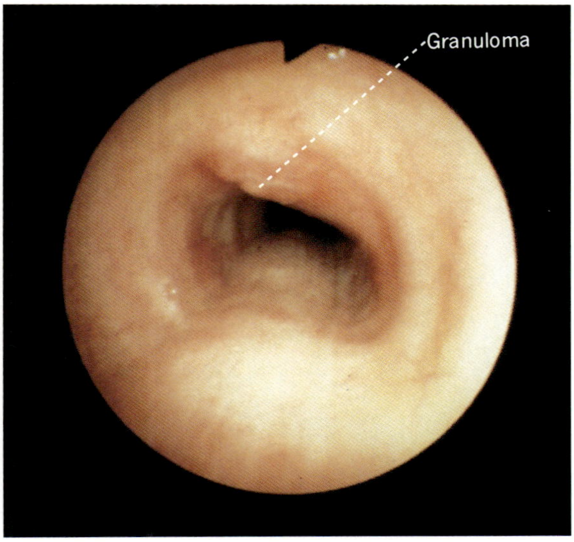

21.4 Bronchoscopic findings of the same region 10 weeks after the anti-tuberculosis therapy described above had begun. While the tumour reduced in size and became flattened, it remained reddened with an irregular surface. Posteroanterior diameter of the trachea diminished further. This is a rare case of tuberculosis of the trachea forming a tumour-like mass.

Case 22: Stenosis of the trachea in a 53-year-old female.

The patient had been well until about 6 months earlier when the cervical lymph nodes swelled; aetiology was unknown. Since then she has presented with increasing dyspnoea.

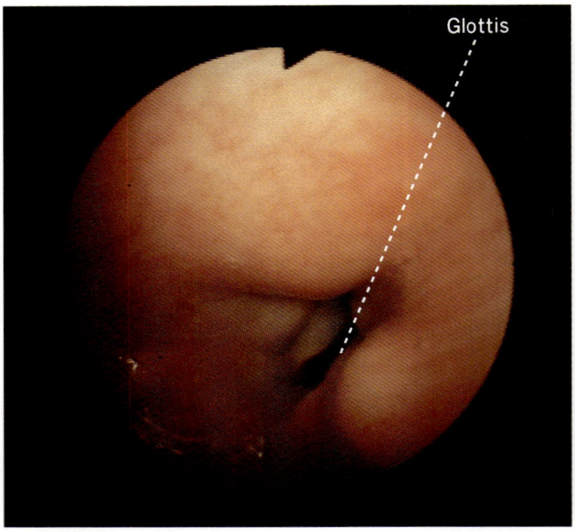

22.1 Bronchoscopic findings at the glottis. Normal findings.

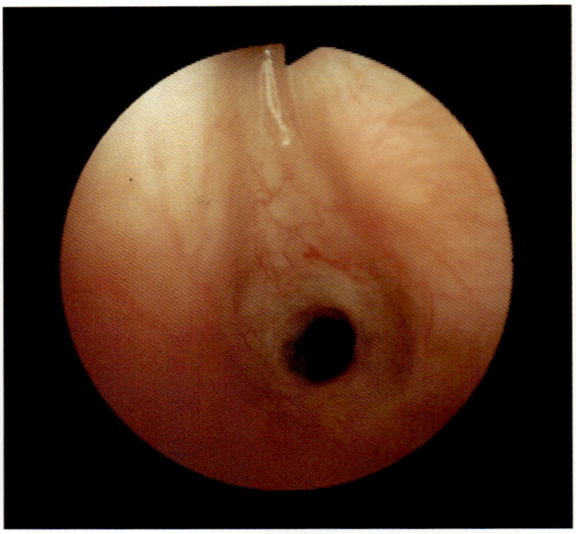

22.2 Bronchoscopic findings just beneath the glottis. The lumen is generally stenotic, accompanying dilatation of the small vessels on the surrounding mucosa.

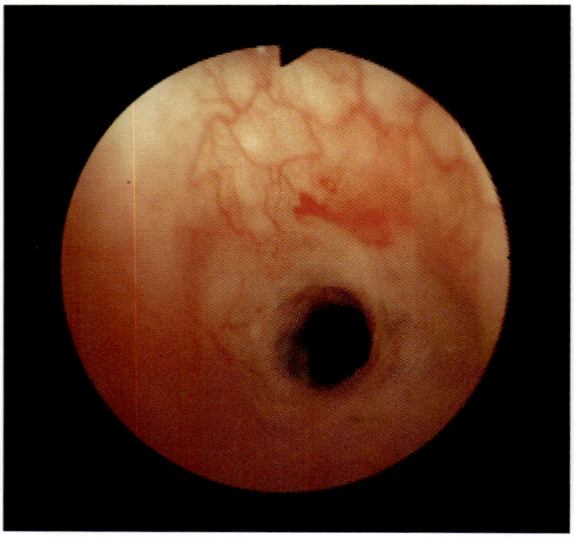

22.3 Close-up of the stenotic site. The stenotic portion, 5 mm in diameter, made it impossible for a fibreoptic bronchoscope to pass through.

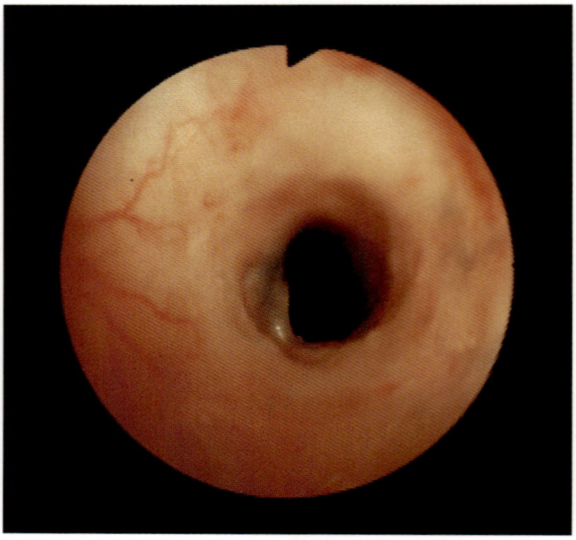

22.4 Further close-up of the stenotic part. Mild anthracosis is present. Stenosis exists 1-2 cm beneath the glottis, leaving the remaining lower portion intact. The aetiology of this case remains unknown and belongs to the so-called 'syndrome of central airway stenosis', presumably related to certain kinds of infection.

Case 23: Stenosis of the trachea and bronchi in a 76-year-old female.

The patient had been well, working as a farmer, until a year ago when she presented with increasing dyspnoea. Chest tomograms and CT scan revealed generalised stenosis, extending from the trachea to the bilateral main bronchi.

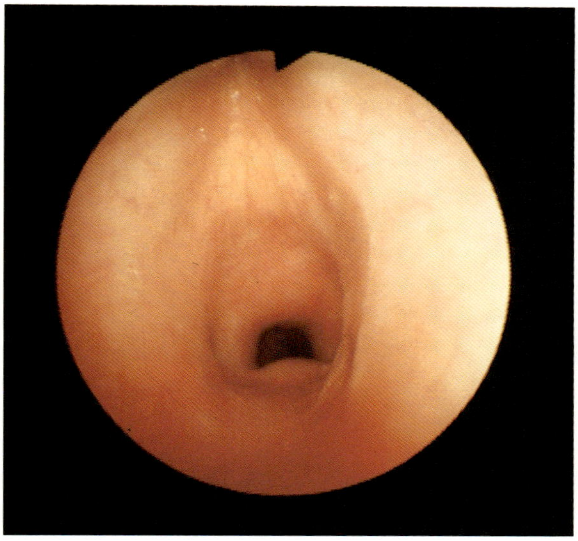

23.1 Bronchoscopic findings just beneath the glottis. The uppermost part of the trachea is extremely narrowed, although its normal configuration is maintained. The mucosa is strikingly reddened.

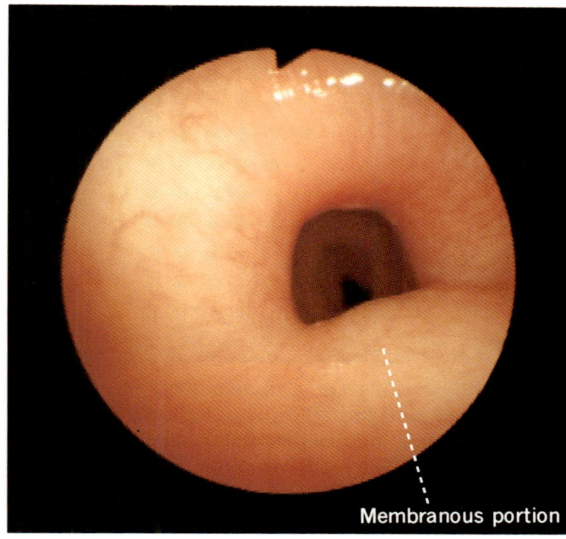

23.2 Close-up of the stenosis. The mucosa is reddened with vascular dilatation. The trachea, in spite of being 7 mm in diameter, retains its own configuration.

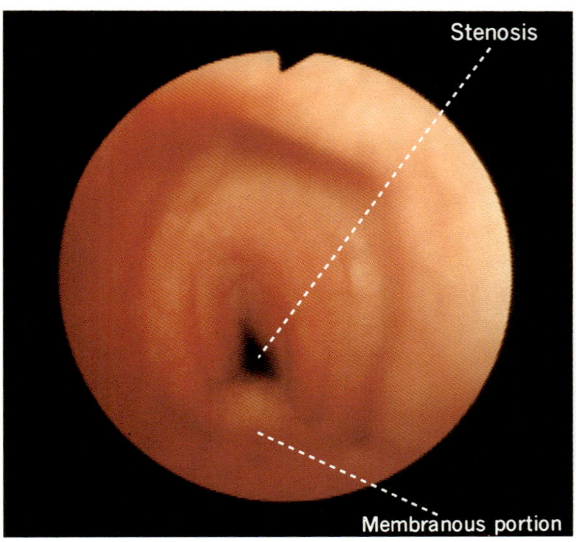

23.3 Further downward view. The mucosa is considerably reddened. The deeper a bronchoscope is inserted, the narrower the diameter of the trachea.

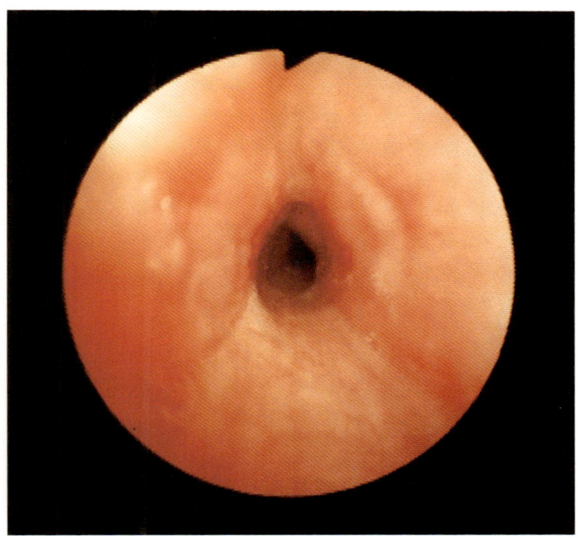

23.4 Even further downward view. The mucosa is irregular and more narrowed; a fibreoptic bronchoscope of usual size can barely pass through. These findings suggest relapsing polychondritis.

Case 26: Sarcoidosis in a 36-year-old male.

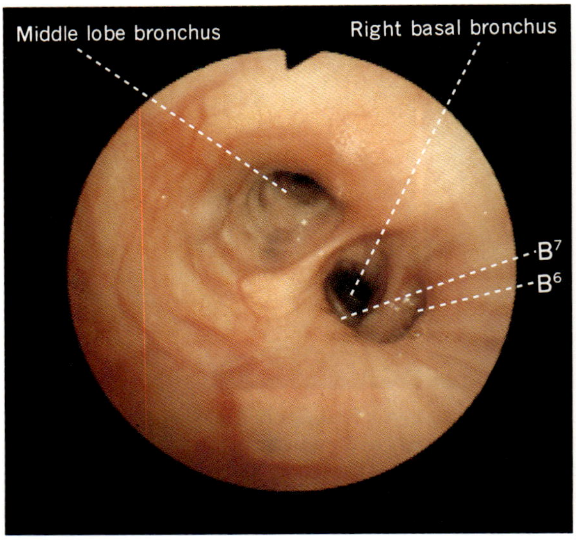

26.1 Bronchoscopic findings in the truncus intermedius. Dilated mucosal vessels, but bifurcations almost intact.

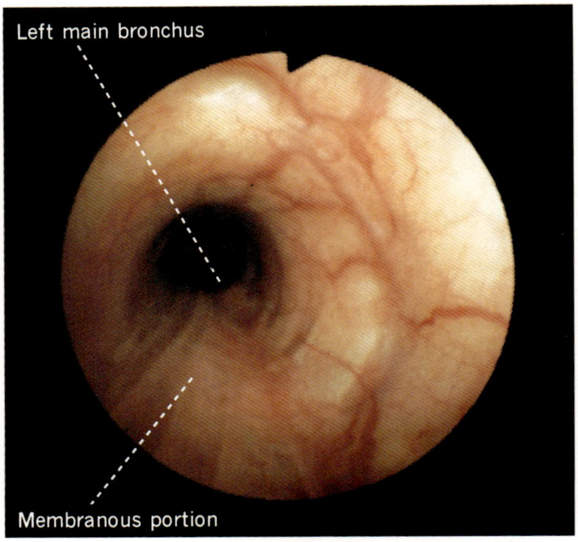

26.2 Bronchoscopic findings in the left main bronchus. The small mucosal vessels are dilated.

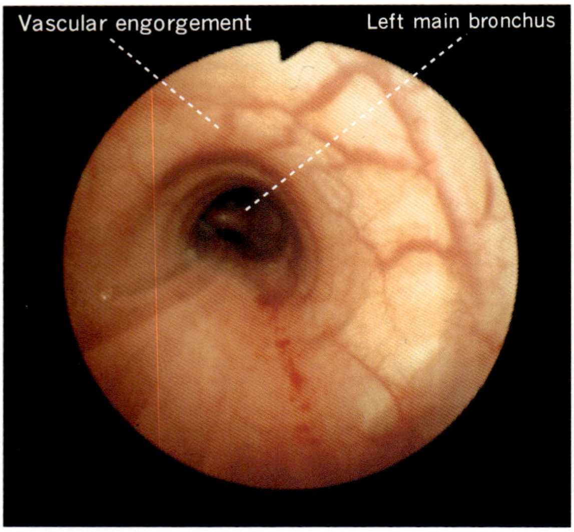

26.3 Further distal view of the left main bronchus. Dilatation of the relatively large vessels as well as small ones, forming the network pattern.

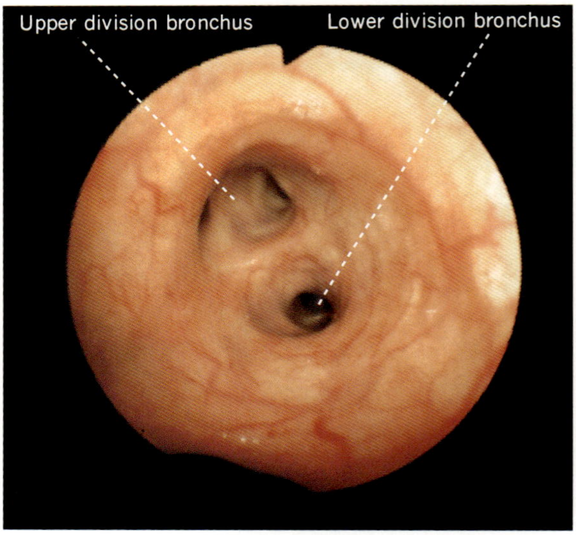

26.4 Bronchoscopic findings in the LUL and LLL bronchi. The bifurcation is somewhat widened, associated with the network pattern of the dilated mucosal vessels.

Case 27: Sarcoidosis in a 24-year-old male.

An asymptomatic patient was referred to us for investigation of bilateral hilar lymphadenopathy shown on his chest radiograph at a public health survey.

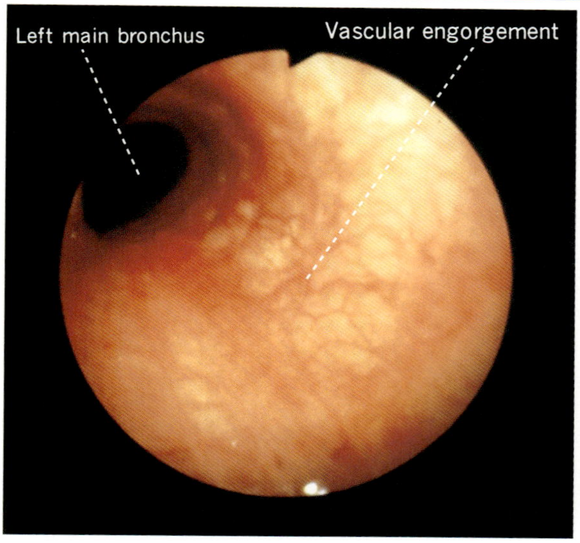

27.1 Bronchoscopic findings in the left main bronchus. The mucosa is rather oedematous, in addition to an obvious network pattern of dilated mucosal vessels.

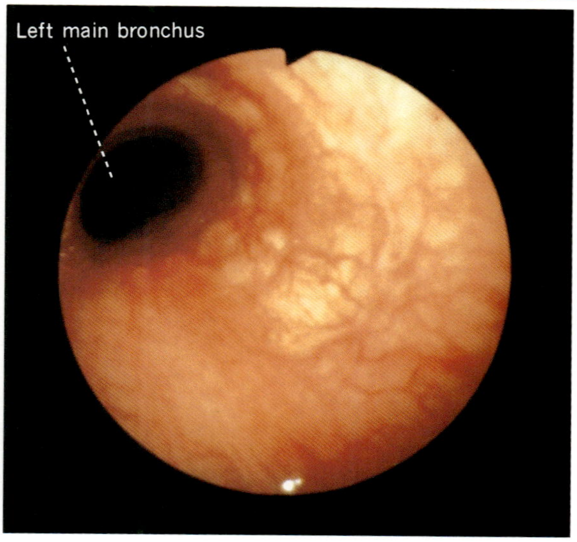

27.2 Further distal view in the left main bronchus. Strikingly dilated vessels, making a network pattern, is one of the most characteristic features of sarcoidosis.

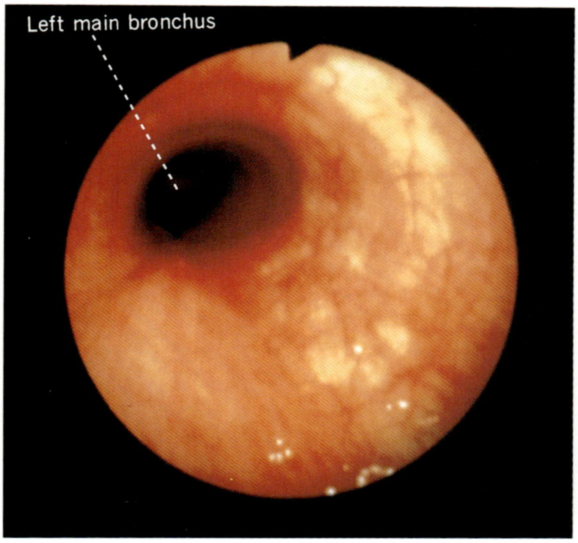

27.3 Bronchoscopic findings of the middle portion of the left main bronchus. Mesh-like dilatation of small mucosal vessels accompanies yellow-white nodules.

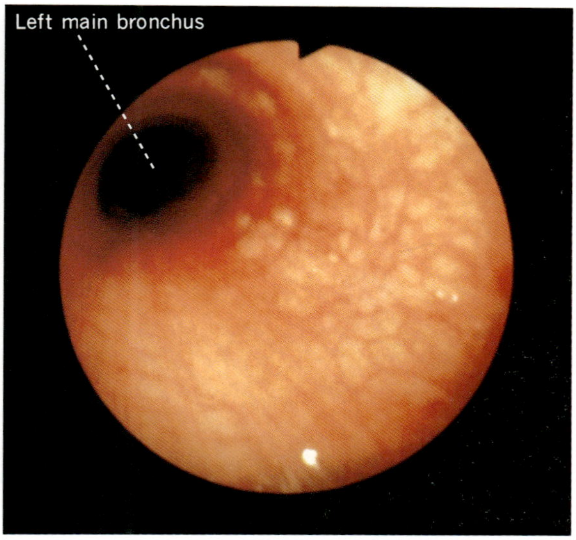

27.4 Bronchoscopic findings at the distal end of the left main bronchus. Mesh-like dilatation of mucosal vessels as well as yellow-white nodules are visible.

Case 28: Sarcoidosis in a 53-year-old female.

An asymptomatic patient with bilateral hilar lymphadenopathy on her chest radiograph during a public health survey. The blood showed high levels of serum angiotensin-converting enzyme.

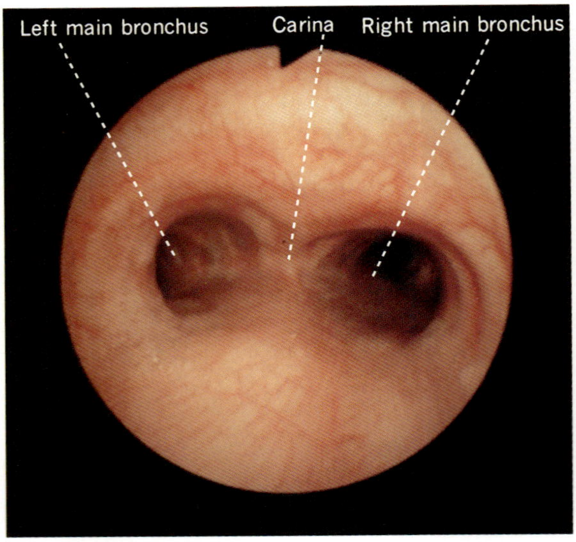

28.1 Bronchoscopic findings at the carina. The disease caused diffuse marked engorgement of the mucosal vessels, including the membranous portion of the trachea, although there was sharp branching of the bifurcation.

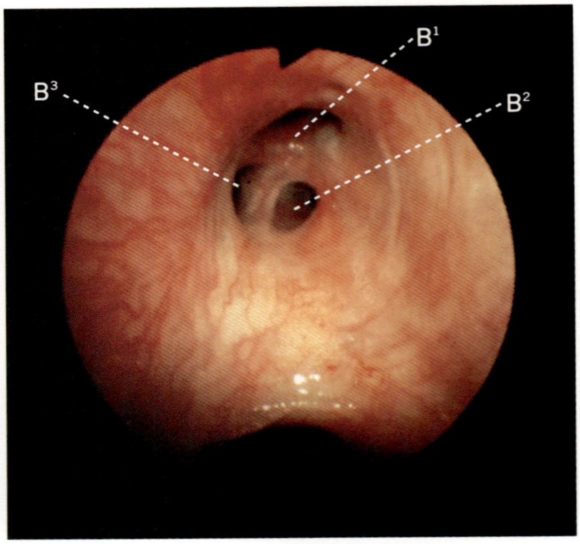

28.2 Bronchoscopic findings in the RUL bronchus. The prominent dilatation of mucosal vessels can be seen.

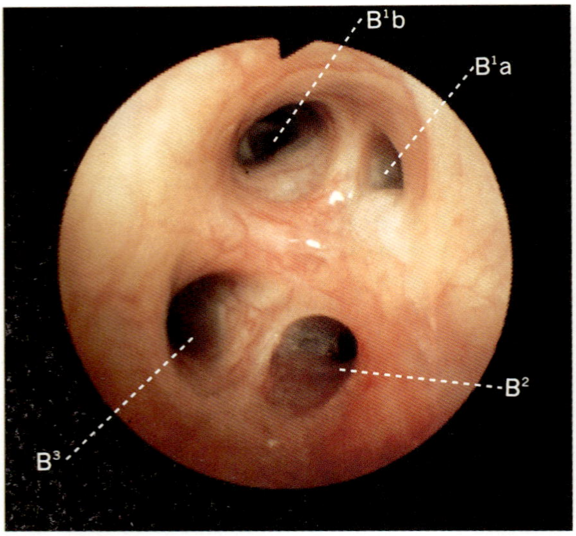

28.3 Close-up of the RUL bronchus. All of the bifurcations appear widened, swollen and oedematous, in addition to engorgement of the mucosal vessels. No stenosis of any bronchial orifice is visible.

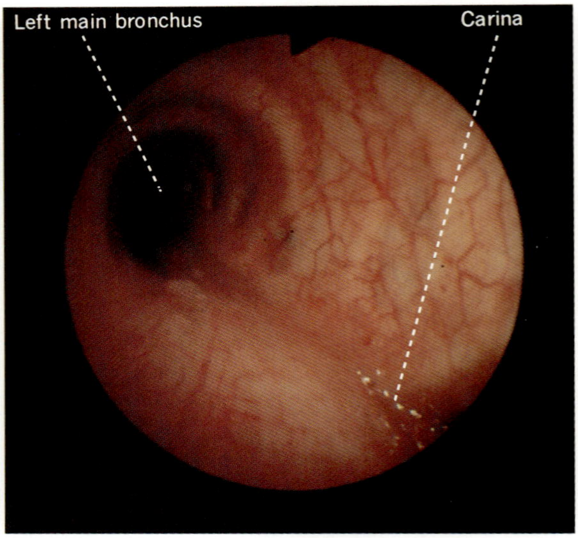

28.4 Bronchoscopic findings in the left main bronchus. Dilated mucosal vessels, forming a network pattern, are generally seen, including the membranous portion.

Case 29: Sarcoidosis in a 29-year-old male.

The patient, free of symptoms, was referred to us for bilateral hilar lymphadenopathy on his chest radiograph taken at a public health survey.

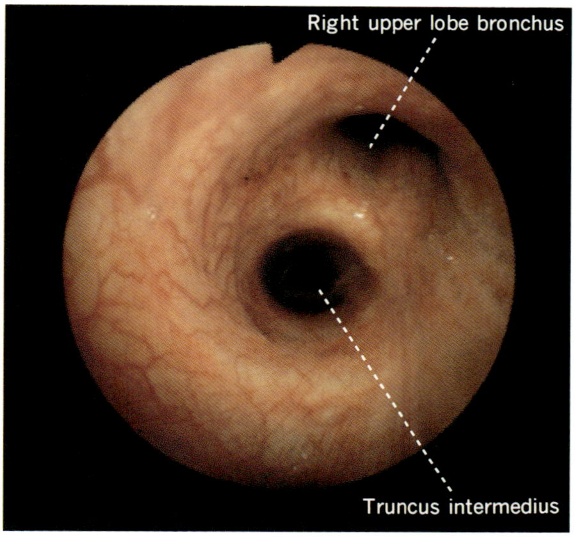

29.1 Bronchoscopic findings in the RUL bronchus and truncus intermedius. The widened, swollen bifurcation shows diffuse engorgement of the mucosal vessels, appearing as a meshwork pattern. These are typical signs of this disease.

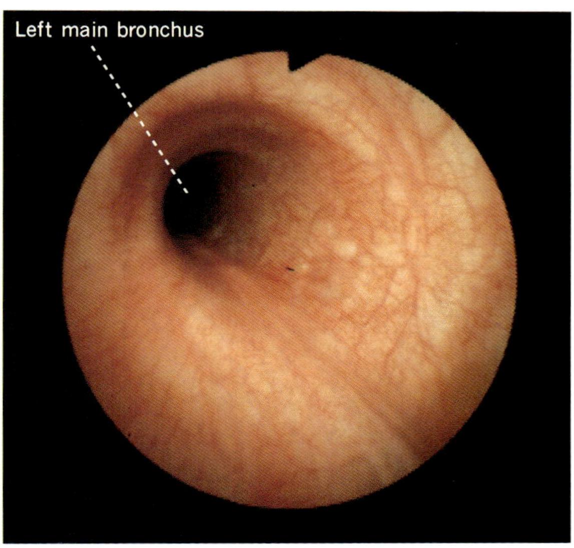

29.2 Bronchoscopic findings in the left main bronchus. The mucosa revealed a prominent mesh-like dilatation of the vessels as well as slight oedema.

Case 33: Sarcoidosis in a 22-year-old female.

This patient presented with a slight non-productive cough. Her chest radiograph during a public health survey revealed bilateral hilar lymphadenopathy. She showed a high level of serum angiotensin-converting enzyme.

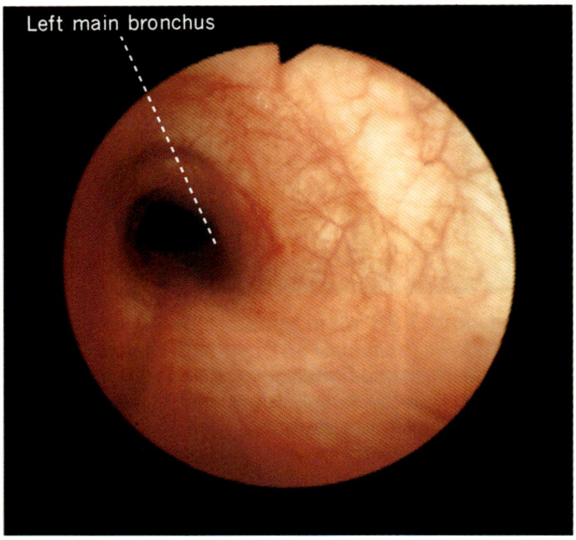

33.1 Bronchoscopic findings in the left main bronchus. Mesh-like dilatation of vessels as well as reddening of the membranous portion are prominent.

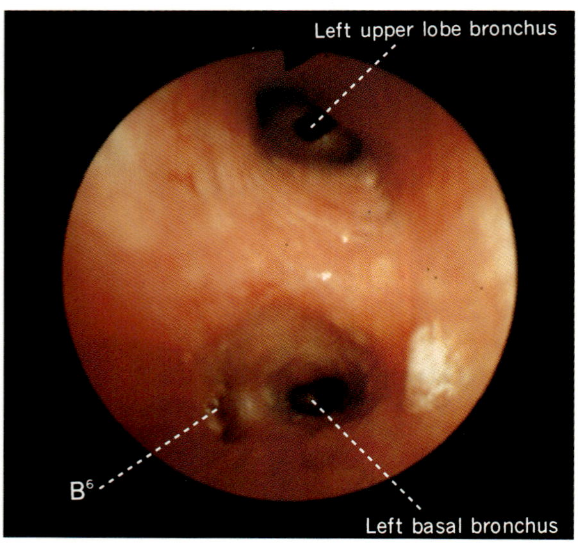

33.2 Bronchoscopic findings in the LUL and LLL bronchi. The bifurcation is widened, associated with oedematous mucosa and vascular dilatation. There are nodules on the irregular wall of the orifice of the RLL bronchus.

4 Other tracheobronchial lesions

Case 34: Tracheobronchopathia osteochondroplastica in a 65-year-old male.

The patient presented with a non-productive cough.

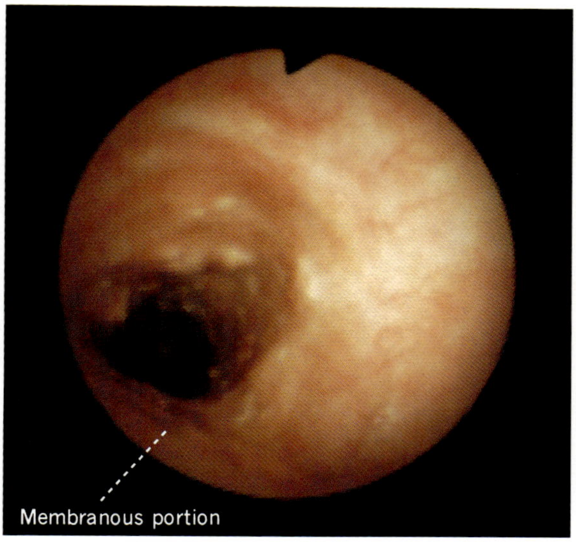

34.1 Bronchoscopic findings in the trachea just beneath the glottis. Nodules are densely present on the bronchial mucosa, except for the membranous portion.

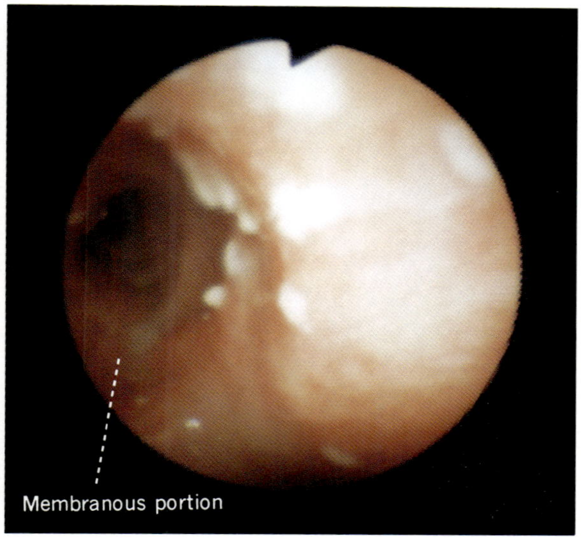

34.2 Close-up of **34.1**. White nodules are scattered on the slightly oedematous mucosa.

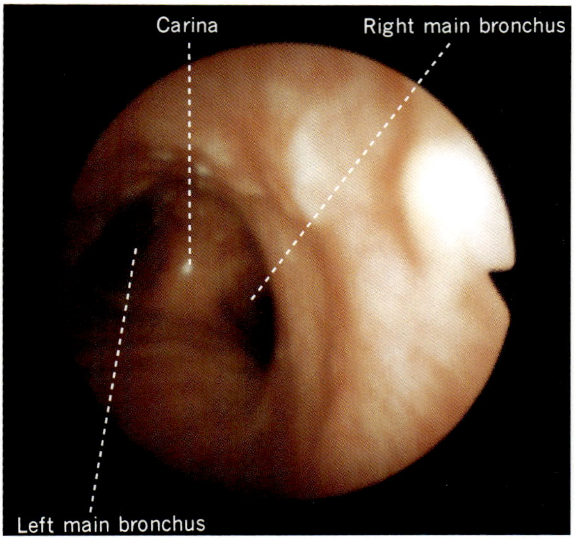

34.3 Bronchoscopic findings in the lower part of the trachea. The carina is widened, surrounded by yellow-white nodules.

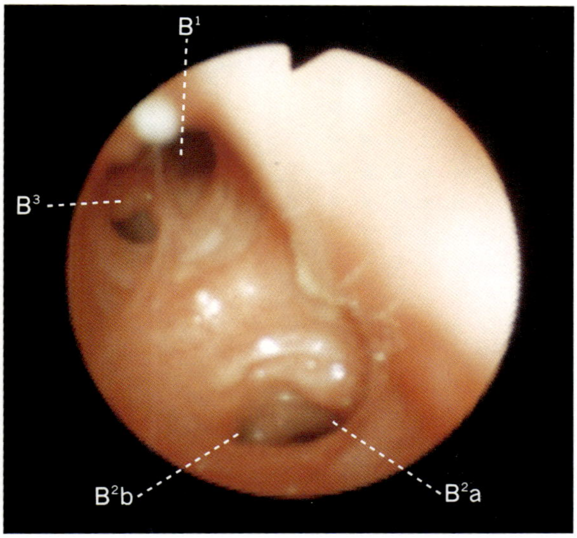

34.4 Bronchoscopic findings in the RUL bronchus. There are nodules at the orifice of B^2 and B^3, although the remaining mucosa is intact.

Case 35: Tracheobronchopathia osteochondroplastica in a 74-year-old male.

The patient, with a history of pulmonary tuberculosis when he was 60 years old, had been treated for chronic bronchitis and/or bronchiectasis for 3 years. He had presented with haemoptysis since March 1981 and was hospitalised in April. Pulmonary function tests revealed that the forced expiratory volume in one second over forced expiratory capacity was 60 per cent, suggesting the presence of an obstructive impairment.

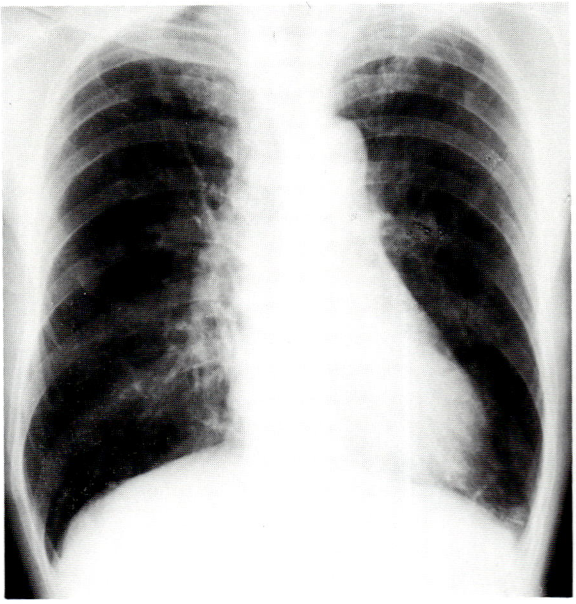

35.1 Posteroanterior chest radiograph. Bilateral apical shadows are suggestive of healed pulmonary tuberculosis. Punctate calcification in the left middle field and a bulla with increased pulmonary markings in the left lower field.

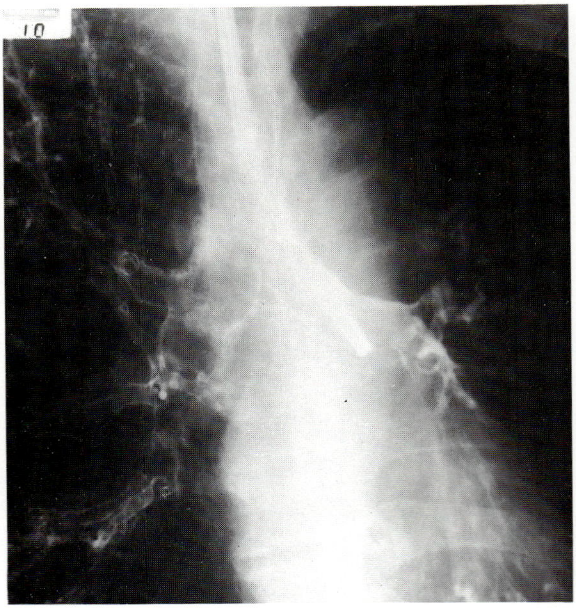

35.2 Bronchogram. The trachea as well as both main bronchi showed an irregularity of the walls and dilatation of the lumen.

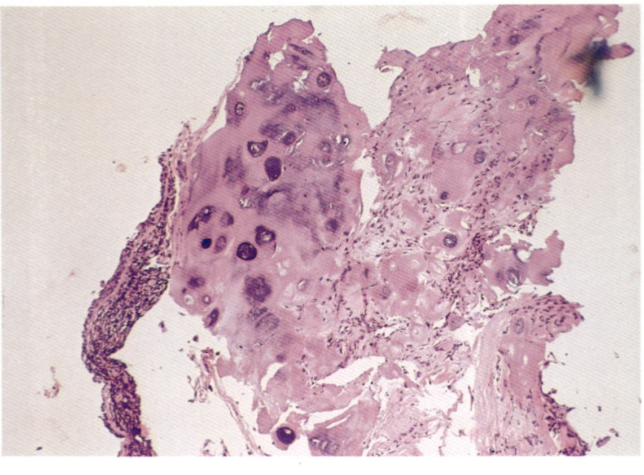

35.3 Histopathology of the specimen biopsied from the left main bronchus. Cartilaginous tissues unrelated to the proper cartilage of the bronchus are covered with bronchial epithelium.

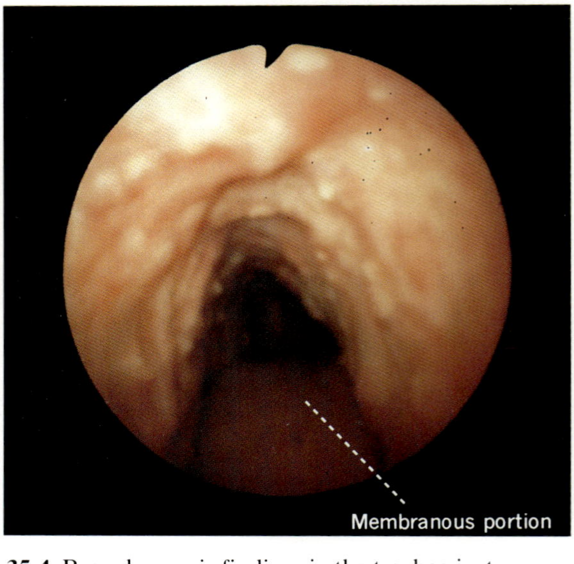

35.4 Bronchoscopic findings in the trachea just beneath the glottis. The mucosal lesion of the trachea is not obvious around here.

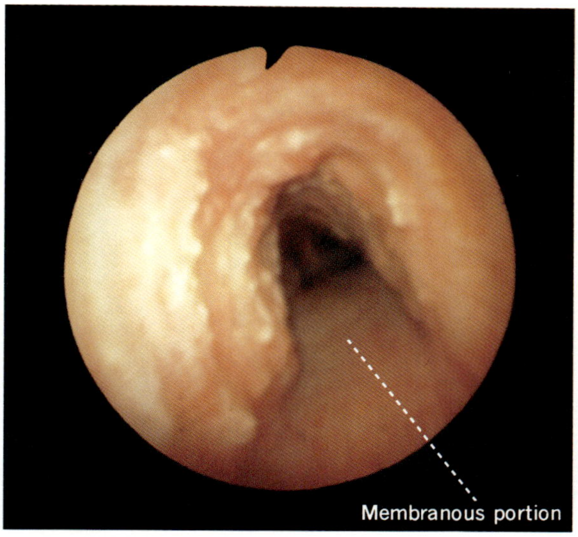

35.5 Bronchoscopic findings in the upper part of the trachea. Prominent nodules all over the bronchial mucosa, except for the membranous portion.

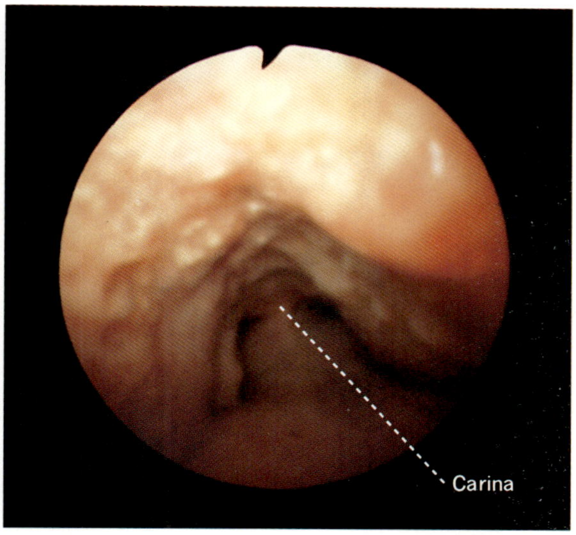

35.6 Bronchoscopic findings in the middle of the trachea. None of the cartilaginous rings is visible.

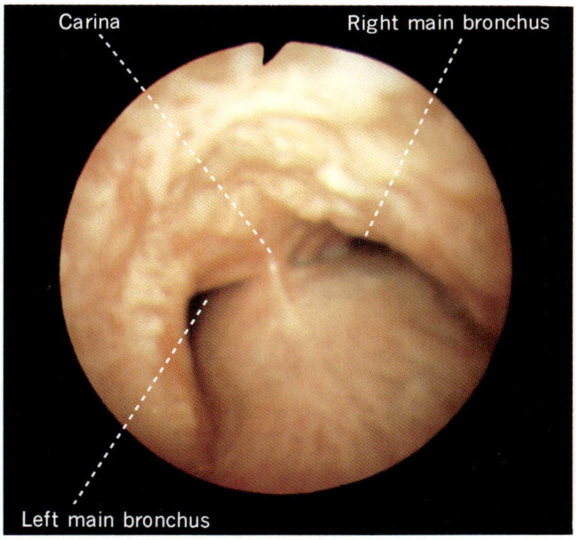

35.7 Bronchoscopic findings at the carina. Irregular mucosal nodules are present everywhere except on the membranous portion. These narrow both main bronchi to some extent.

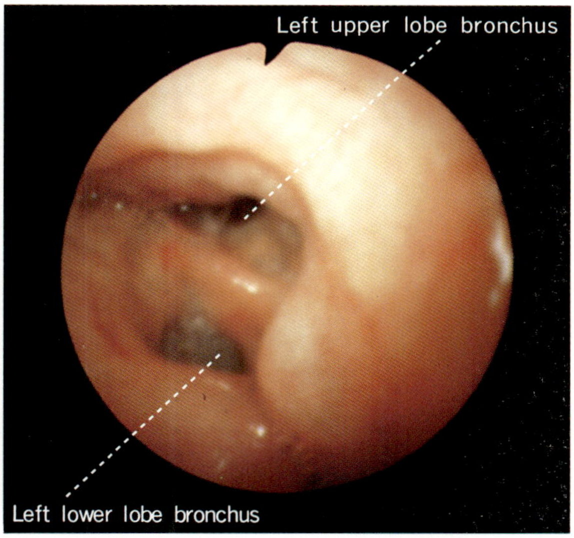

35.8 Bronchoscopic findings in the LUL and LLL bronchi. Intramural nodular lesions are prominent, accompanying the widened bifurcation.

Case 36: Tracheobronchopathia osteochondroplastica in a 65-year-old male.

The patient with no subjective symptoms was referred to us for further evaluation of healed pleurisy on the left side.

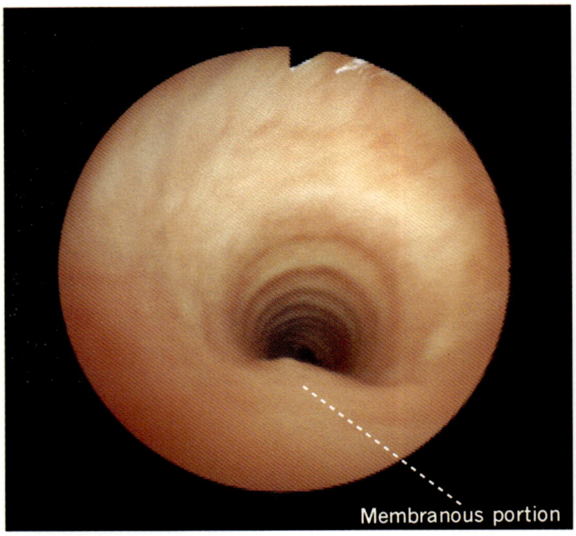

36.1 Bronchoscopic findings in the trachea just beneath the glottis. The colour of the mucosa is intact. A nodule is seen above the nearest cartilage ring.

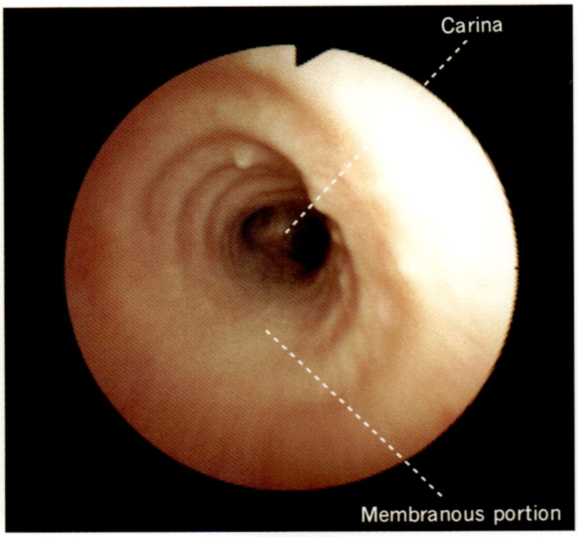

36.2 Further distal view of the trachea. Nodules are present on the anterior and right walls.

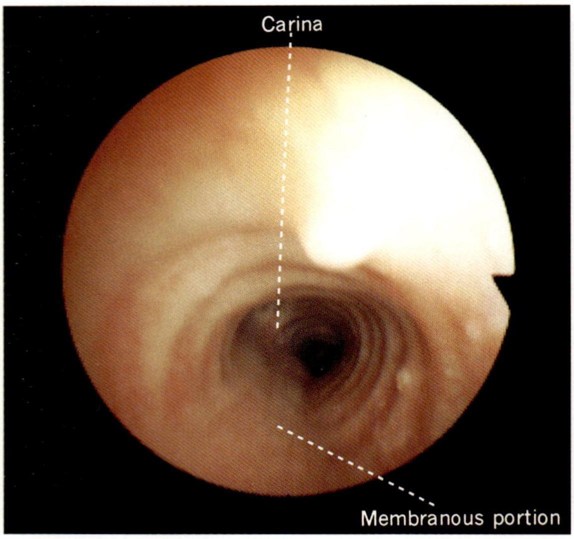

36.3 Several scattered nodules, sparing the membranous portion.

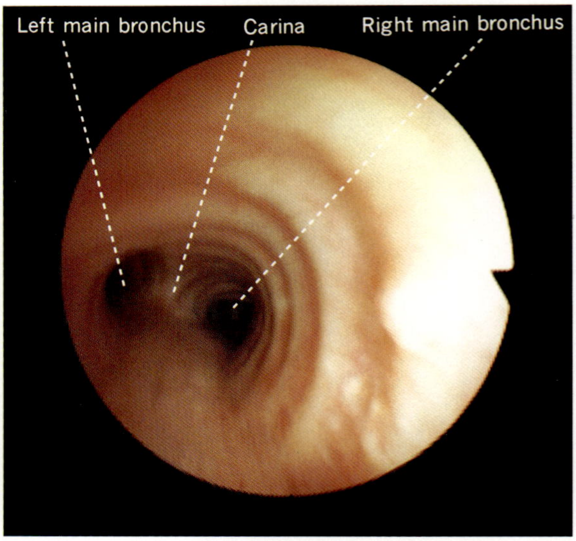

36.4 Close-up of lower part of the trachea. No abnormalities are visible around this area, including the carina.

Case 37: Tracheobronchopathia osteochondroplastica in a 63-year-old female.

This patient had primary lung cancer (adenocarcinoma, 4 cm in diameter, in S^9), which was revealed at investigation. She was asymptomatic.

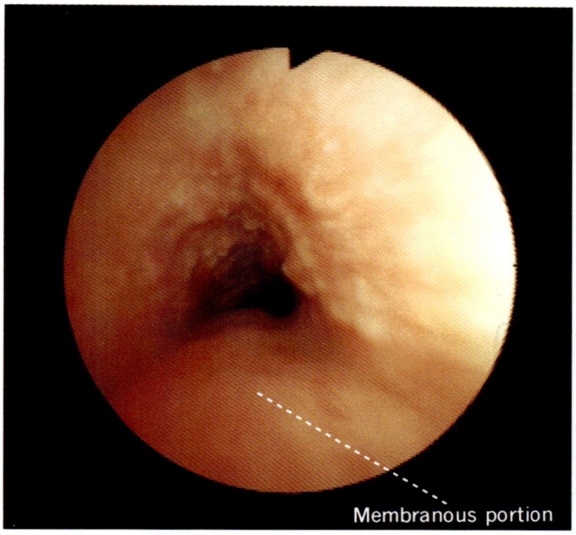

37.1 Bronchoscopic findings in the upper part of the trachea. Nodules are densely distributed on the bronchial wall, except for the membranous portion.

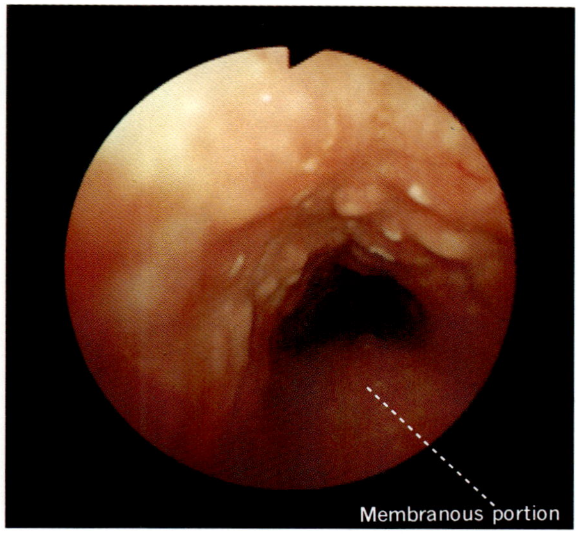

37.2 Bronchoscopic findings in the mid-portion of the trachea. Multiple nodules with a yellow-white surface are present diffusely, except on the membranous portion. Closer observation revealed nodules lining the middle of the membranous portion. This is a rare case.

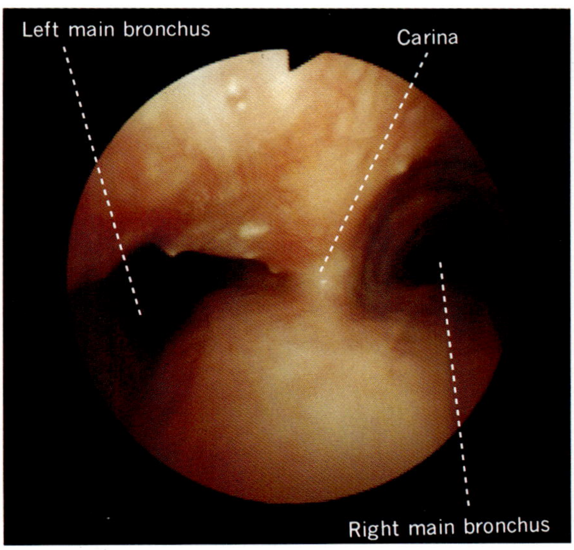

37.3 Bronchoscopic findings at the carina. The bifurcation is widened. Nodules can be seen at the orifices of both main bronchi, where the membranous portion has remained normal.

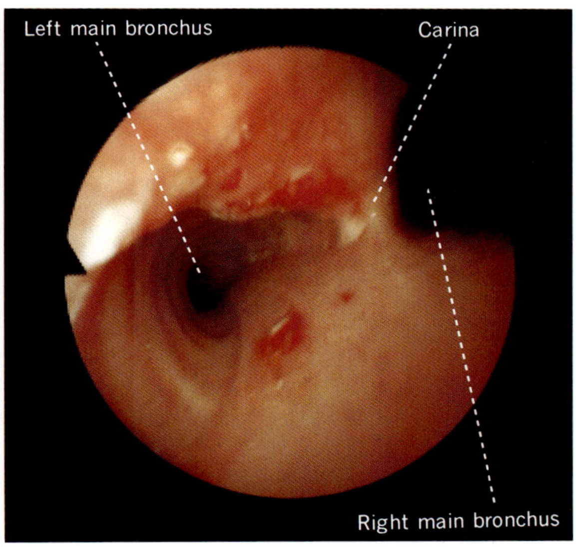

37.4 Bronchoscopic findings in the left main bronchus. On its anterior wall there are nodular lesions, which enabled us to deduce that this patient did not suffer from tracheopathia but tracheo-bronchopathia.

Case 38: Tracheobronchopathia osteochondroplastica in a 57-year-old male.

This patient owned a public bath in Tokyo. He had used wood chips as fuel for 30 years. He complained of having a productive cough for several years and was treated for chronic bronchitis by his own doctor.

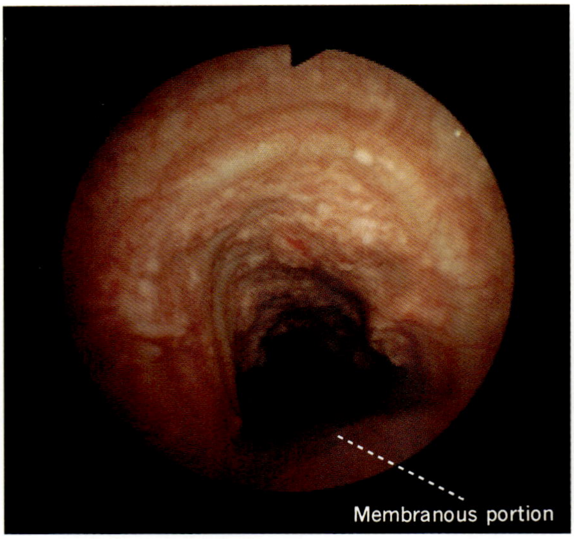

38.1 Bronchoscopic findings in the trachea just beneath the glottis. Many irregular protruding lesions are seen, sparing the membranous portion. Vascular dilatation is also marked.

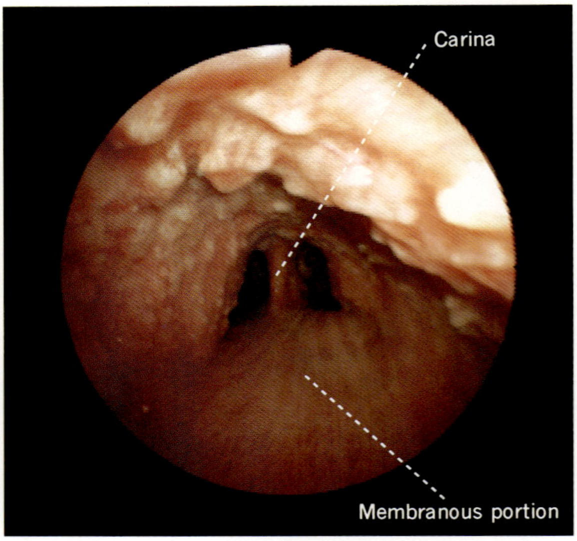

38.2 Bronchoscopic findings in the mid-portion of the trachea. The surface of the protruding lesion is irregular and unrelated to tracheal cartilages.

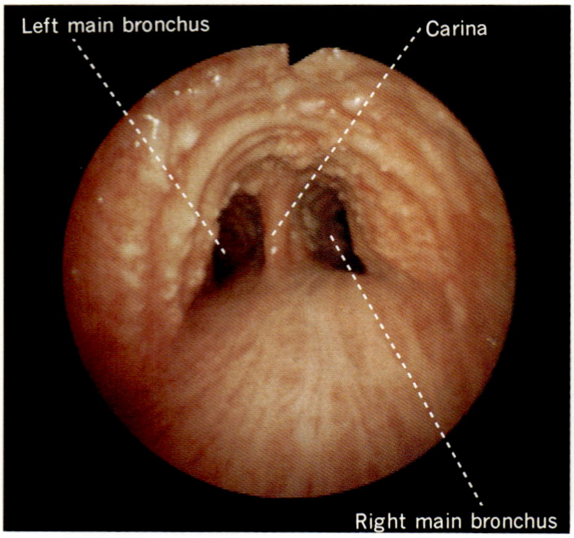

38.3 Bronchoscopic findings in the lower part of the trachea and carina. The same lesions are seen in all areas, except in the membranous portion.

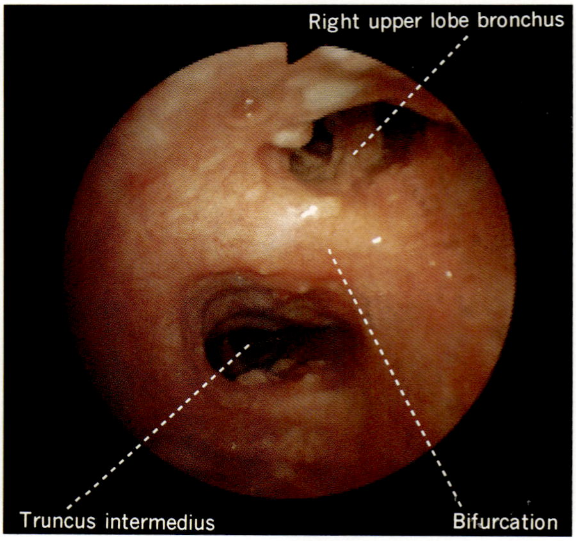

38.4 Bronchoscopic findings of the RUL bronchus and truncus intermedius. Bifurcation is strikingly widened and oedematous, accompanying dilated vessels and protruding yellow-white lesions.

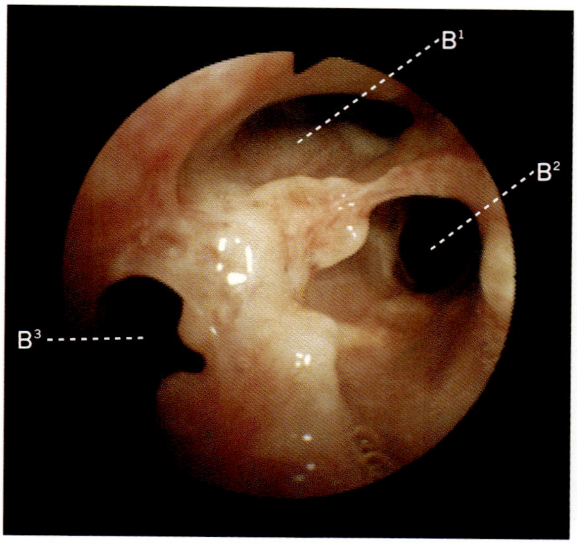

38.5 Bronchoscopic findings in the RUL bronchus. Many white nodular lesions are seen at the centre of the bifurcations.

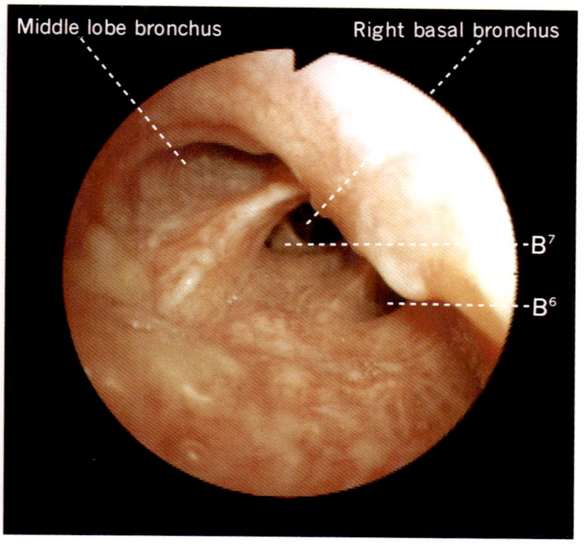

38.6 Bronchoscopic findings in the RML and RLL bronchi. The mucosa is reddened, associated with vascular engorgement and a nodular surface relatively flat.

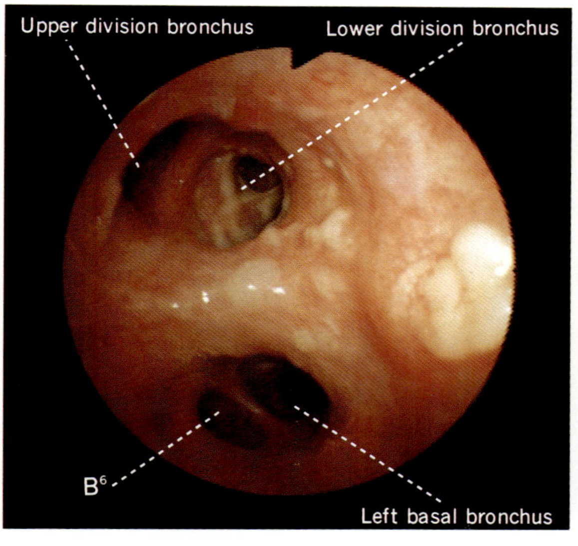

38.7 Bronchoscopic findings of the LUL and LLL bronchi. The bifurcation is widened. Dilated mucosal vessels and many yellow-white nodules are visible.

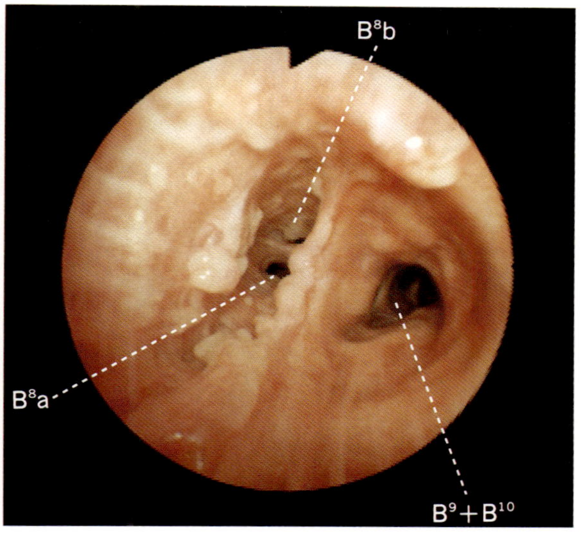

38.8 Bronchoscopic findings in the left basal bronchus. There are many nodular lesions, particularly around the orifice of B^8.

Case 39: Wegener's granulomatosis in a 39-year-old male.

This patient presented with cough, fever and abnormal shadows on his chest radiograph. Histopathological examination of the mucosa of the paranasal sinus confirmed diagnosis of this lesion. Effective steroid therapy resulted in a marked improvement of intrapulmonary and endobronchial lesions.

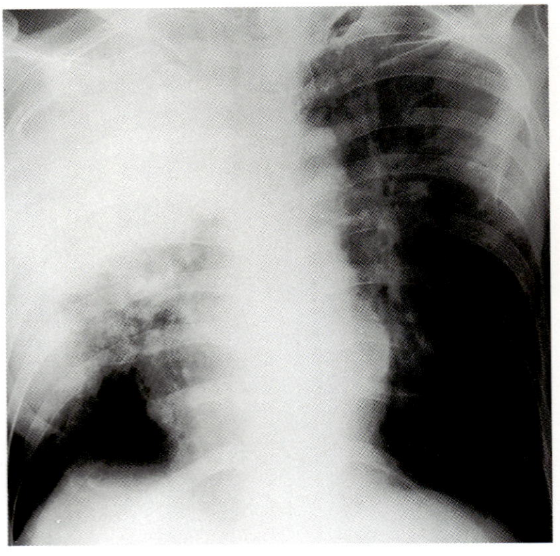

39.1 Posteroanterior chest roentgenogram. Radio-opaque lesions are distributed in the right upper and middle fields as well as in the left upper field.

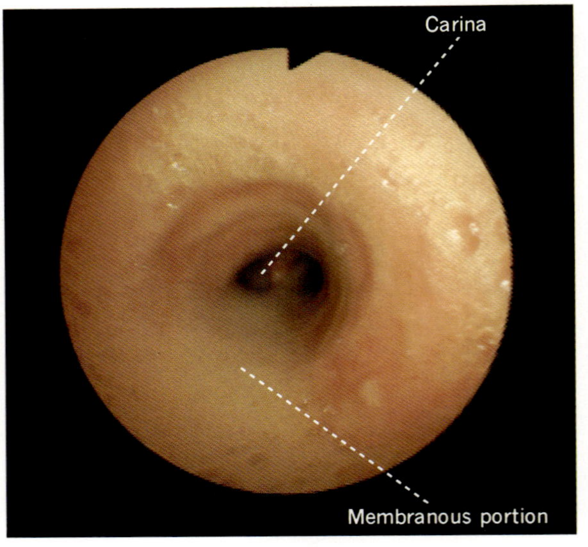

39.2 Bronchoscopic findings in the trachea just beneath the glottis. Copious serous secretion is visible.

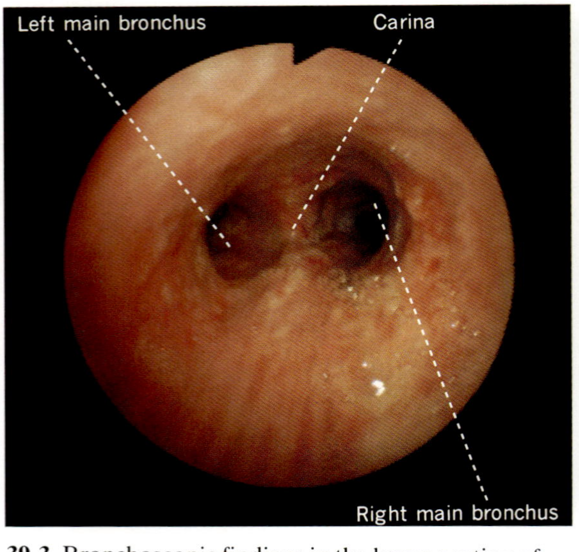

39.3 Bronchoscopic findings in the lower portion of the trachea. The mucosa generally showed reddening and secretion, in addition to multiple protruding lesions with irregular surfaces.

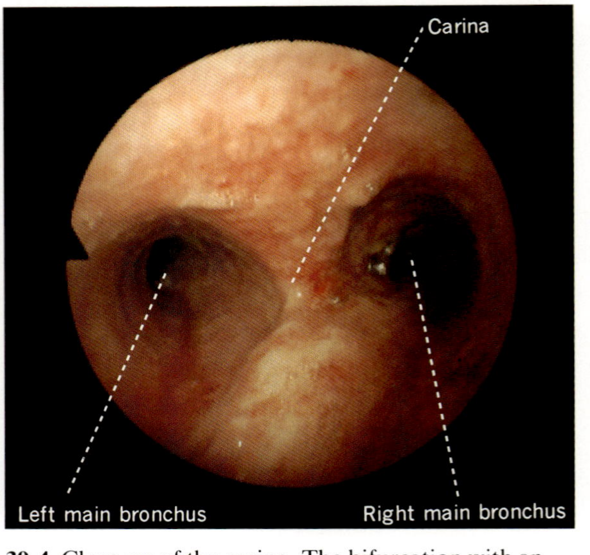

39.4 Close-up of the carina. The bifurcation with an irregular surface caused by nodules or granulomatous lesions is widened and oedematous.

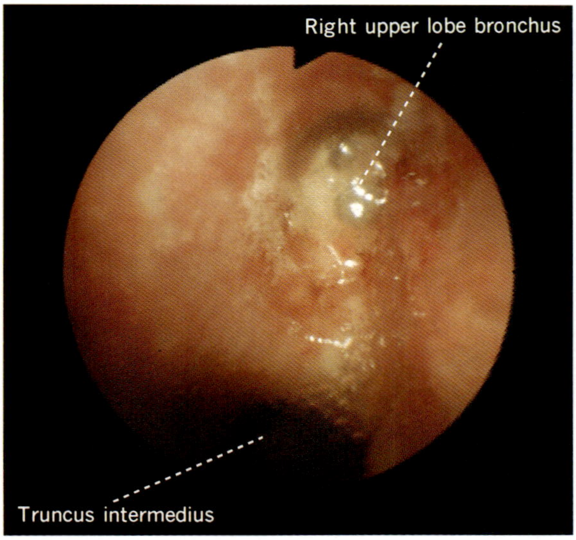

39.5 Bronchoscopic findings in the RUL bronchus and truncus intermedius. The bifurcation is widened and oedematous. The RUL bronchus is completely occluded by mucopurulent secretion and granulation tissue.

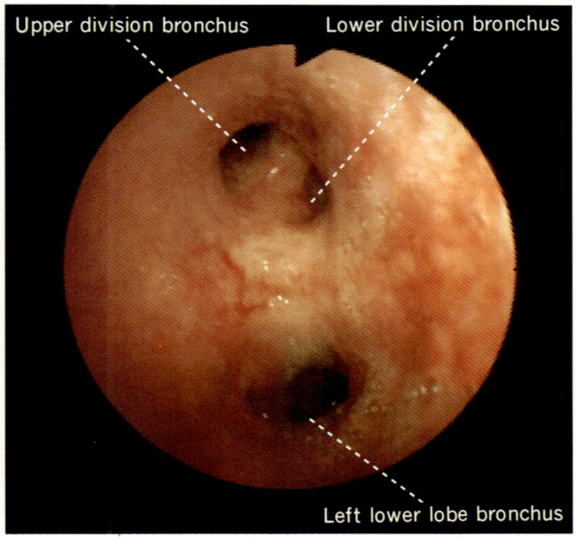

39.6 Bronchoscopic findings in the LUL and LLL bronchi. Bifurcation is strikingly widened and oedematous. The mucosa is generally irregular because of granulomatous lesions, accompanying secretion and dilated vessels.

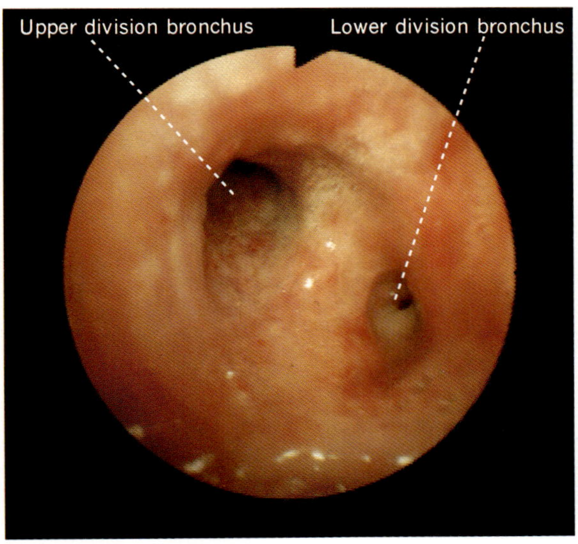

39.7 Bronchoscopic findings in the LUL bronchus. The bifurcation is widened and oedematous. The mucosa is irregular and associated with vascular engorgement.

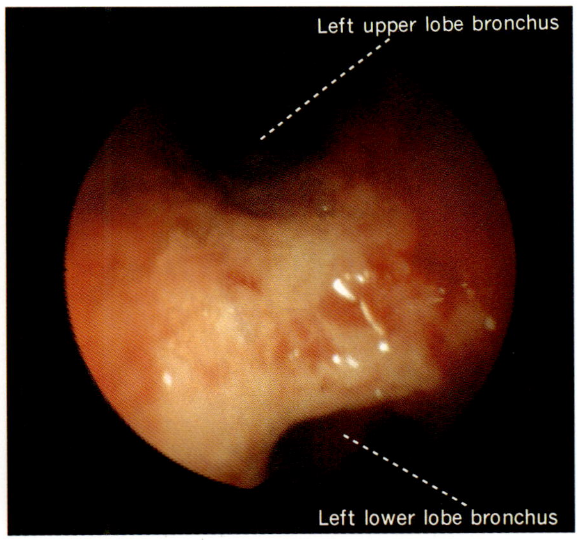

39.8 Close-up of **39.6**. The spur with an irregular surface, covered with white necrotic tissue, is markedly widened.

Case 40: Amyloidosis of trachea and bronchi in a 68-year-old male.

This patient was admitted to the Department of Otolaryngology in our hospital because of pharyngeal amyloidosis. He was asymptomatic and his chest radiograph showed no abnormalities.

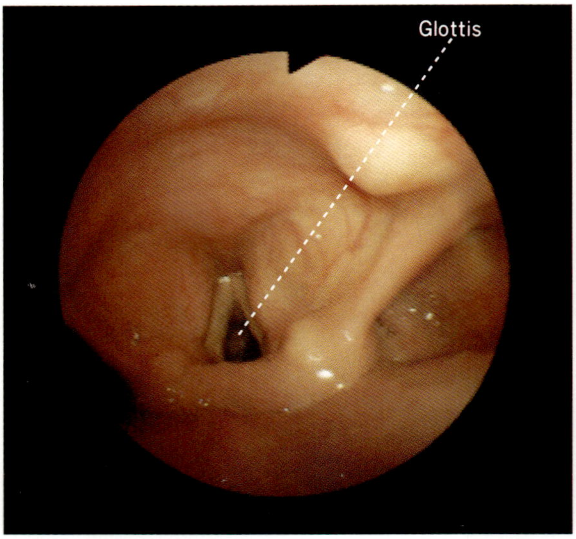

40.1 Bronchoscopic findings at the glottis. Nodules made up of amyloid are visible.

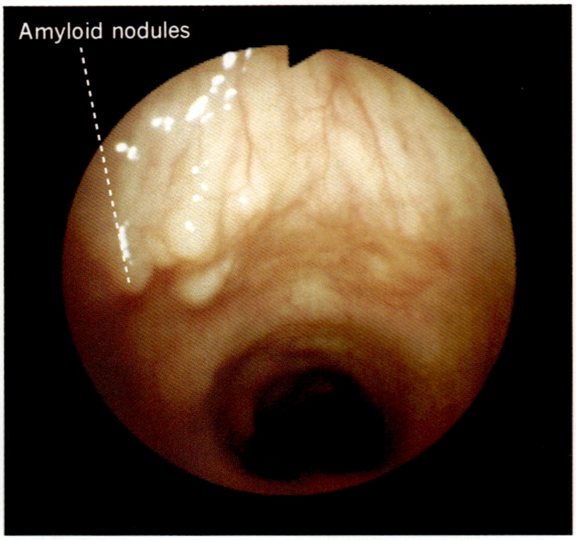

40.2 Bronchscopic findings in the trachea just beneath the glottis. There are several amyloid nodules with smooth surfaces at the upper left.

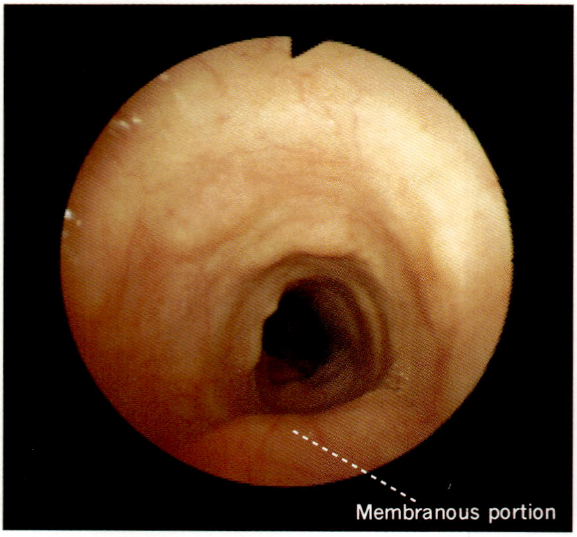

40.3 Bronchoscopic findings in the upper part of the trachea. Nodular lesions are present everywhere, including in the membranous portion.

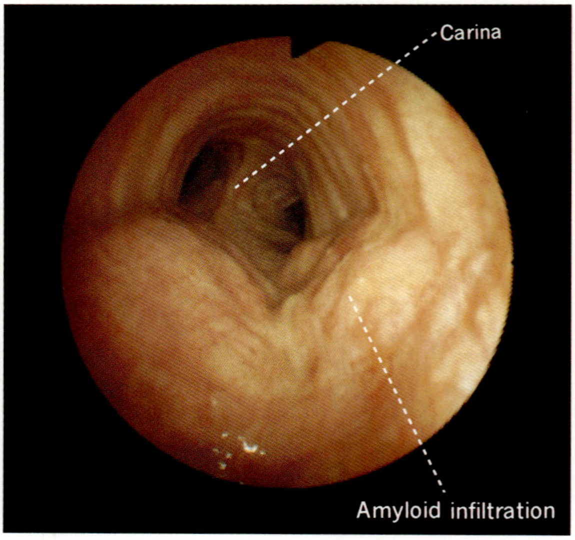

40.4 Bronchoscopic findings in the mid-portion of the trachea. There are nodules on the membranous portion and on the right-sided wall. Although small mucosal vessels may be dilated, the colour of the mucosa is almost normal.

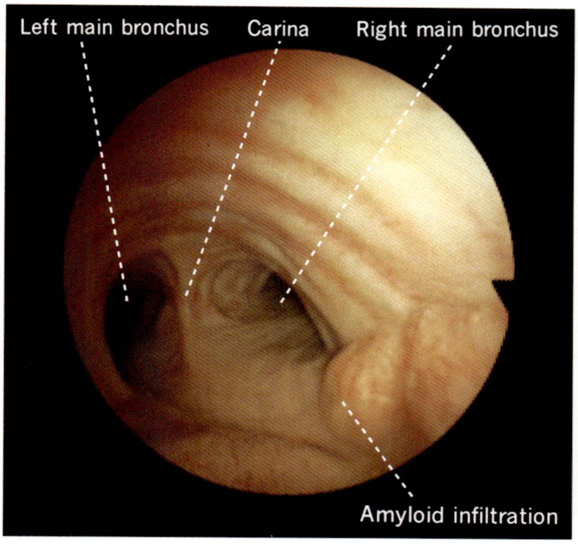

40.5 Bronchoscopic findings at the carina. A band-like protruding lesion is seen on the right wall. The branching angle of the carina is still sharp.

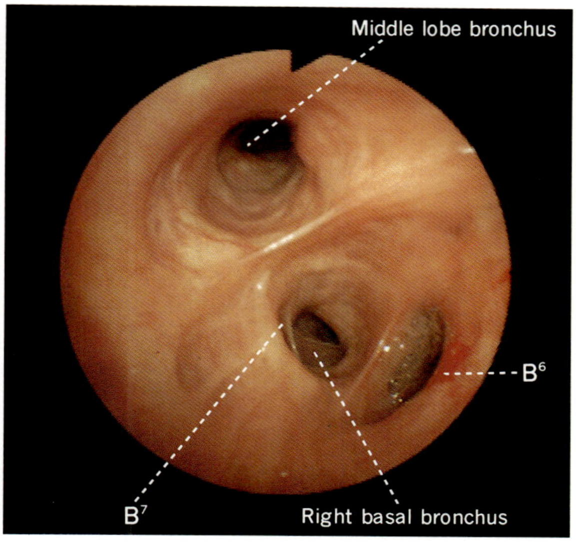

40.6 Bronchoscopic findings in the RML and RLL bronchi. The bifurcation appears sharp-edged. However, the mucosa is rather reddened, in addition to a small protrusion at the orifice of the RML bronchus.

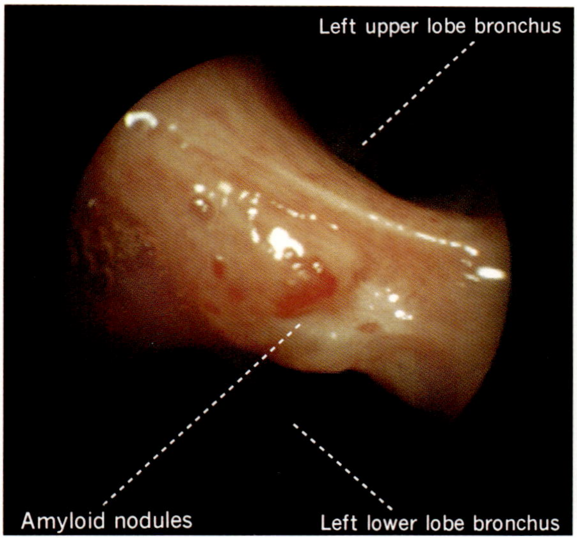

40.7 Bronchoscopic findings in the LUL and LLL bronchi. The bifurcation is prominently widened. There exists a nodule with an irregular surface at the orifice of the LLL bronchus, on which biopsy was carried out for pathological diagnosis.

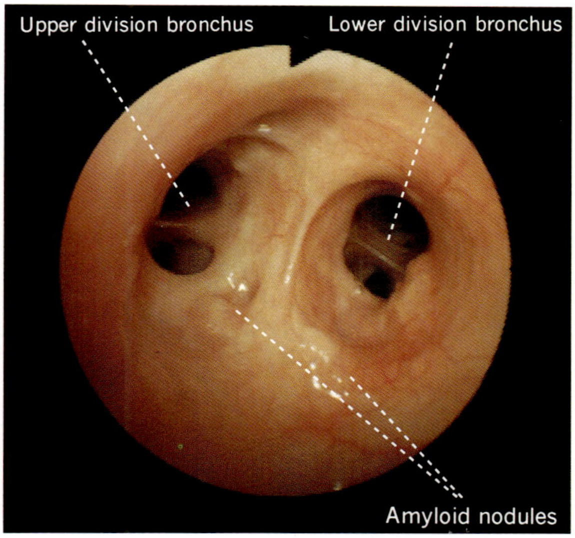

40.8 Bronchoscopic findings in the LUL bronchus. In spite of sharp-edged bifurcation, nodules can be seen at the orifices of B^3 and B^5 as well as on the bifurcation into the upper and lower division bronchi. Note vascular engorgement.

Case 41: Pulmonary tuberculosis (cavitary change) in a 50-year-old male.

The patient had suffered from diabetes mellitus for 10 years and in September 1980, 16 units of insulin per day were prescribed. Because of low-grade fever since November and abnormalities on his chest radiographs, he was hospitalised with a diagnosis of pulmonary tuberculosis in December. Sputum examination revealed presence of Mycobacterium (Gaffky 5).

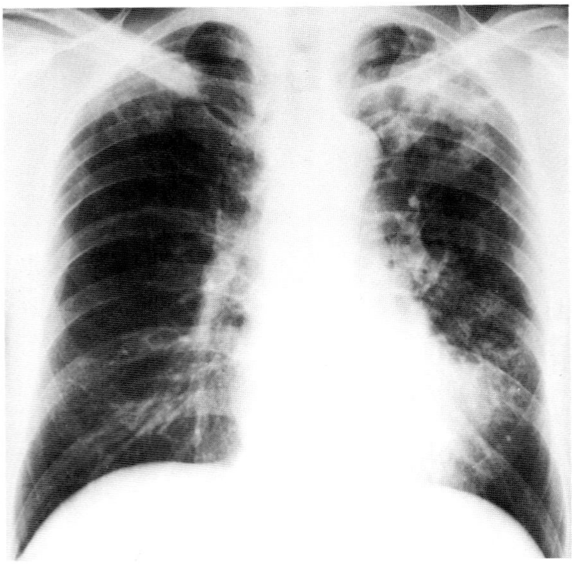

41.1 Posteroanterior chest radiograph 3 months after initiation of antituberculosis therapy. Infiltration and cavitation are seen in the upper fields of both lungs. The left heart border is obliterated, suggesting a silhouette sign.

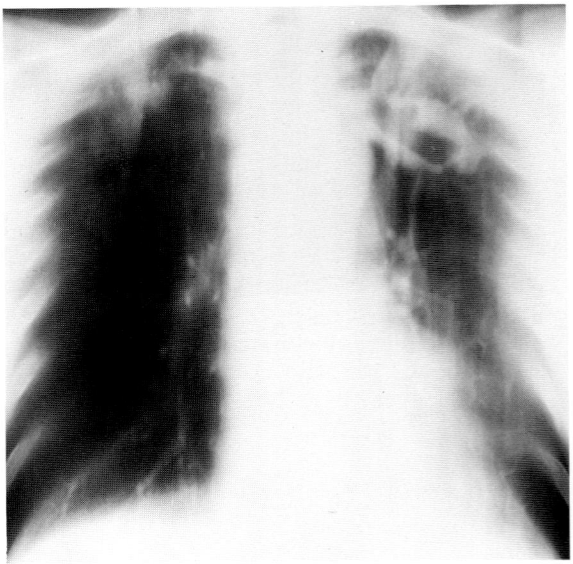

41.2 Chest tomogram (7 cm from the back). A large cavity is seen in the left apex.

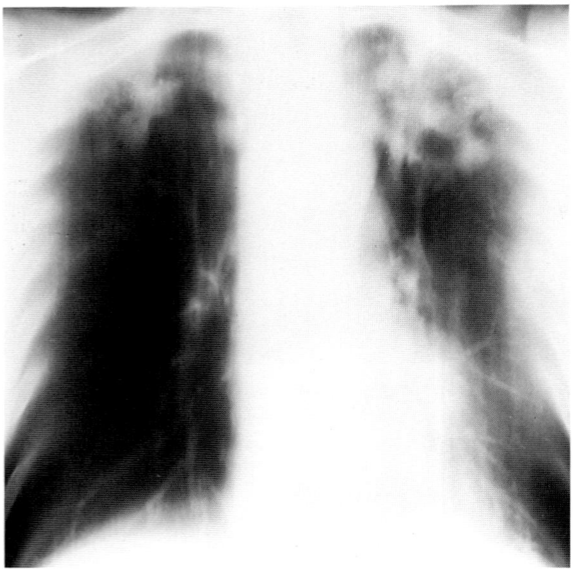

41.3 Chest tomogram (8 cm from the back). A tumour-like shadow is seen in the right apex.

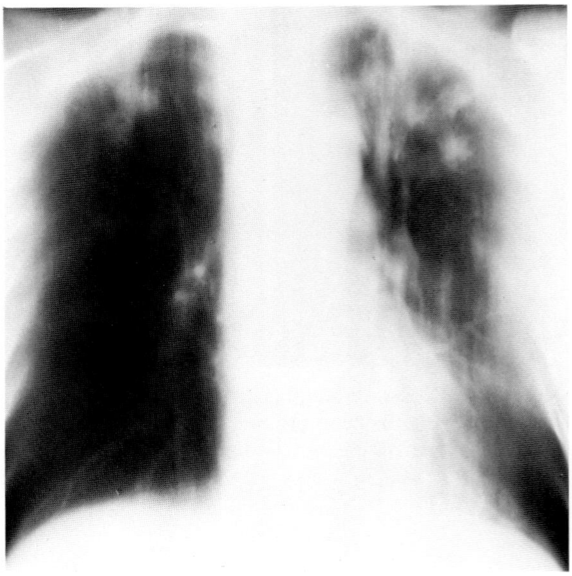

41.4 Chest tomogram (9 cm from the back). Infiltration and tumour-like shadows are visible in both apices, accompanying a small cavity on the right.

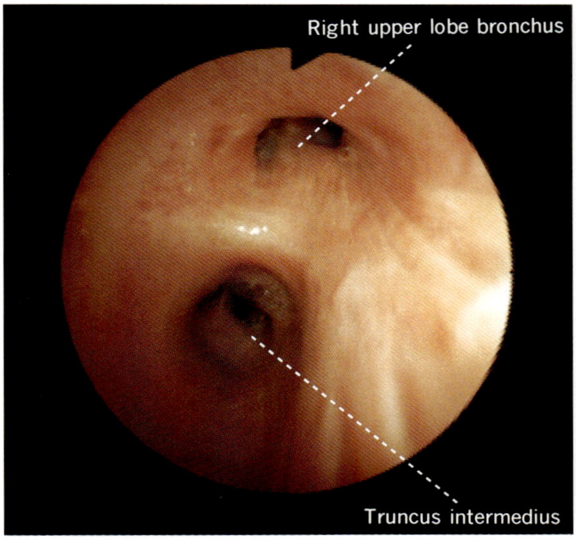

41.5 Bronchoscopic findings in the RUL bronchus and truncus intermedius. The bifurcation is slightly widened and mucosal vessels are dilated. In addition, anthracotic changes are present around the orifice of B^3.

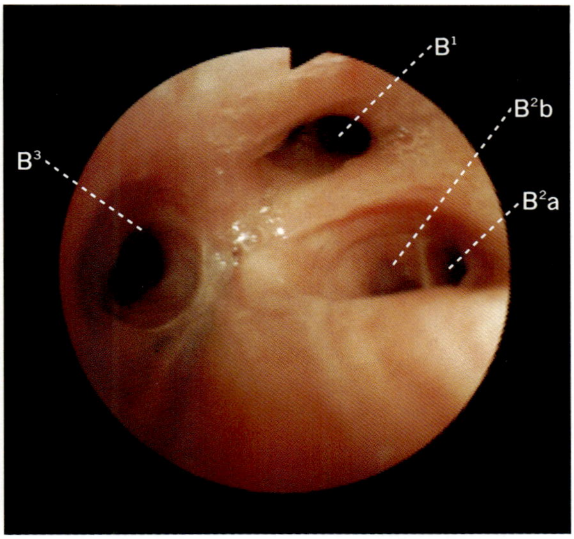

41.6 Bronchoscopic findings in the RUL bronchus. Anthracotic changes continuing from the orifices of B^3 to B^3b. The bifurcations appear rather widened.

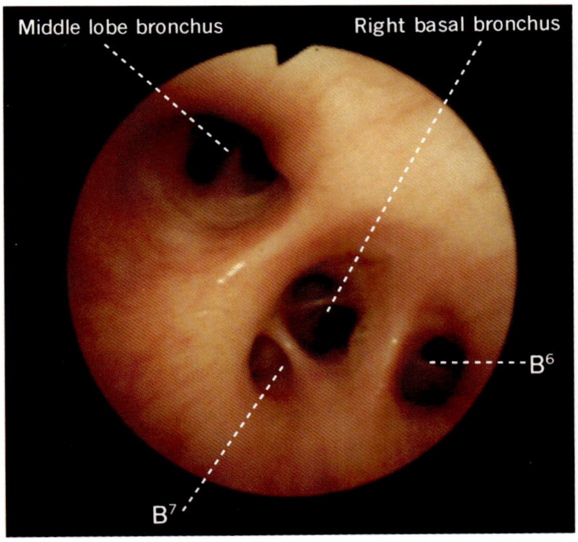

41.7 Bronchoscopic findings in the RML and RLL bronchi. Bifurcations are more or less widened and the mucosal vessels are strikingly engorged.

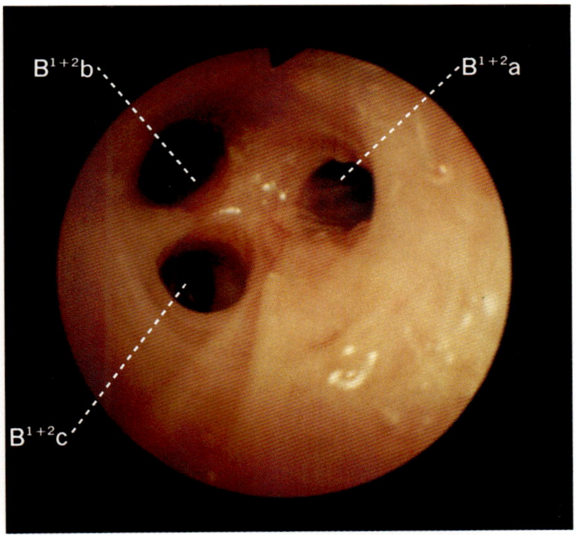

41.8 Bronchoscopic findings in left upper division bronchus. Each bifurcation shows prominent widening and reddening.

Case 42: Haemoptysis (pulmonary tuberculosis) in a 66-year-old female.

This patient presented with significant haemoptysis in April 1981. This continued for 3 days although the volume was low. She had no fever or cough. At 20 years of age abnormalities on her chest radiograph were pointed out, but she chose to ignore them.

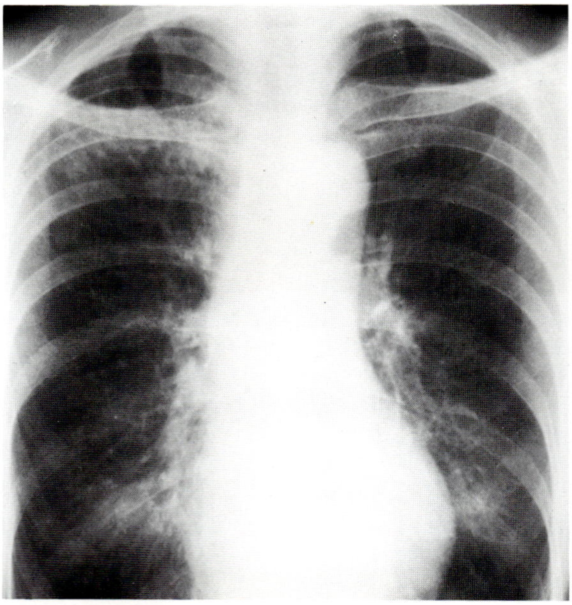

42.1 Posteroanterior chest radiograph. In addition to an infiltrative shadow in the right apex and downward deviation of the minor fissure, the right heart border is obliterated, suggesting a silhouette sign.

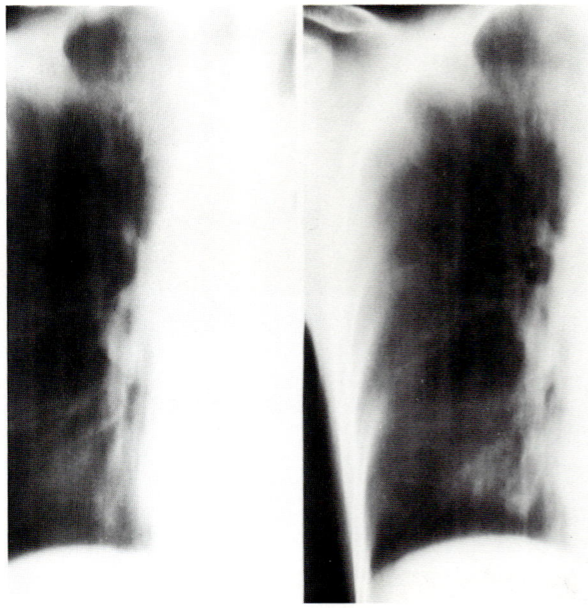

42.2 Chest tomogram (right: 7 cm from the back; left: 8 cm from the back). Infiltrate in S^1 and ground glass-like appearance in the lower lung field.

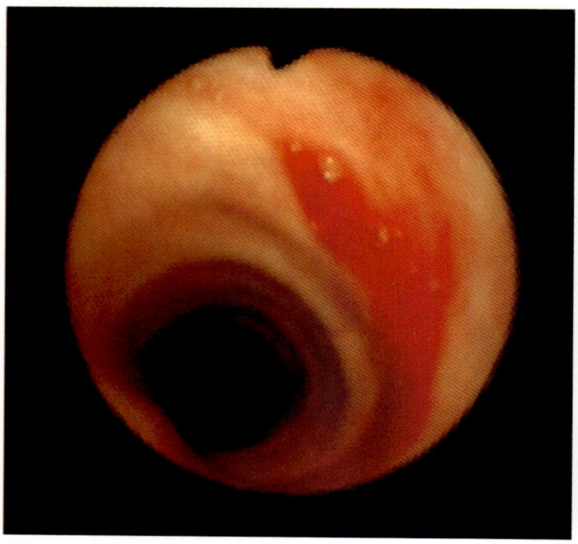

42.3 Bronchoscopic findings in the trachea just beneath the glottis, while she still had haemoptysis. Bloody sputum is seen on the mucosa in the subglottic region.

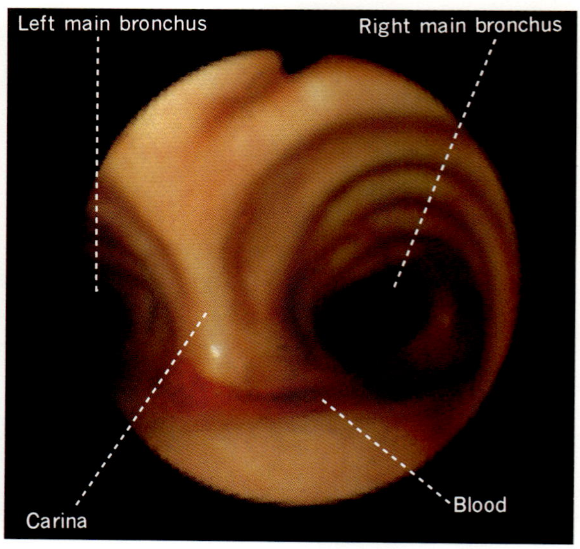

42.4 Bronchoscopic findings at the carina. Blood is coming from the right main bronchus.

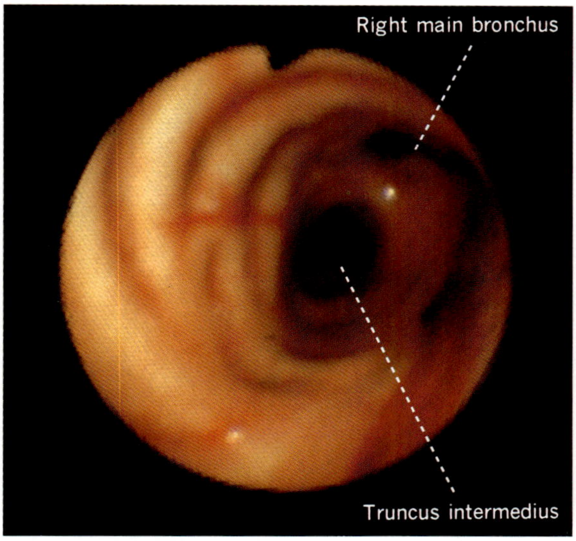

42.5 Bronchoscopic findings in the RUL bronchus and truncus intermedius. Blood is coming from the RUL bronchus.

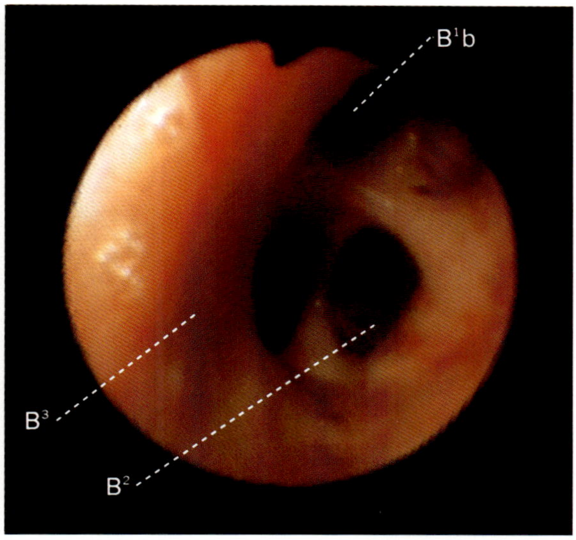

42.6 Bronchoscopic findings in the RUL bronchus. Bloody sputum covering all the orifices of segmental bronchi makes its original source unclear.

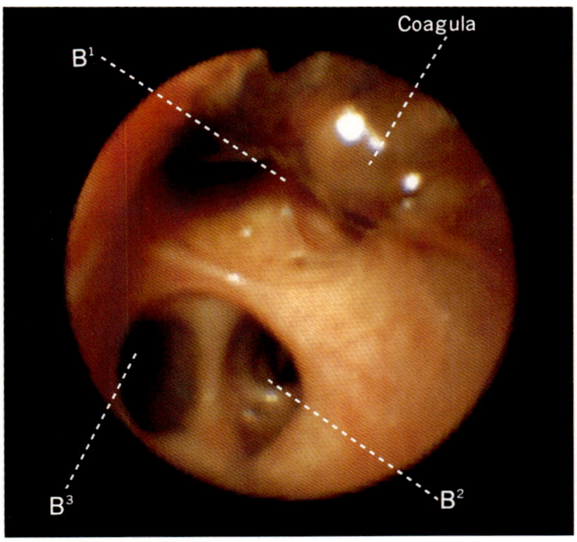

42.7 Lavage and suction showed blood clot at the orifice of B^1.

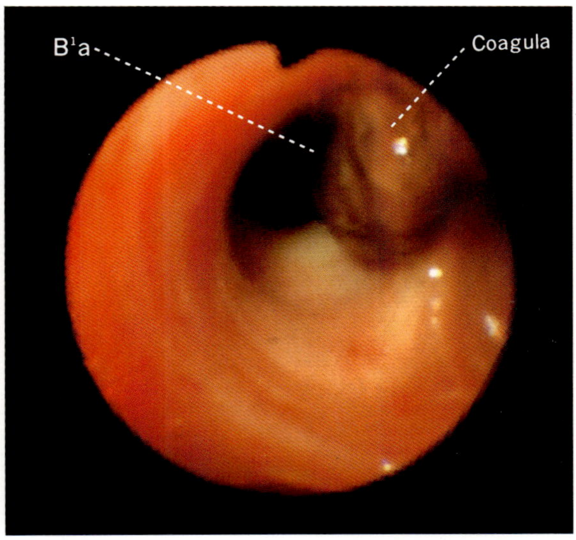

42.8 Repeated lavage followed by removal of part of the coagulated blood made it clear that bleeding occurred from B^1a. The bleeding stopped immediately after a thrombin solution was injected through a polyethylene tube into the bronchi. Examination of the aspirate revealed human type mycobacterium tuberculosis.

Case 43: Healed pulmonary tuberculosis in a 66-year-old female.

The patient, who had a history of treatment for pulmonary tuberculosis 30 years ago, often presented with flu-like symptoms, sometimes with a cough and sputum production.

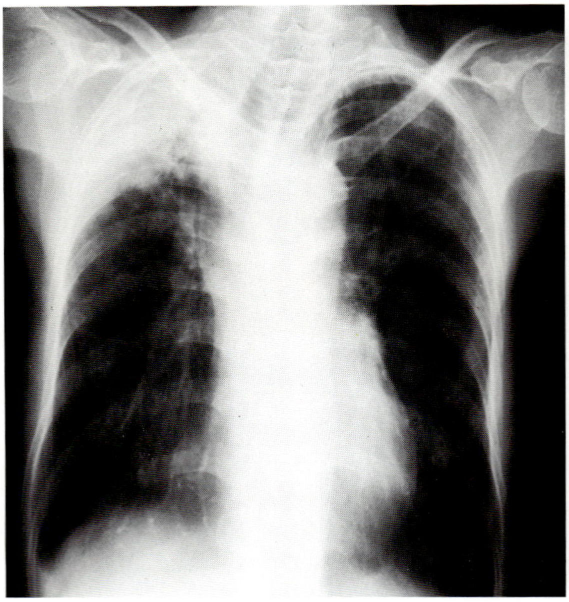

43.1 Posteroanterior chest radiograph. The right upper lobe shows loss of volume, forming almost complete atelectasis. The trachea is deviated to the right and the right hilum has moved upwards.

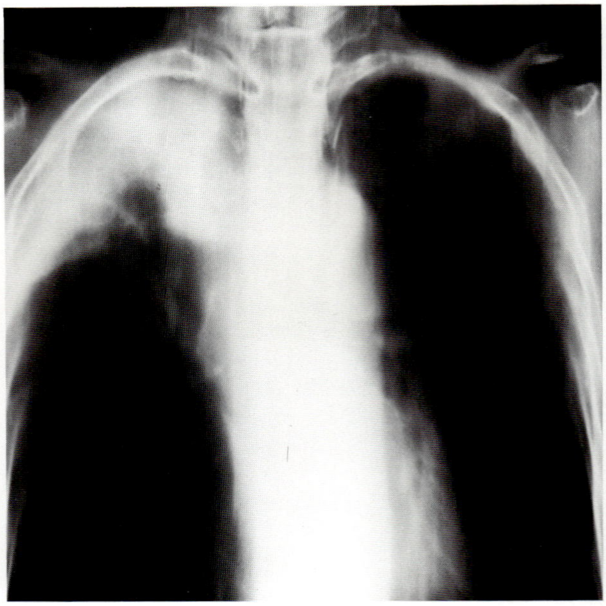

43.2 Chest tomogram (7 cm from the back). Shrinkage of right upper lobe is visible. Calcified shadow is seen on the wall of the LLL bronchus.

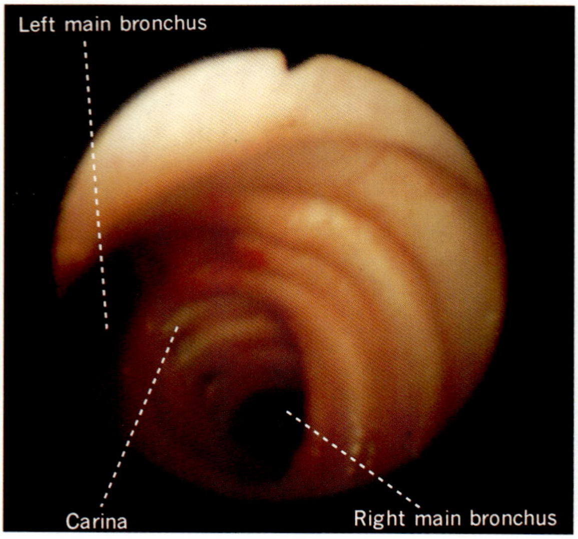

43.3 Bronchoscopic findings in the trachea. Deformed trachea shows atrophic change of the mucosa, which exaggerates tracheal cartilages. A few pits are present on the mucosa of the right main bronchus.

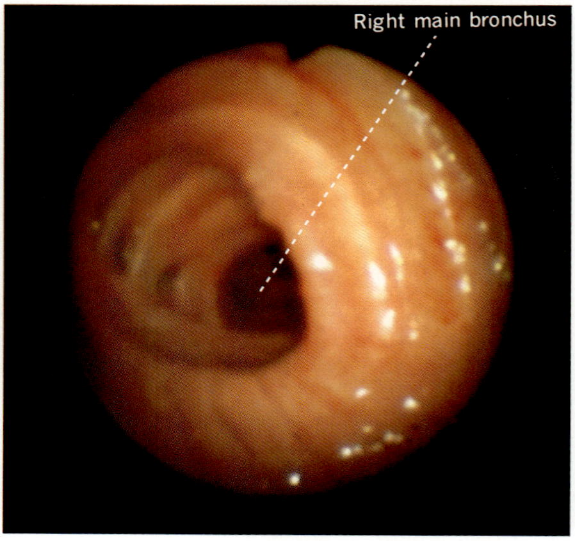

43.4 Bronchoscopic findings in the right main bronchus. The orifice of the bronchus is stenotic and deviated.

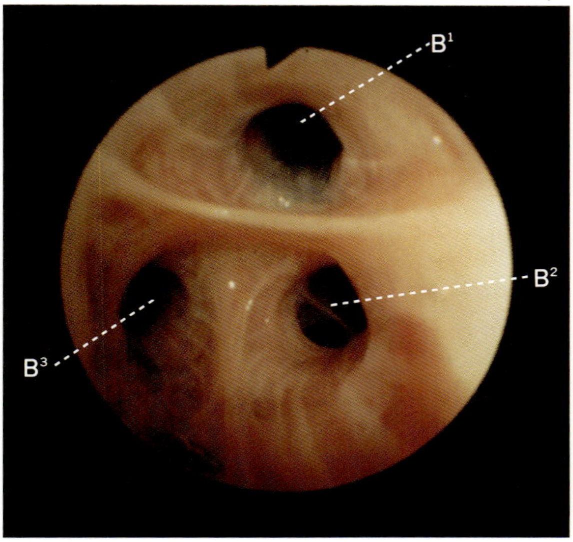

43.5 Bronchoscopic findings in the RUL bronchus. Marked anthracotic changes are visible at the orifice of B^1, associated with engorgement of the contiguous mucosal vessels.

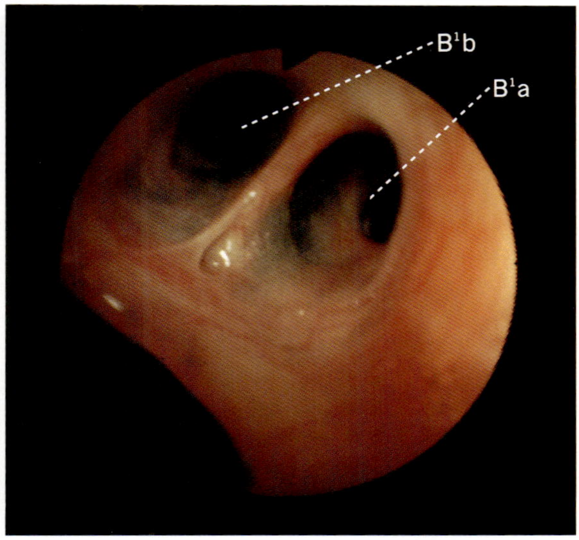

43.6 Bronchoscopic findings in B^1. Prominent anthracotic changes are visible at the orifices of B^1a and B^1b.

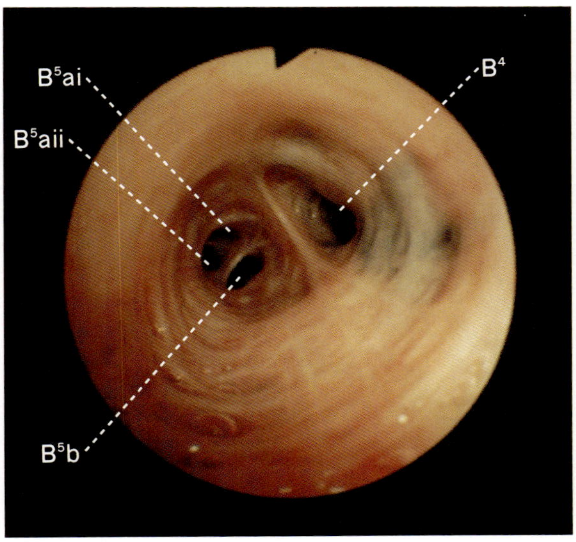

43.7 Bronchoscopic findings in the RML bronchus. The mucosa is strikingly atrophic as well as irregular.

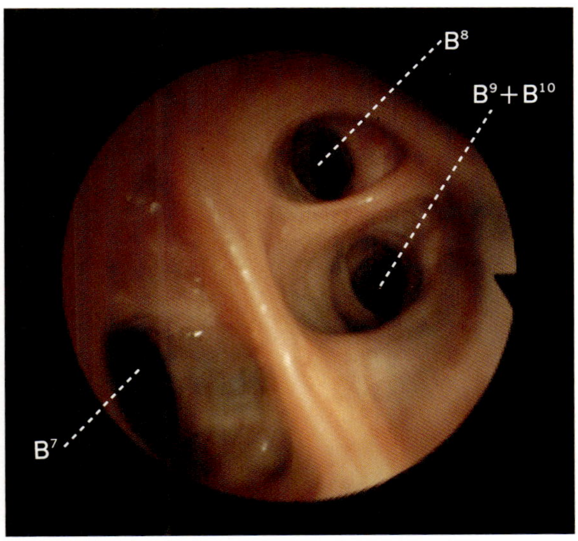

43.8 Bronchoscopic findings in the right basal bronchus. The mucosal atrophy of the spurs among B^7, B^8, B^9, and B^{10} is obvious, exaggerating the tracheal cartilages.

Case 44: Tuberculosis of intrathoracic lymph nodes in a 19-year-old male.

The patient presented with fever, skin rash, massive pleural effusion with ascites, and lymph node swelling of the neck and mediastinum.

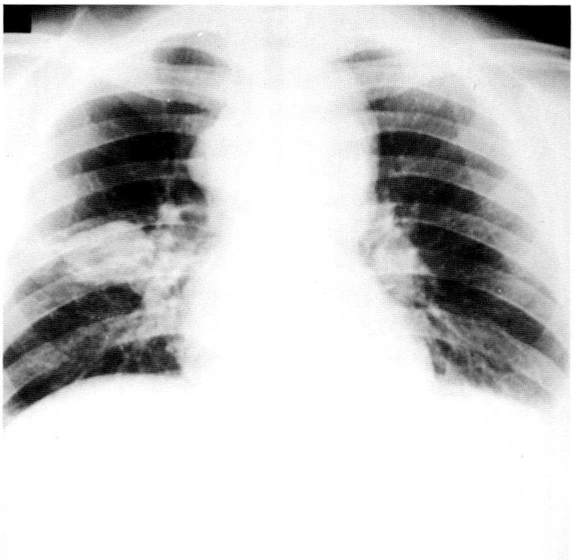

44.1 Posteroanterior chest radiograph. Lymph node swelling of the mediastinum and a tumour-like shadow in the right middle field are present. Also note bilateral pleural fluid and diaphragmatic elevation caused by ascites.

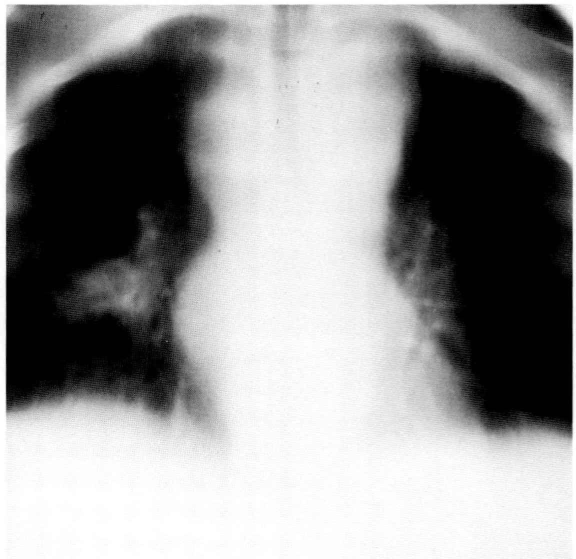

44.2 Chest tomogram (6 cm from the back). There is lymph node swelling in the mediastinum and a tumour-like shadow with cavitation in right S^6.

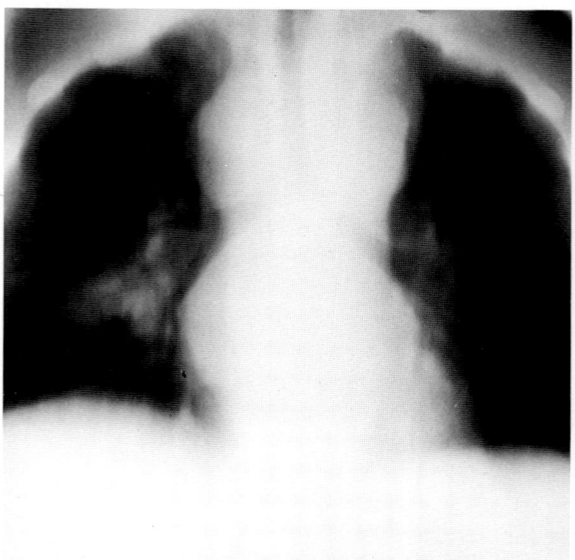

44.3 Chest tomogram (9 cm from the back). Lymphadenopathy of the mediastinum and hila is visible.

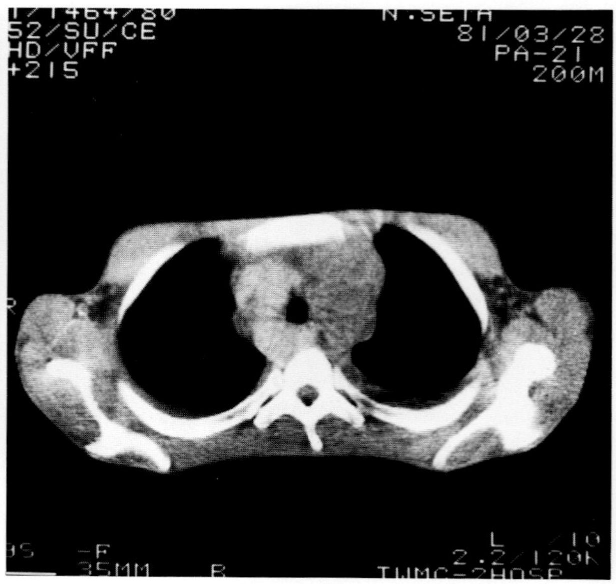

44.4 Chest CT scan with contrast enhancement. In addition to right-sided aortic arch, swelling of the paratracheal lymph nodes on both sides is obvious.

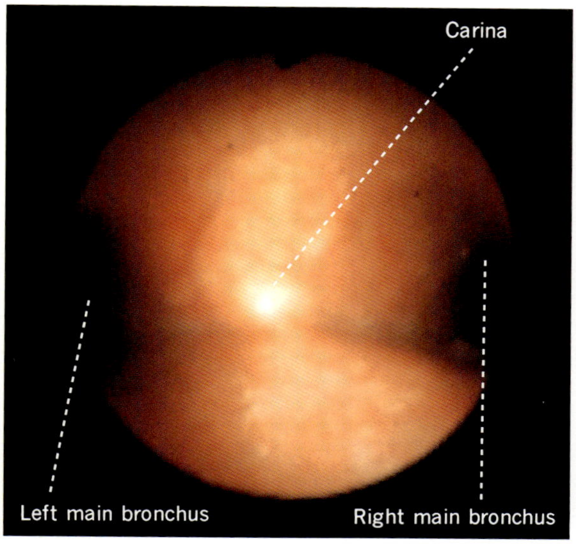

44.5 Bronchoscopic findings of the carina. The bifurcation is widened, with reddened and swollen mucosa.

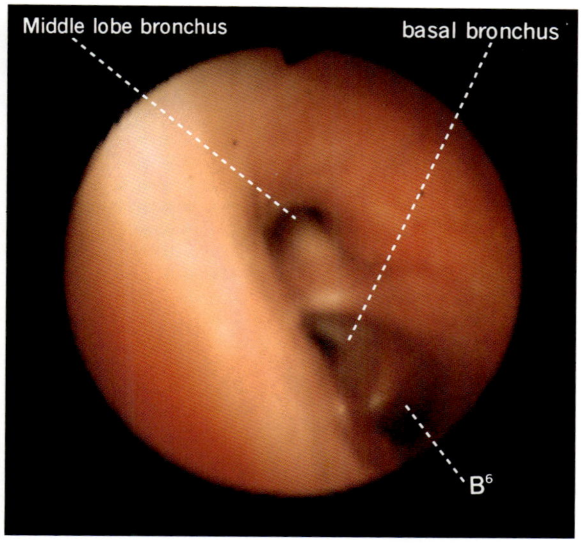

44.6 Bronchoscopic findings in the truncus intermedius. It was compressed from the mediastinal side, resulting in stenosis of the lumen. The orifice of the RML bronchus is also compressed extramurally. The mucosa is reddened as well as swollen.

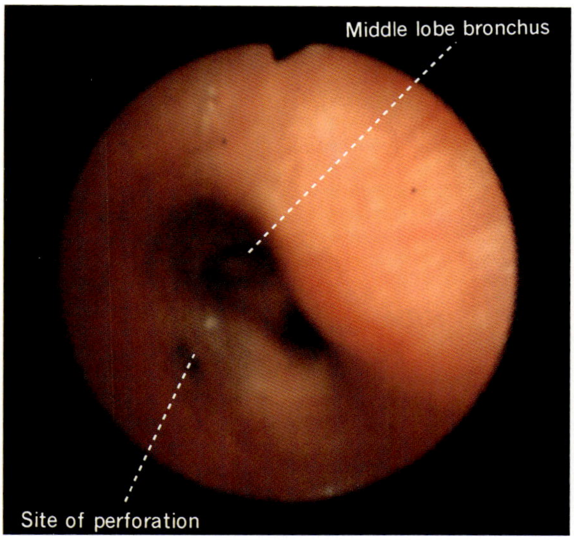

44.7 Bronchoscopic findings in the **RML** bronchus. On the mediastinal side there can be seen a black spot, indicating an anthracotic change. It has been proved, however, that this represents the perforation of mediastinal lymph nodes, resulting in spreading of tuberculosis. The orifice of the RML bronchus is narrowed because of compression caused by the swollen lymph nodes.

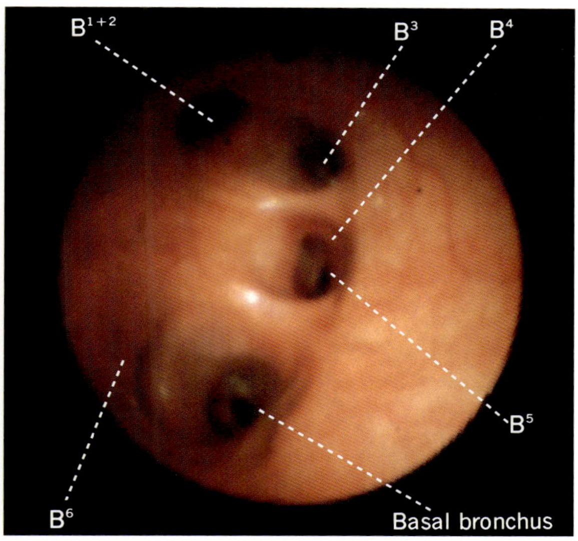

44.8 Bronchoscopic findings in the LUL and LLL bronchi. The medial wall of the main bronchus protrudes in some degree because of swollen mediastinal lymph nodes. The mucosa is reddened with dilated mucosal vessels. This is a case with anomalous branching of the bronchi, in which the lingular bronchus is located on the carina between the LUL and LLL bronchi. The patient responded well to antituberculosis therapy.

Case 45: Pulmonary tuberculosis (early stage) in a 23-year-old female.

The patient had been well until her periodical medical check up in May 1981, when abnormal shadows were found on her chest radiograph. Erythrocyte sedimentation rate 15 mm/h, C-reactive protein negative. Sputum examination failed to detect Mycobacterium.

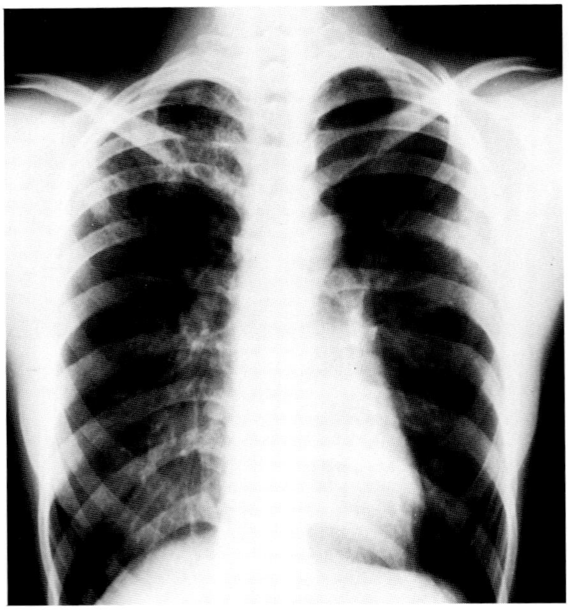

45.1 Posteroanterior chest radiograph. Infiltrates are visible in the right upper lung field and in left S^2a. Elevation of the right hilum is also visible.

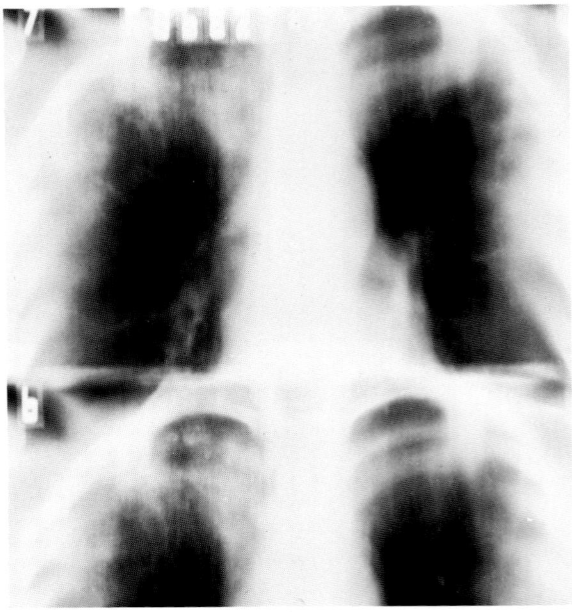

45.2 Chest tomogram (top: 7 cm from the back, bottom: 6 cm from the back). Infiltrative shadows are visible in right S^1, S^2 and in left S^3a, accompanying minute calcification.

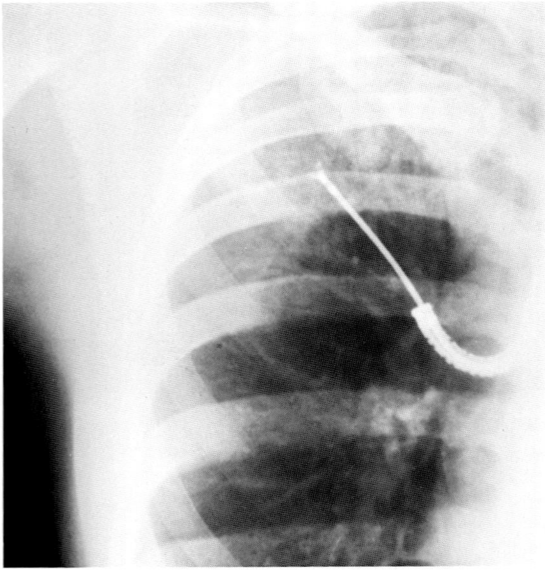

45.3 Transbronchial lung biopsy (TBLB) was carried out to obtain a definite diagnosis because mycobacterium was not detected in her sputum. This film shows TBLB being done on right B^1b, using a flexible forceps.

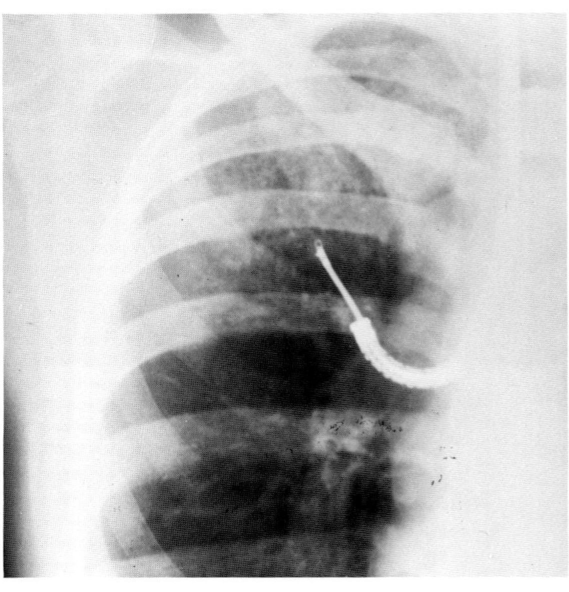

45.4 TBLB is being performed on right B^2b.

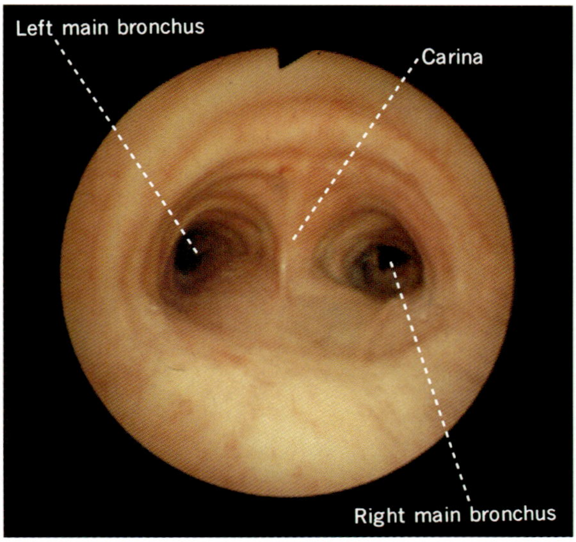

45.5 Bronchoscopic findings at the carina. The mucosa appears intact, although slight reddening is visible.

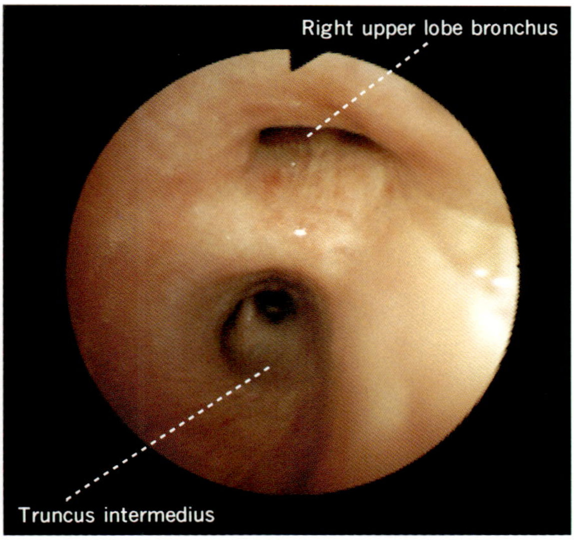

45.6 Bronchoscopic findings in the RUL bronchus and truncus intermedius. The mucosa is oedematous and there is vascular engorgement.

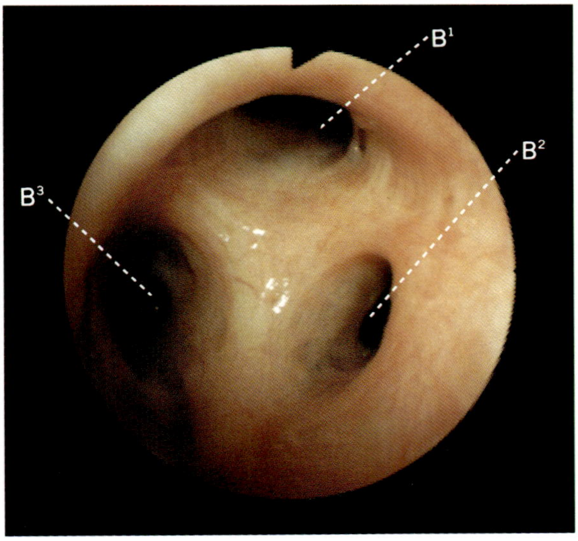

45.7 Bronchoscopic findings in the RUL bronchus. The bifurcations of the segmental and subsegmental bronchi look widened, swollen and reddened, with dilated mucosal vessels.

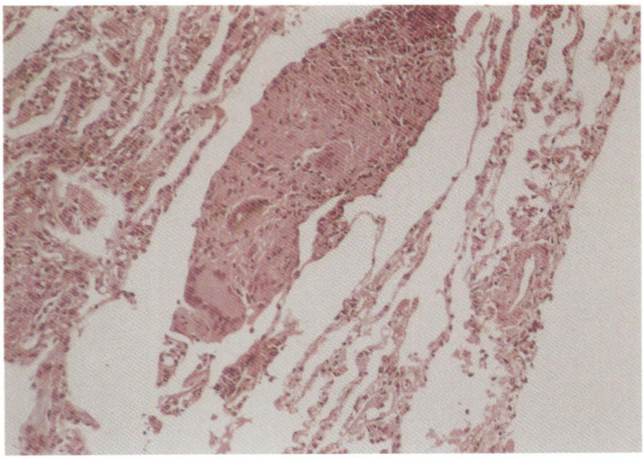

45.8 Histopathology findings of the biopsied lung. An epithelioid cell granuloma with Langhans' giant cells is visible.

Case 46: Miliary tuberculosis in a 78-year-old female.

The patient had been well until 2 weeks before when she presented with fever and slight dyspnoea. She was admitted to hospital for further examination and treatment in November 1980. On admission she complained of a non-productive cough. Repeated examination of sputum and gastric juice failed to detect Mycobacterium.

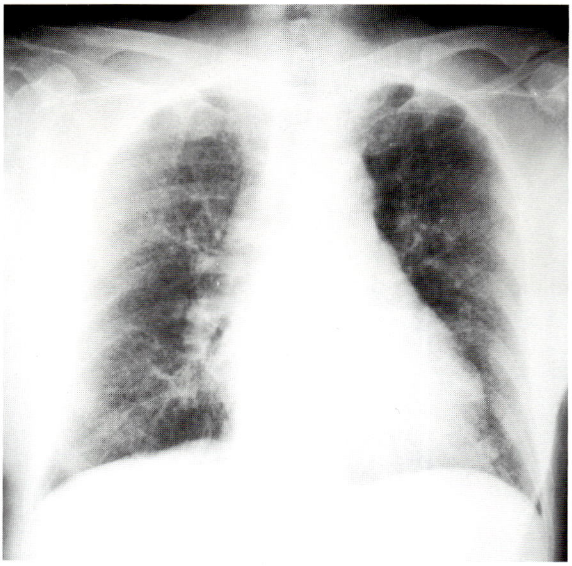

46.1 Posteroanterior chest radiograph on admission. Disseminated miliary shadows are demonstrated all over the lung fields.

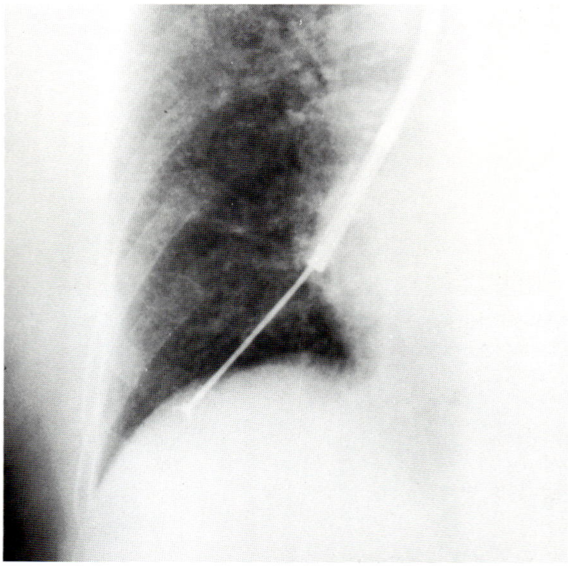

46.2 Transbronchial lung biopsy (TBLB) is being performed in right B^8b under fluoroscopy, using a flexible forceps.

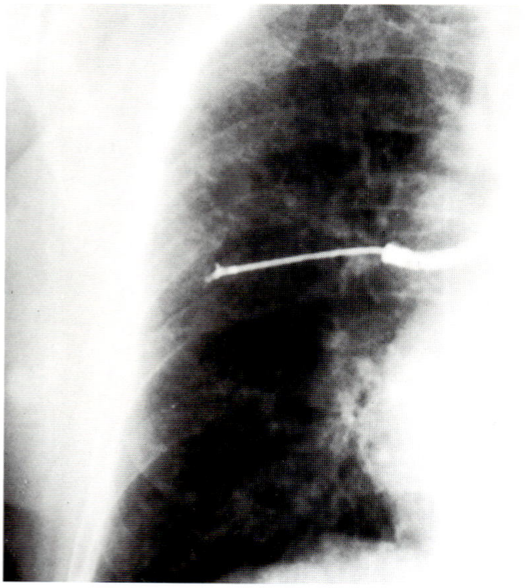

46.3 TBLB is being performed in right B^3a.

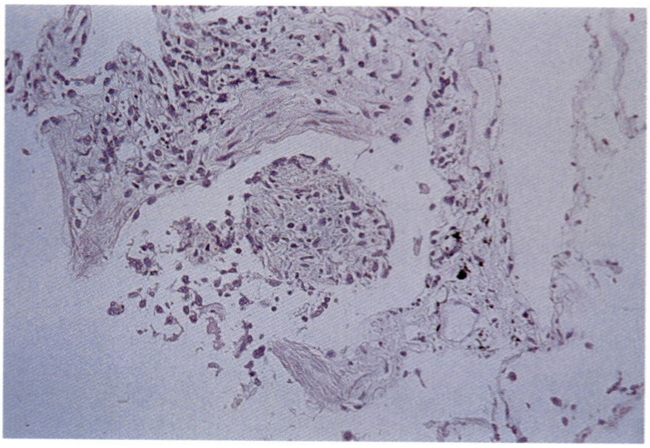

46.4 Histopathology of the biopsied lung (200x). An epithelioid cell granuloma is shown, although Mycobacterium was not detected.

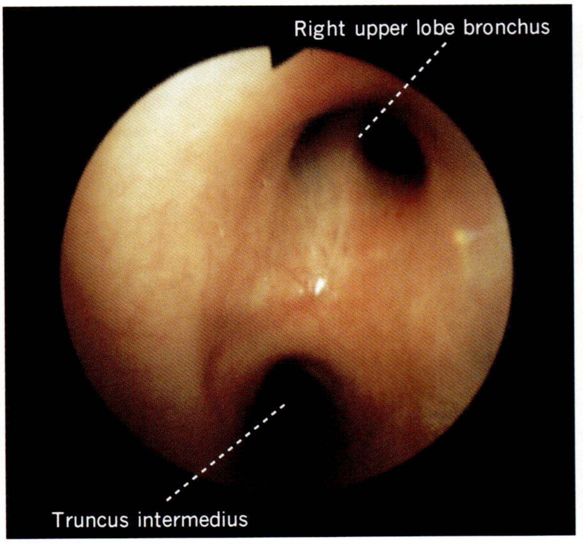

46.5 Bronchoscopic findings in the RUL bronchus and truncus intermedius. The bifurcation is slightly widened and swollen, with dilated mucosal vessels in part.

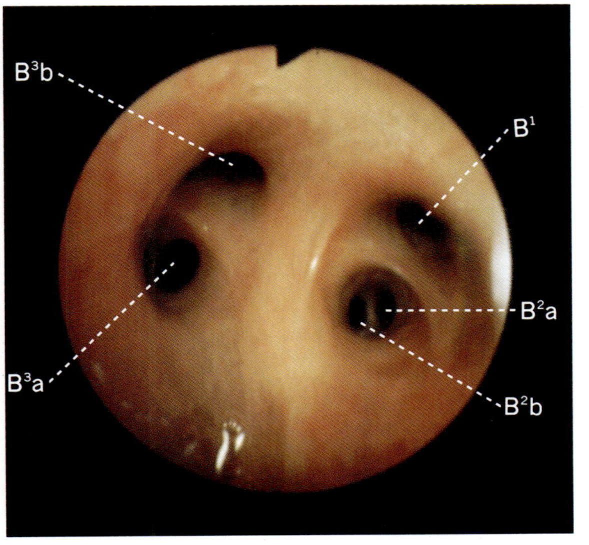

46.6 Bronchoscopic findings in the RUL bronchus. In spite of irregular mucosa, the bifurcations are almost intact.

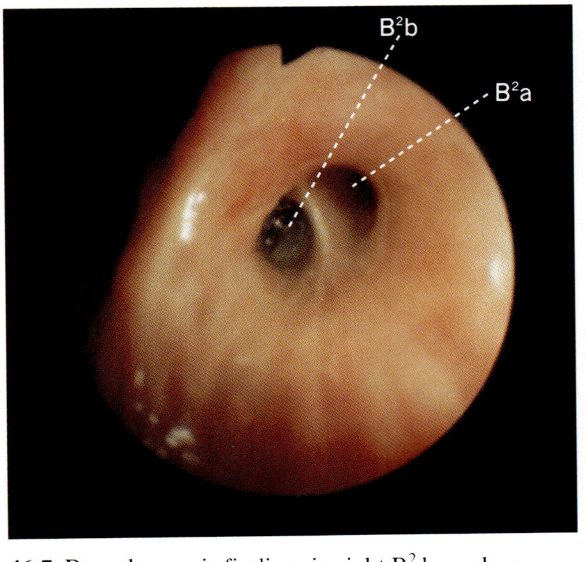

46.7 Bronchoscopic findings in right B^2 bronchus. The bifurcations appear oedematous to some degree.

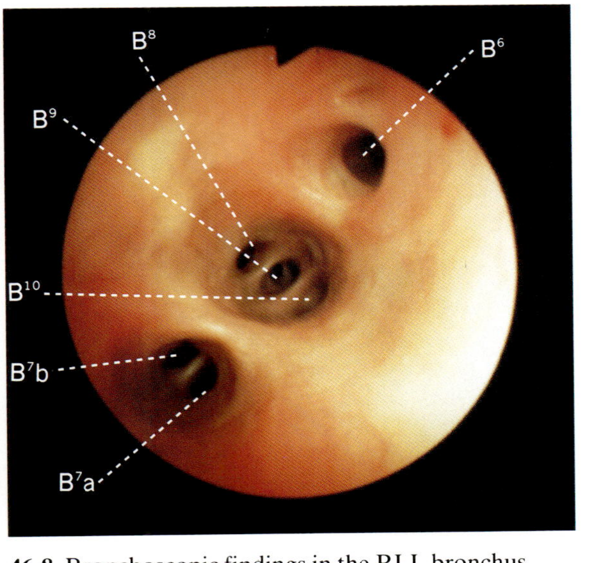

46.8 Bronchoscopic findings in the RLL bronchus. The mucosa is slightly reddened and the bifurcations between segmental bronchi appear widened.

6 Primary lung cancer (small cell carcinoma)

Case 47: Small cell carcinoma in a 67-year-old female.

The patient was referred to us for evaluation of abnormalities on her chest radiograph in March 1981. Biopsy of the bronchial wall revealed small cell carcinoma. She responded well to radiotherapy combined with chemotherapy.

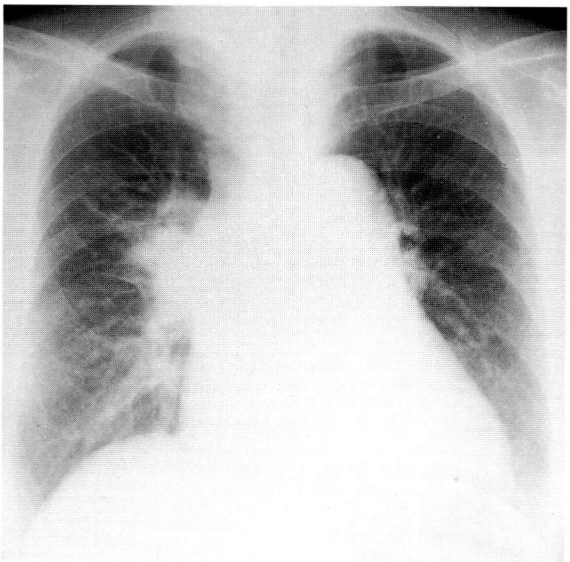

47.1 Posteroanterior chest radiograph. A tumour-like shadow is located in the right hilum. The carina is widened, suggesting metastasis to mediastinal lymph nodes.

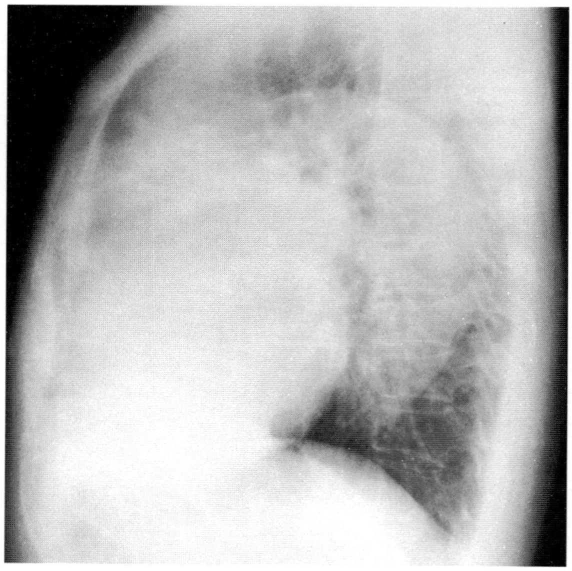

47.2 Lateral chest radiograph. The abnormal shadow starts at the carina and spreads to the anterior mediastinum, obliterating the upper heart border completely.

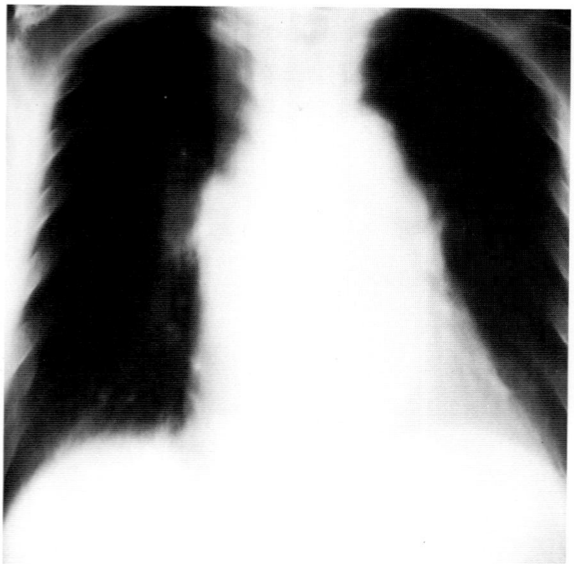

47.3 Chest tomogram (6 cm from the beck). Enlargement of the mediastinum and bilateral hilar lymphadenopathy are visible.

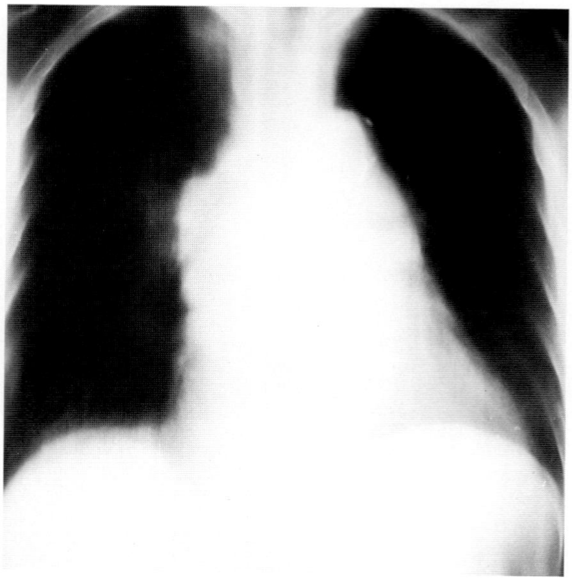

47.4 Chest tomogram (8 cm from the back). Widening of the carina and bilateral hilar lymphadenopathy are visible.

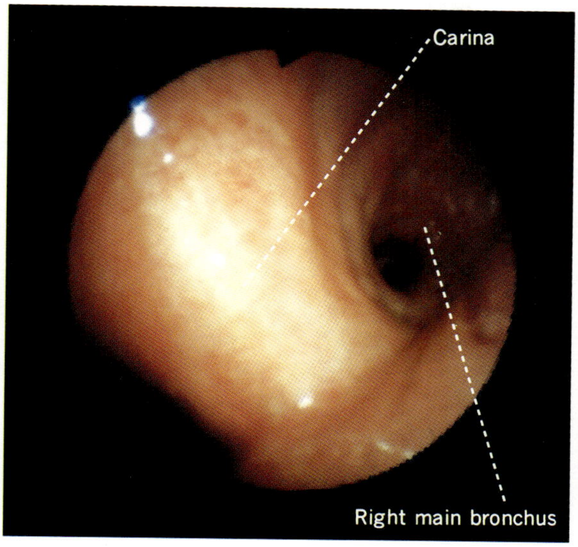

47.5 Bronchoscopic findings at the carina. The bifurcation is widened as well as reddened and swollen.

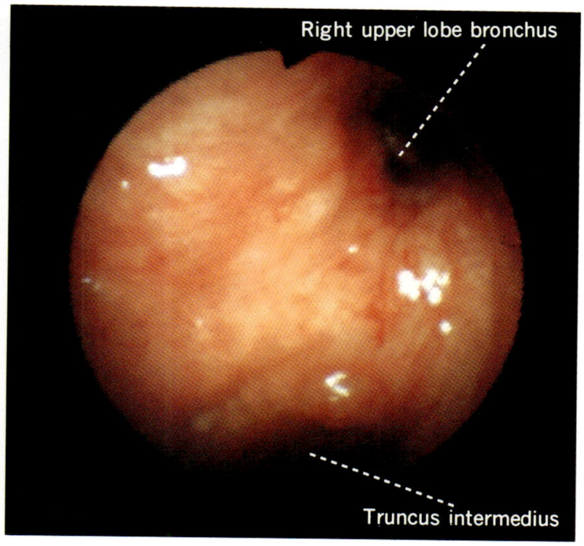

47.6 Bronchoscopic findings in the RUL bronchus and truncus intermedius. The mucosa of the bifurcation, with irregular surface and vascular dilatation, is obviously invaded with carcinoma.

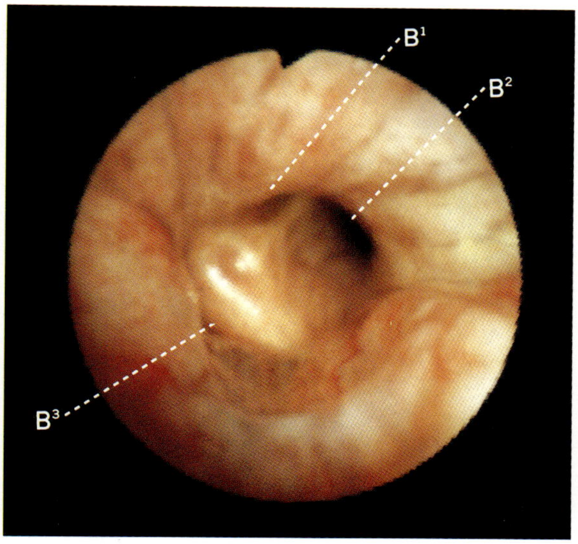

47.7 Bronchoscopic findings in the RUL bronchus. Marked reddening and swelling of the mucosa and narrowing of the bronchial lumen are present. With prominent vascular engorgement, the orifices of B^1, B^2 and B^3 are stenotic. Biopsy of the bronchial wall led to a definite diagnosis of small cell carcinoma.

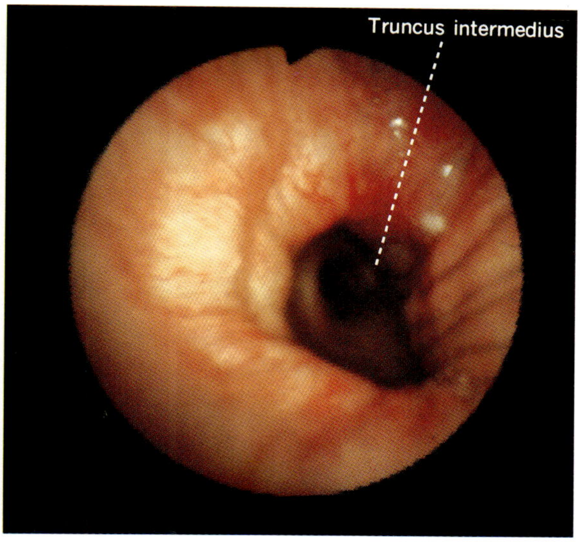

47.8 Bronchoscopic findings in the truncus intermedius. The irregularities of the wall and the dilated results are the result of invasion by carcinoma. The membranous portion is spared.

Case 48: Small cell carcinoma is a 58-year-old female.

This patient had smoked 9,000 cigarettes per year. She presented with a productive cough from 1977. From March 1981 the cough worsened and abnormalities were found on her chest radiograph. She was admitted in April 1981.

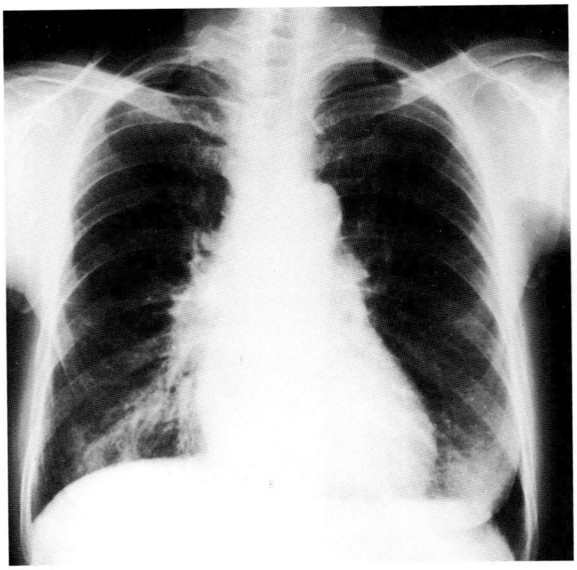

48.1 Posteroanterior chest radiograph. Increased vascular markings and enlarged right hilum are visible. The right diaphragm is slightly obscured, suggesting a silhouette sign.

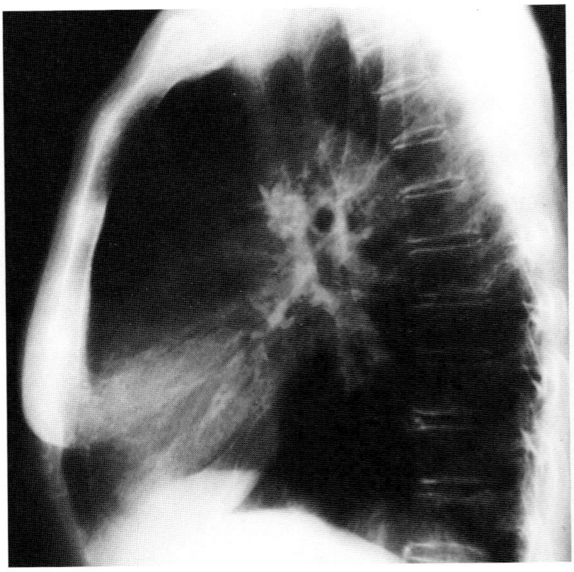

48.2 Lateral chest Xray. Increased radiolucency of the substernal and retrocardiac spaces indicates the presence of pulmonary emphysema. A mass shadow with irregular contours is located at the base of B^{10}.

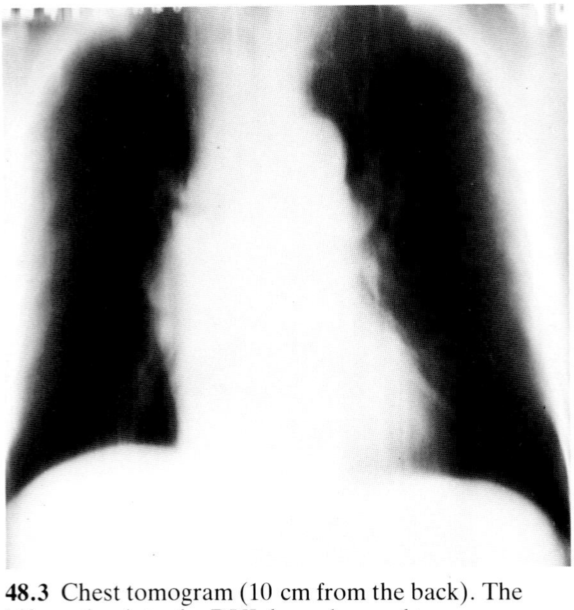

48.3 Chest tomogram (10 cm from the back). The bifurcation into the RUL bronchus and truncus intermedius is compressed by the swollen lymph nodes or the tumour, causing almost total obstruction of the truncus intermedius.

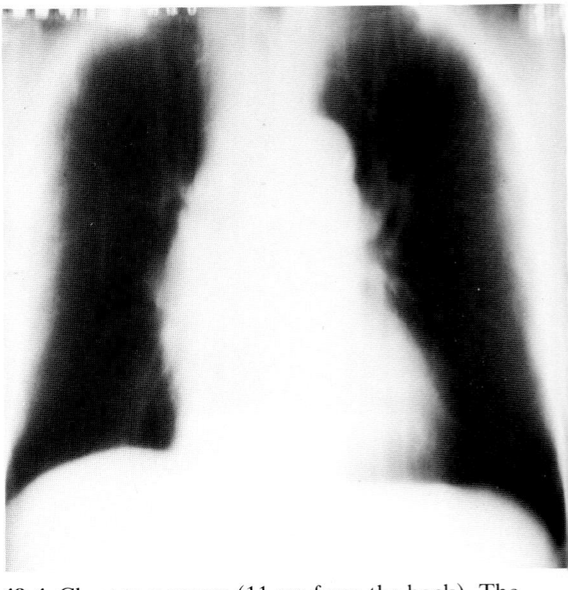

48.4 Chest tomogram (11 cm from the back). The mass shadow, 3-4 cm in diameter, protrudes into the truncus intermedius.

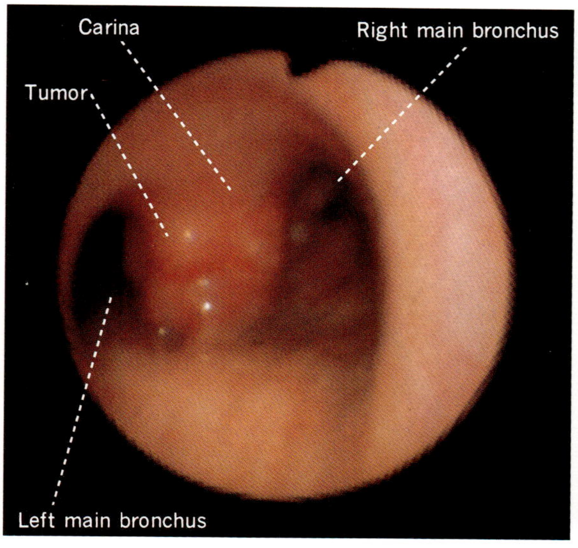

48.5 Bronchoscopic findings at the carina. The bifurcation is replaced by a nodular mass.

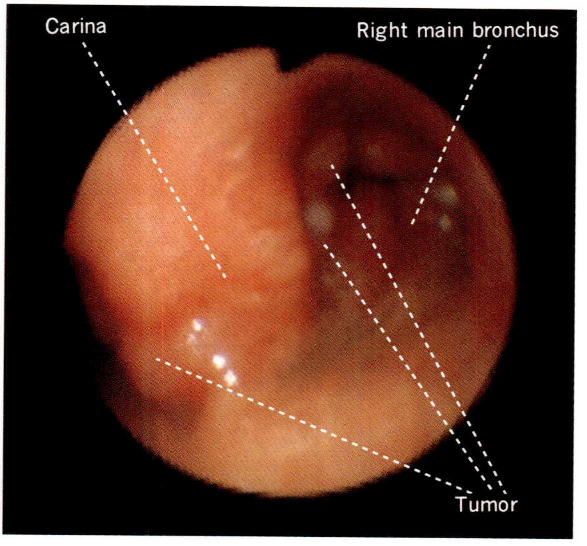

48.6 Close-up of **48.5** showing the nodular mass, with reddened and oedematous mucosa.

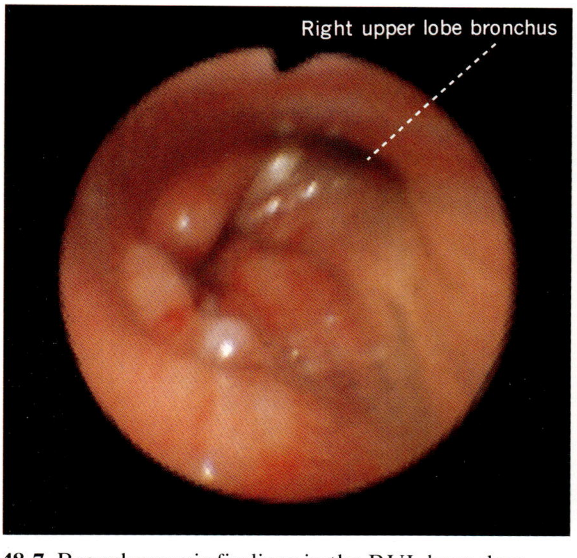

48.7 Bronchoscopic findings in the RUL bronchus and truncus intermedius. The truncus intermedius is almost occluded by the nodular mass.

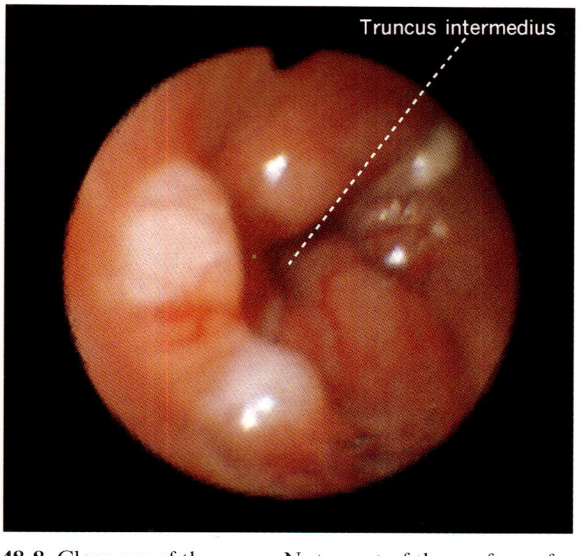

48.8 Close-up of the mass. Note part of the surface of the nodular mass is white through which small vessels are visible. Air flows via the spaces between multiple nodules. Biopsy of this mass confirmed it to be small cell carcinoma.

Case 49: Small cell carcinoma in a 60-year-old male.

The patient, a farmer, had been well until December 1981, when he started to complain of nocturnal cough. He was referred in January 1982 for further examination, when abnormalities were found on his chest radiograph.

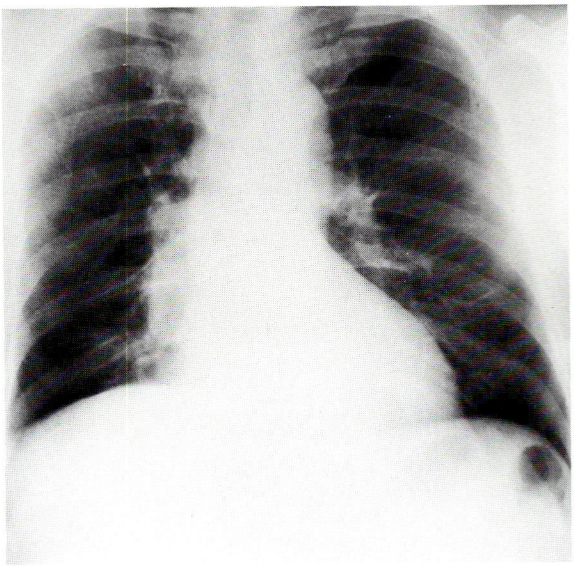

49.1 Posteroanterior chest radiograph. The right hilum deviates downwards and the minor fissure is depressed by two intercostal spaces. Neither the right heart border nor the right diaphragm are obliterated, although the right costophrenic angle is.

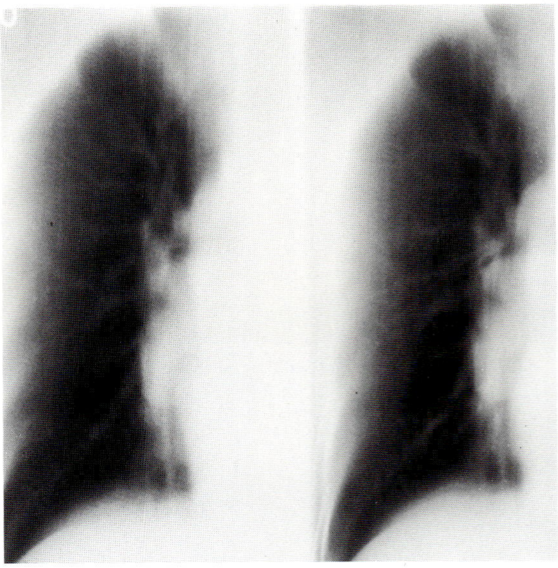

49.2 Chest tomogram (left: 10 cm from the back; right: 11 cm from the back). The mass shadow, 4 x 3 cm in diameter, is around the orifice of the right basal bronchus.

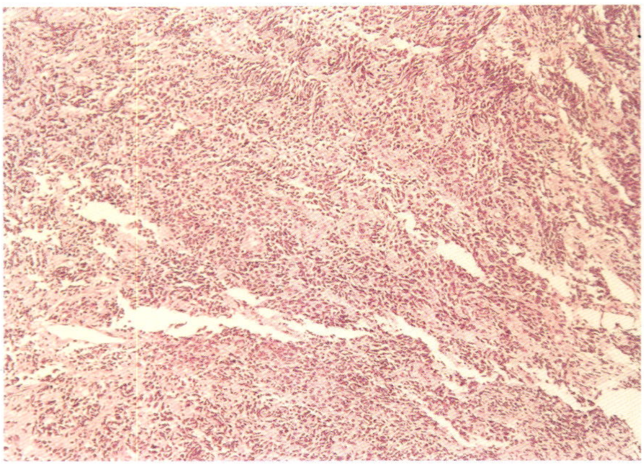

49.3 Histopathology showing small cell carcinoma.

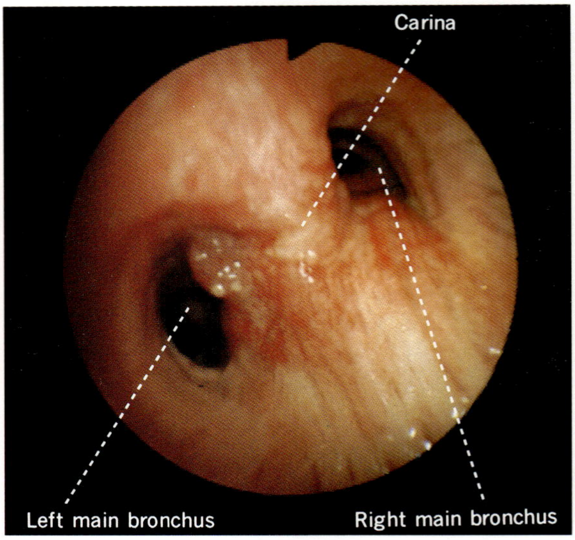

49.4 Bronchoscopic findings at the main carina. The widened bifurcation is invaded with carcinoma, with prominent vascular dilatation.

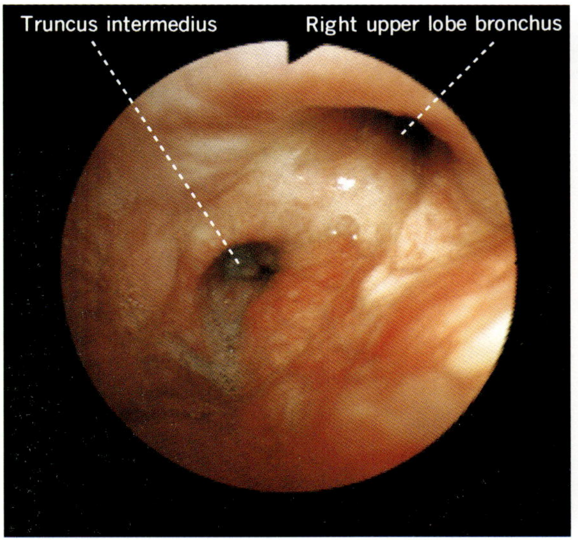

49.5 Bronchoscopic findings in the RUL bronchus and truncus intermedius. The bifurcation is widened and strikingly invaded with carcinoma.

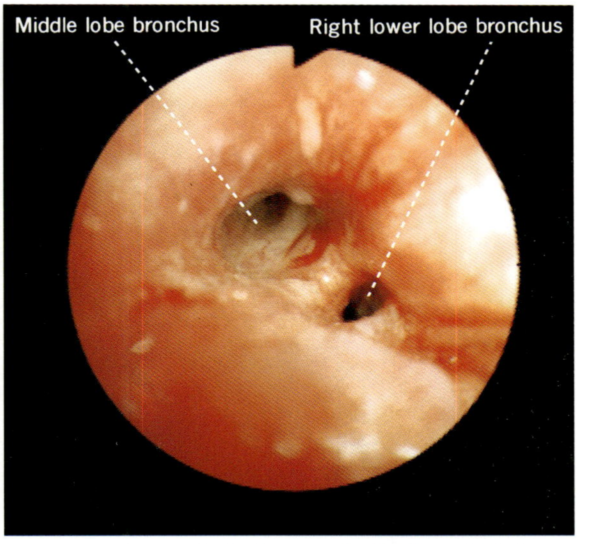

49.6 Bronchoscopic findings in the RML and RLL bronchi. The spurs are oedematous and widened by tumour invasion, narrowing all the orifices of bronchi.

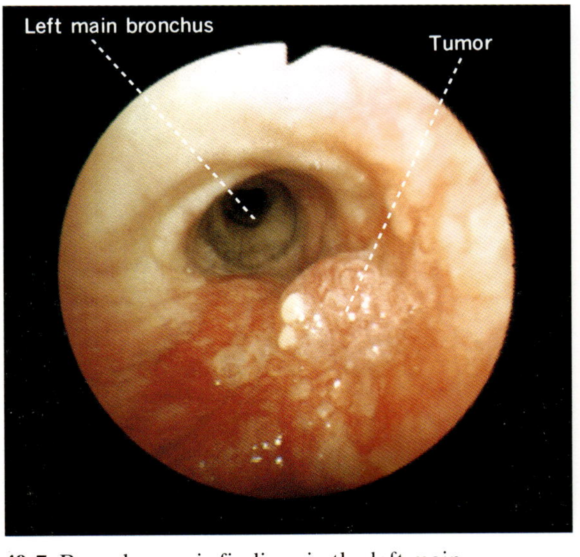

49.7 Bronchoscopic findings in the left main bronchus. At the orifice of the main bronchus a tumour with dilated vessels on its surface, part of which is covered with necrotic white tissue, is clearly visible.

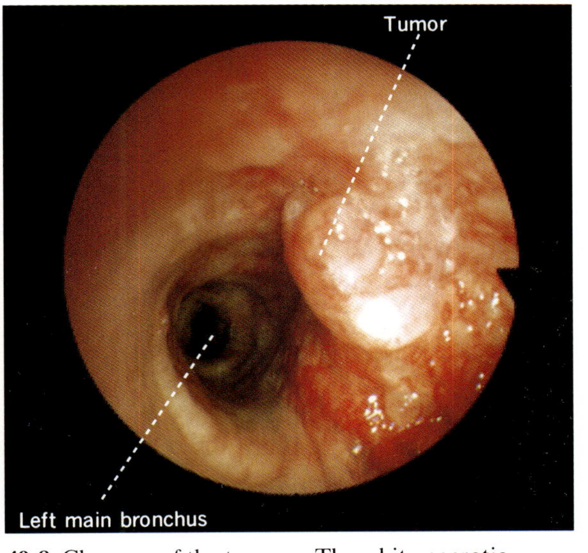

49.8 Close-up of the tumour. The white necrotic tissue covers the tumour, which is surrounded by mucosa with prominently dilated vessels.

Case 50: Small cell carcinoma in a 67-year-old male.

This patient's small cell lung carcinoma originated from the right middle lobe, and metastatised to the brain.

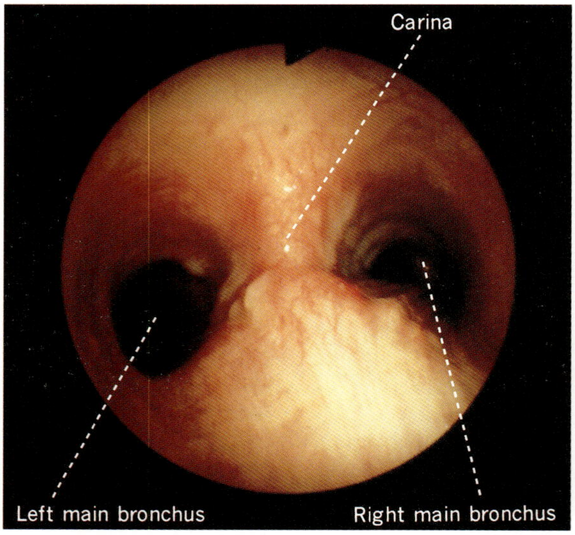

50.1 Bronchoscopic findings at the main carina. Multiple protruding lesions with vascular engorgement are seen particularly on the membranous portion, including the posterior part of the carina. The bifurcation is widened and swollen.

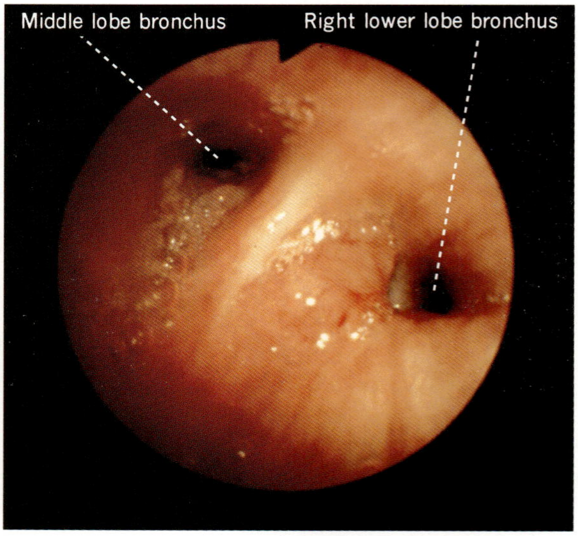

50.2 Bronchoscopic findings in the RML and RLL bronchi. The spur, to which some secretion is attached, is widened by tumour invasion, narrowing each bronchial orifice.

Case 51: Small cell carcinoma in a 68-year-old male.

This patient had small cell carcinoma of the left upper lobe. Chest radiograph revealed incomplete atelectasis of left upper lobe.

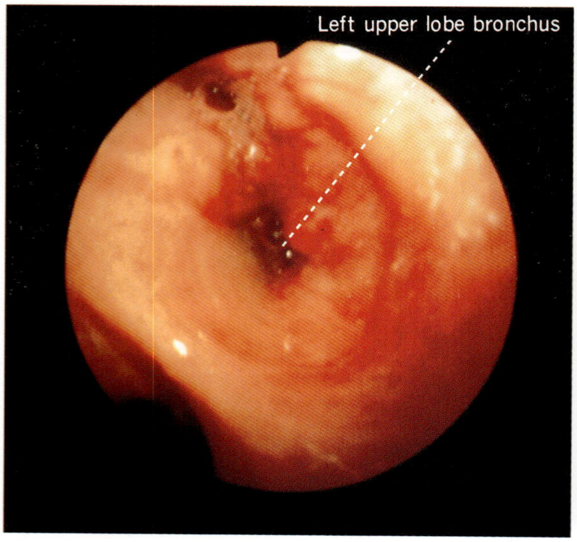

51.1 Bronchoscopic findings in the LUL bronchus. Both the left upper and lower division bronchi are occluded with the tumour, which barely permits air bubbles to escape.

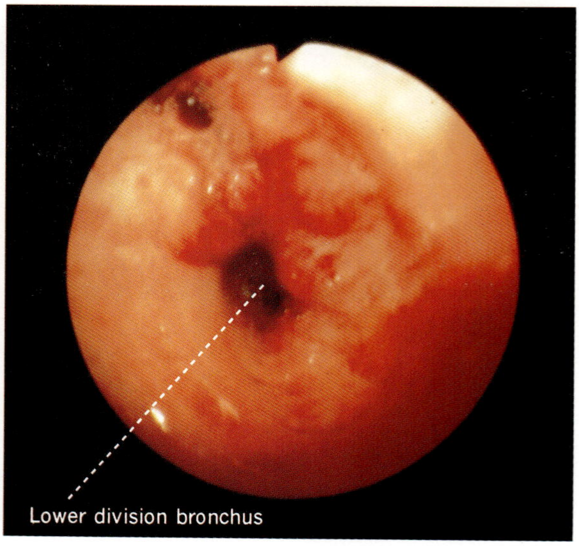

51.2 Close-up of **51.1**. The orifice of the lower division bronchus is hardly visible through the irregular-surfaced tumour.

Case 52: Small cell carcinoma in a 54-year-old male.

This patient had small cell carcinoma of the right upper lobe. Atelectasis of the right upper lobe is visible on his chest roentgenogram.

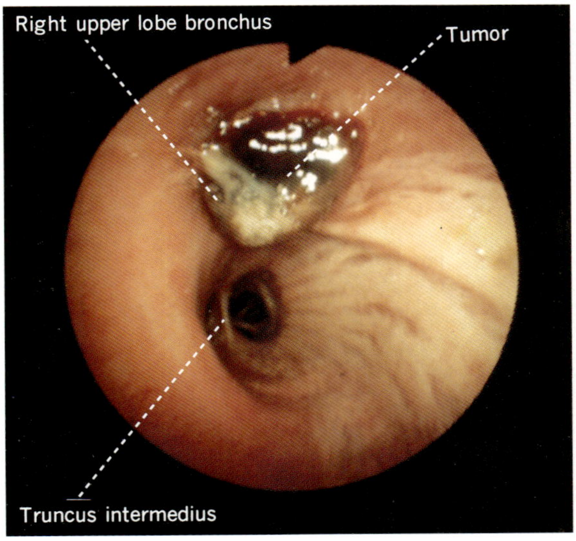

52.1 Bronchoscopic findings in the RUL bronchus and truncus intermedius. The RUL bronchus is totally obstructed by the tumour which is covered with coagulated blood.

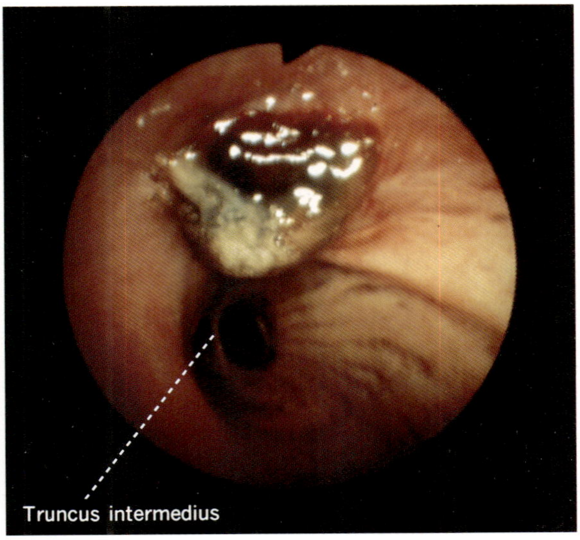

52.2 Close-up view of the tumour. White necrotic tissue is visible among the coagulated blood. The surrounding mucosa is reddened.

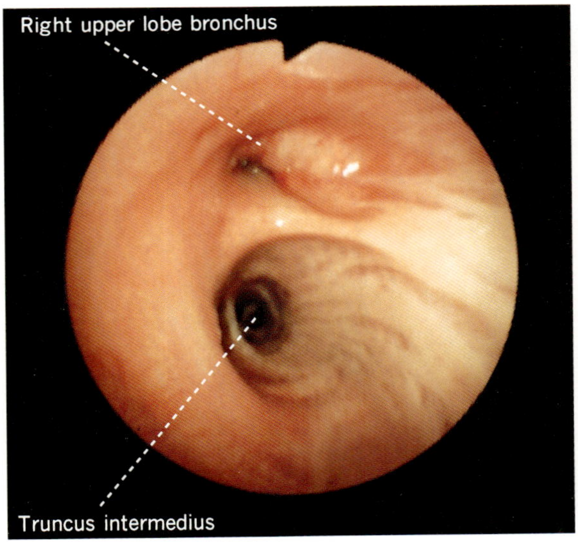

52.3 Bronchoscopic findings in the same area after a course of chemotherapy. The tumour diminished and the coagulated blood disappeared.

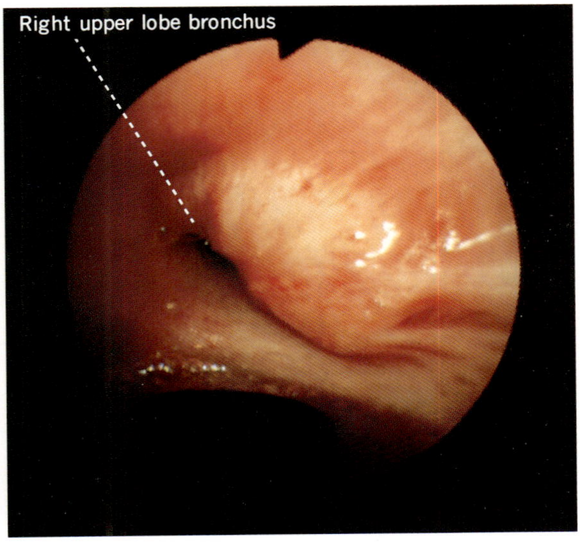

52.4 Close-up of the tumour. It has decreased in size, allowing increased aeration of the upper lobe.

Case 53: Small cell carcinoma in a 53-year-old male.

This patient had small cell lung carcinoma. The primary lesion is located in left B^6. The tumour responded to radiotherapy and chemotherapy.

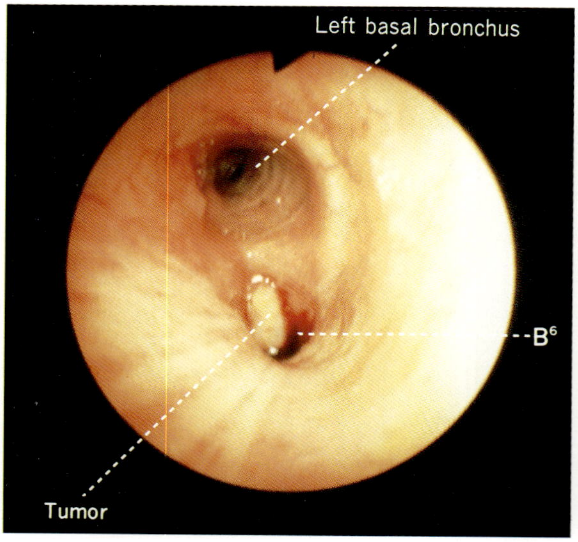

53.1 Bronchoscopic findings in the LLL bronchus. At the orifice of B^6 there exists a white tumour, whose invasion narrows the orifice of the left basal bronchus as well.

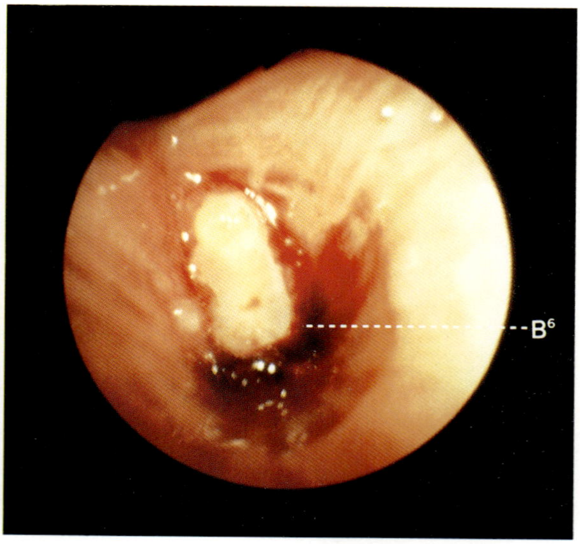

53.2 Close-up of the tumour. The orifice of B^6 is mostly occluded by the tumour covered with white necrotic tissue, which bleeds easily.

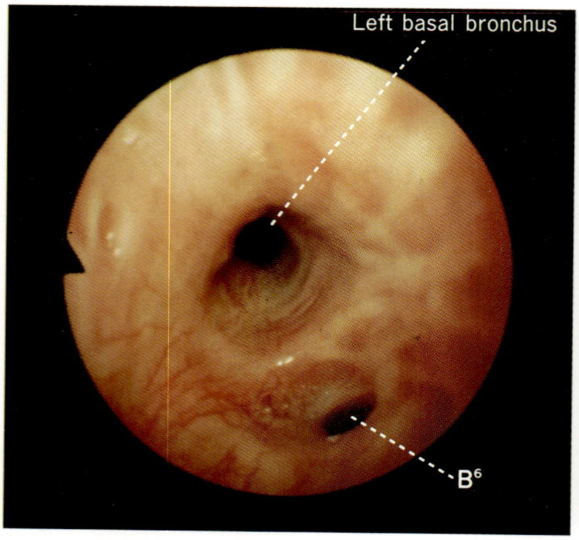

53.3 Bronchoscopic findings of the same region after four courses of chemotherapy. The orifice of B^6 is patent, despite the vascular engorgement.

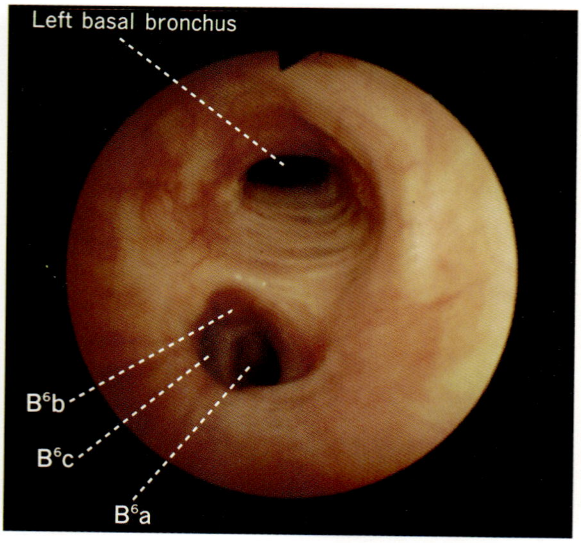

53.4 Close-up of B^6. The bifurcations of B^6 into subsegmental bronchi appear relatively sharp-edged and the orifices of subsegmental bronchi are visible, although the mucosal vessels are engorged around the orifice of the basal bronchus.

Case 54: Small cell carcinoma in a 73-year-old male.

This is a case with small cell carcinoma originating from the truncus intermedius, complicated by total collapse of the right middle and lower lobes.

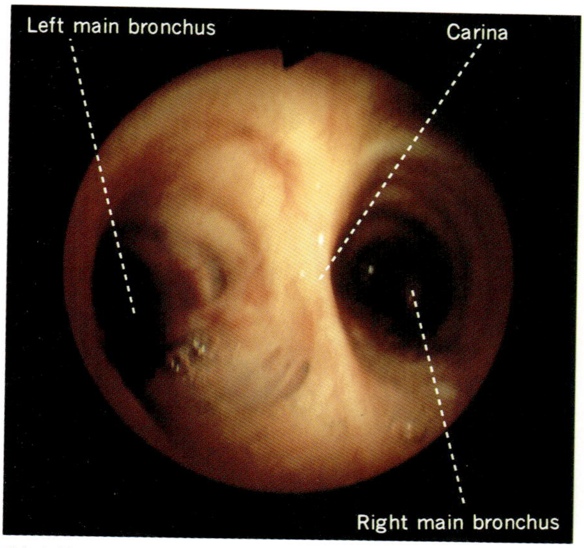

54.1 Bronchoscopic findings at the carina. The bifurcation remains sharp-edged.

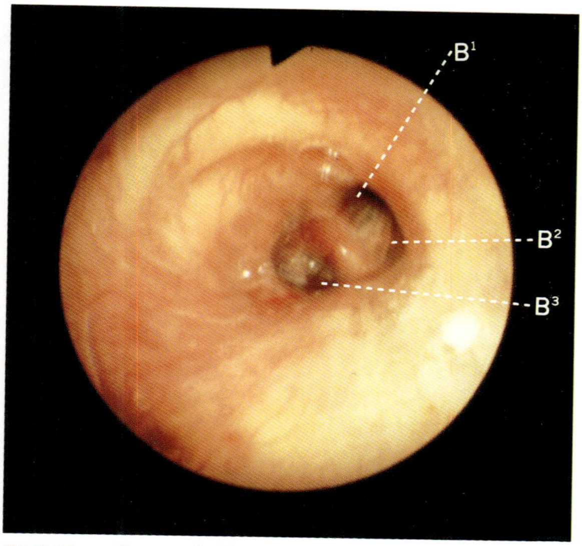

54.2 Bronchoscopic findings of right main bronchus. The bifurcation into the RUL bronchus and truncus intermedius is widened and swollen. The truncus intermedius is completely occluded, with prominent vascular dilatation.

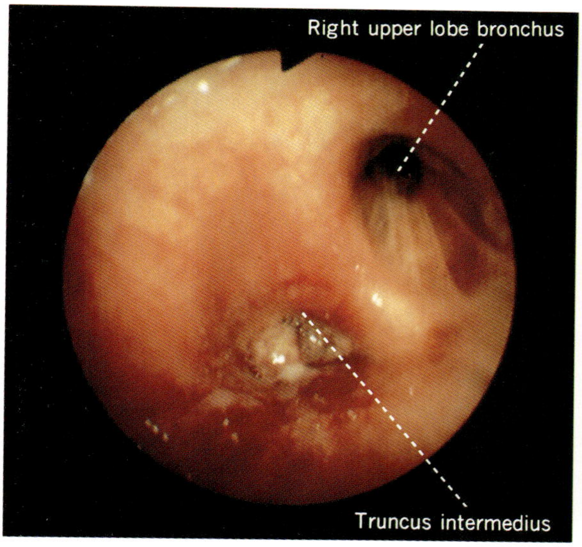

54.3 Close-up of the bifurcation into the RUL bronchus and truncus intermedius. It is oedematous and widened, with total occlusion of the truncus intermedius.

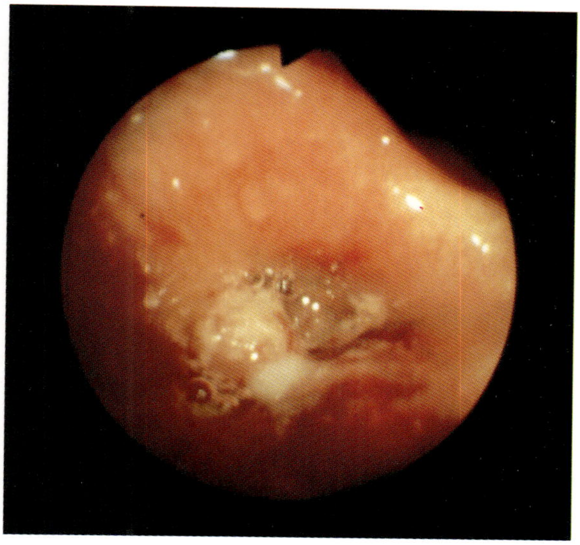

54.4 Close-up of the tumour. The mucosa is reddened as well as oedematous. Part of the tumour is covered with white necrotic tissue. The emerging air bubble implies minimal patency of the bronchus.

Case 55: Small cell carcinoma in a 67-year-old female.

The patient was a heavy smoker without a history of significant illness. She had small cell lung carcinoma which arose from the LUL bronchus.

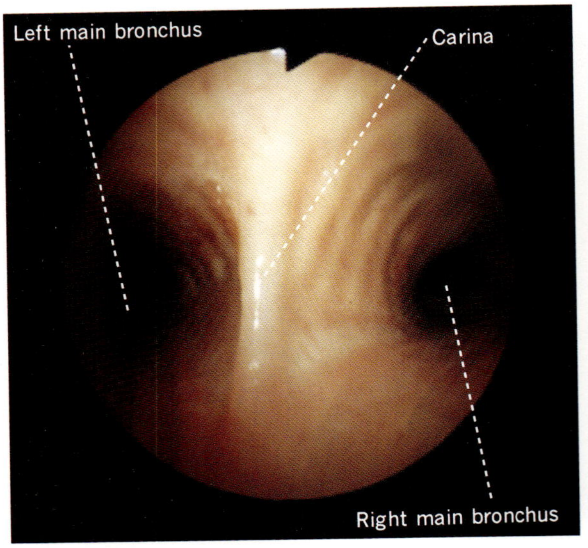

55.1 Bronchoscopic findings at the carina. The bifurcation is oedematous and widened to a mild degree.

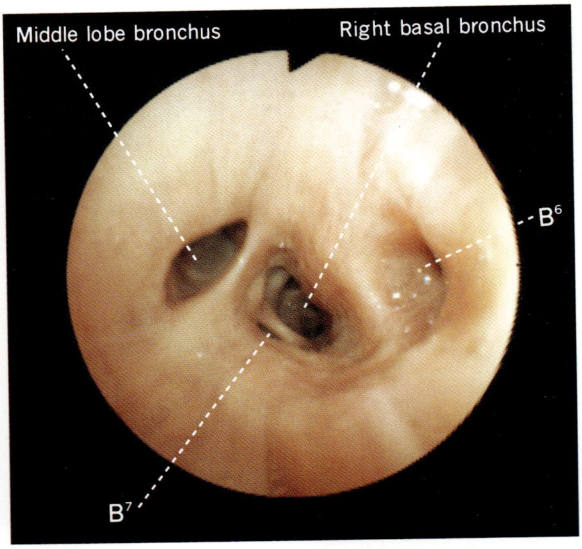

55.2 Bronchoscopic findings in the RML and RLL bronchi. The orifice of B^6 appears oedematous with widening of the spur. The orifice of the basal bronchus is also swollen, suggesting tumour invasion.

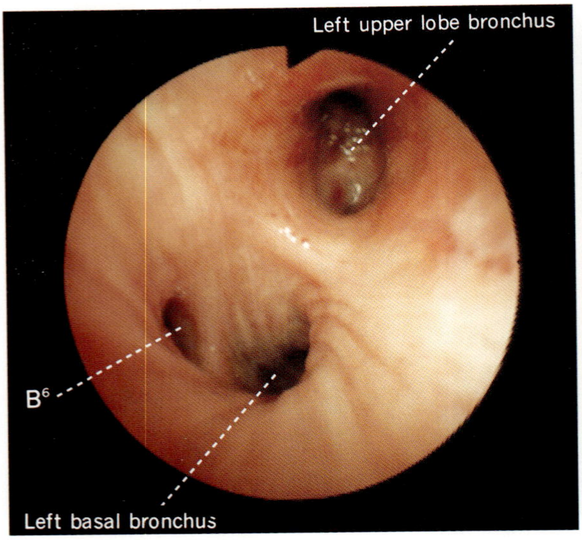

55.3 Bronchoscopic findings in the LUL and LLL bronchi. The bronchial bifurcations are oedematous and widened and the orifice of the LUL bronchus is quite red.

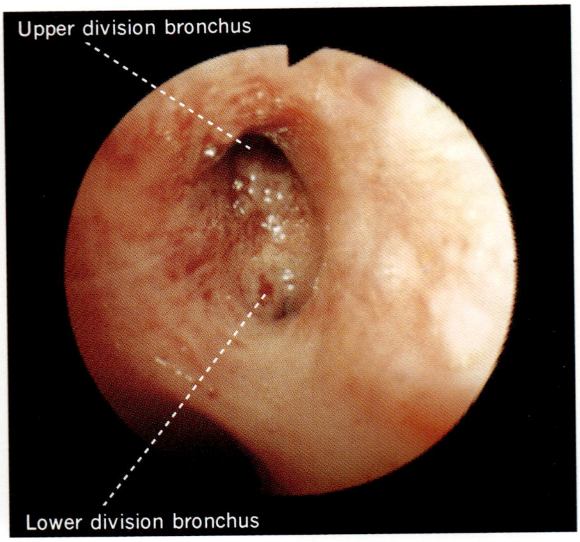

55.4 Bronchoscopic findings in the LUL bronchus. The reddened mucosa of the orifice bleeds easily.

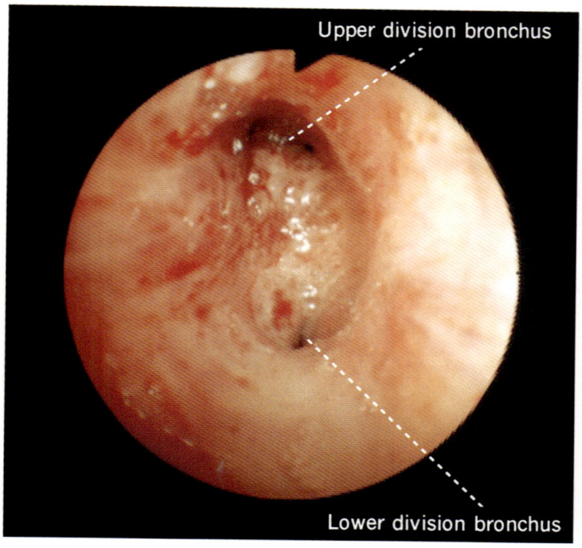

55.5 Close-up of the LUL bronchus. The tumour continues from the left wall of the orifice to each division of the bronchus, narrowing the orifices to a great extent.

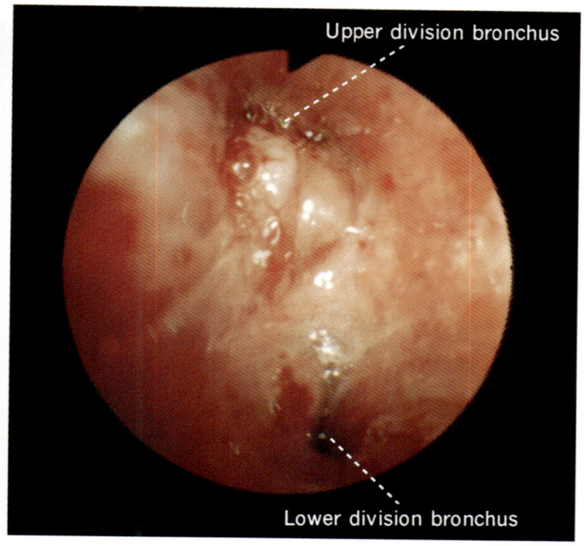

55.6 Close-up of the tumour. There is a nodular tumour narrowing the orifice of the lower division bronchus to the size of a pinhole. Air bubbles are coming out of the upper division bronchus, indicating its minimal patency.

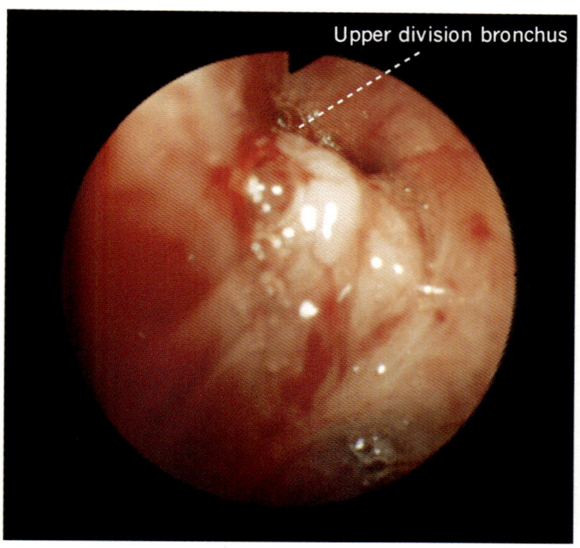

55.7 Close-up of the left upper division bronchus. The orifice is covered with a white tumour, through which air bubbles escape.

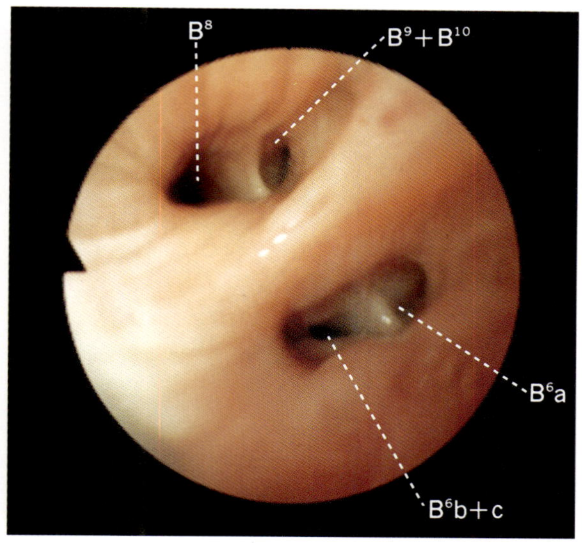

55.8 Bronchoscopic findings in the LLL bronchus. Orifices of B^6 and the basal bronchus appear oedematous, with widened bifurcation of B^6.

7 Primary lung cancer (squamous cell carcinoma)

Case 56: Epidermoid carcinoma in an 80-year-old male.

The patient had been well until April 1981, when he began to complain of a cough as well as a low-grade fever which came on in the evenings.

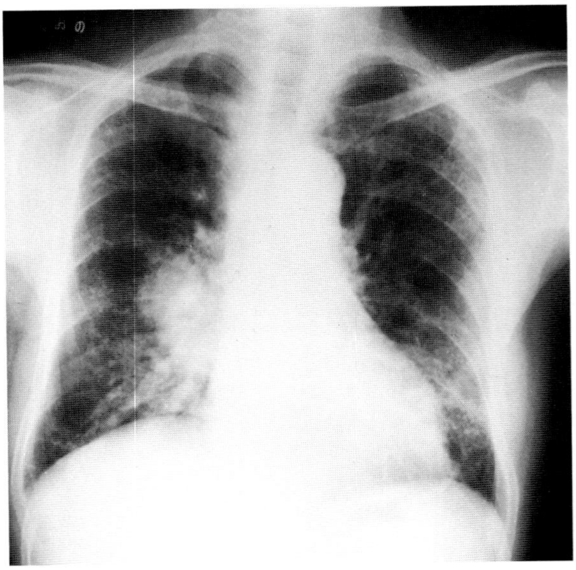

56.1 Posteroanterior chest radiograph. In addition to a reticular pattern throughout the lungs, a tumour-like shadow is visible over the right hilum and in S^6.

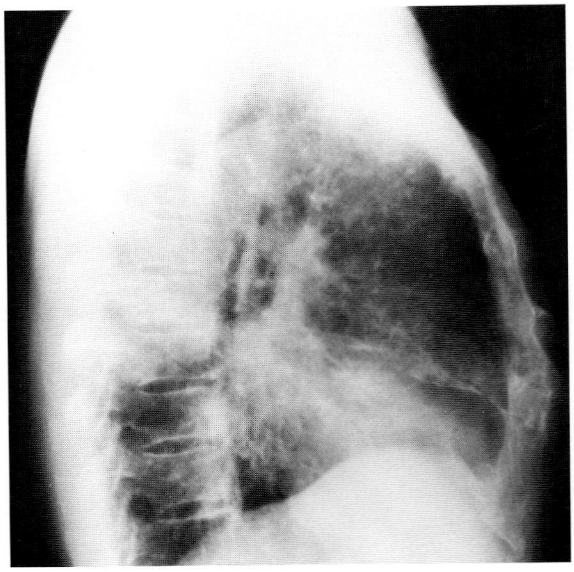

56.2 Lateral chest radiograph. Apart from the diffuse reticulonodular pattern, a mass shadow with relatively homogenous density is seen over the hilum and in S^6.

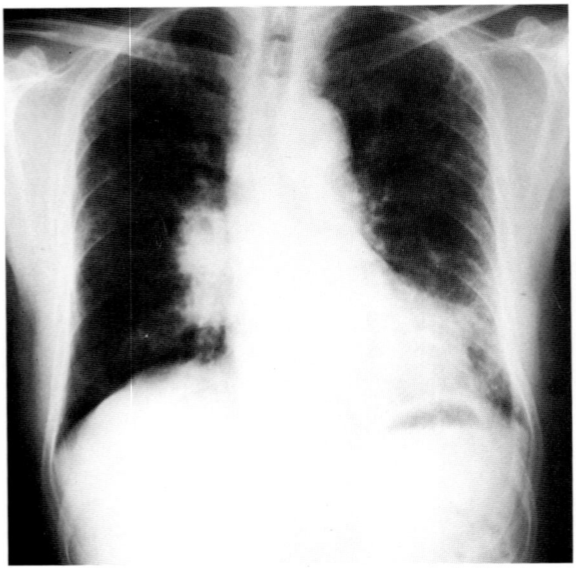

56.3 Posteroanterior chest radiograph 7 weeks later. After instilling anticancer drugs into the tumour five times, the shadow reduced in size considerably.

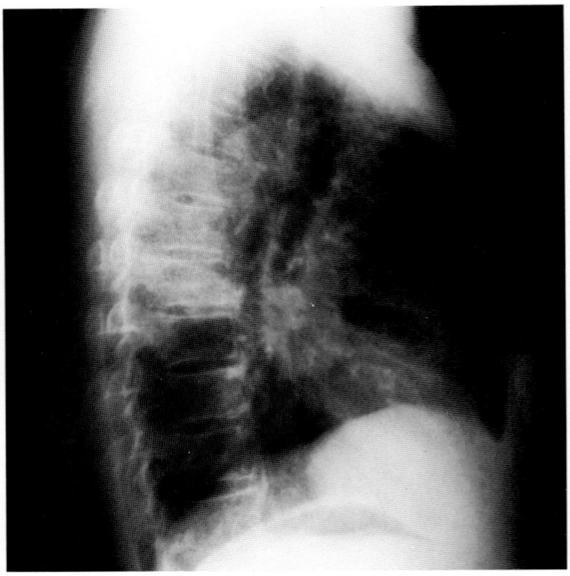

56.4 Lateral chest radiograph 7 weeks later. The tumour mass has decreased in size.

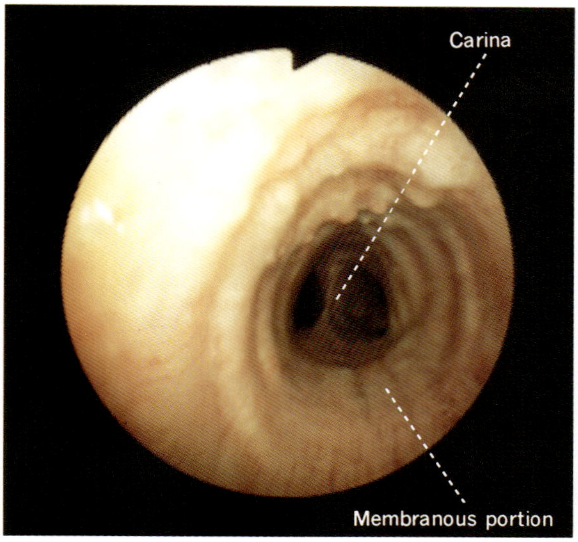

56.5 Bronchoscopic findings in the trachea just beneath the glottis. Multiple protruding lesions are distributed over the anterior half of the left wall, indicating tumour invasion.

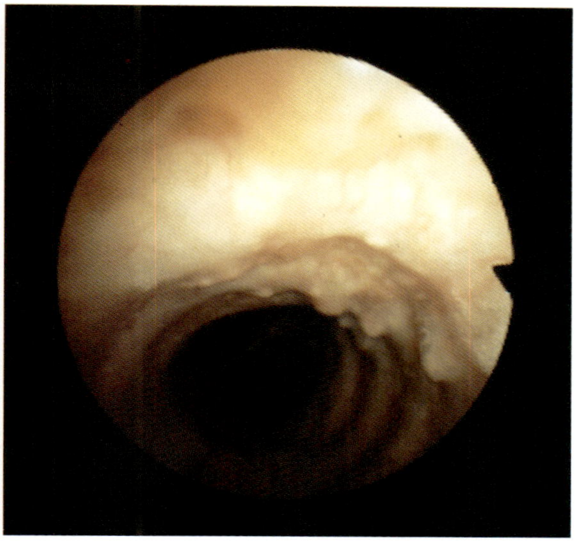

56.6 Close-up of **56.5**. Protruding lesions are slightly reddened and differ in size.

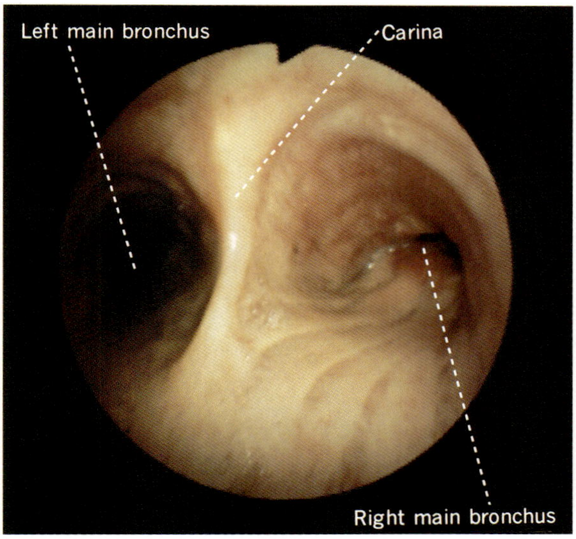

56.7 Bronchoscopic findings at the carina. Although the bifurcation remains sharp-edged, the mucosa around the orifice of the RUL bronchus is generally reddened, excluding the membranous portion. The truncus intermedius is narrowed by the protruding tumour in the membranous portion.

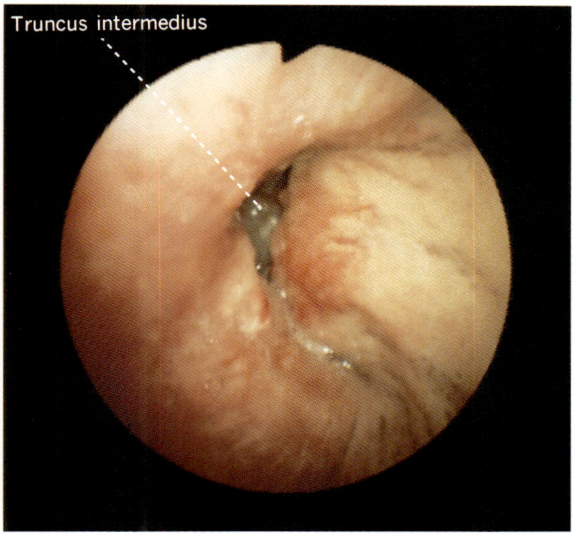

56.8 Close-up of the stenosis of the truncus intermedius. The membranous portion with irregular surface and dilated vessels protrudes into the lumen. The surrounding mucosa is also oedematous because of tumour invasion, although the bronchus remains slightly patent. Black necrotic tissue partly covers the mucosal surface.

Case 57: Epidermoid carcinoma (well differentiated) in a 75-year-old male.

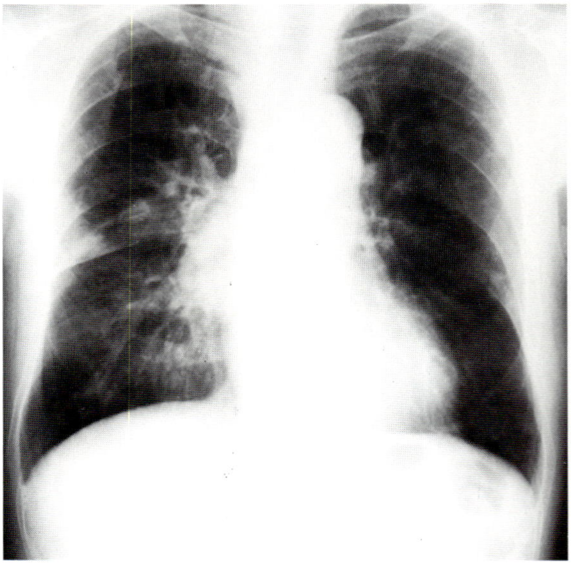

57.1 Posteroanterior chest radiograph. Enlargement of the right hilum and atelectasis of right S^3a is visible. Small cavity lesions, 0.5-1 cm in diameter, are scattered throughout the lungs.

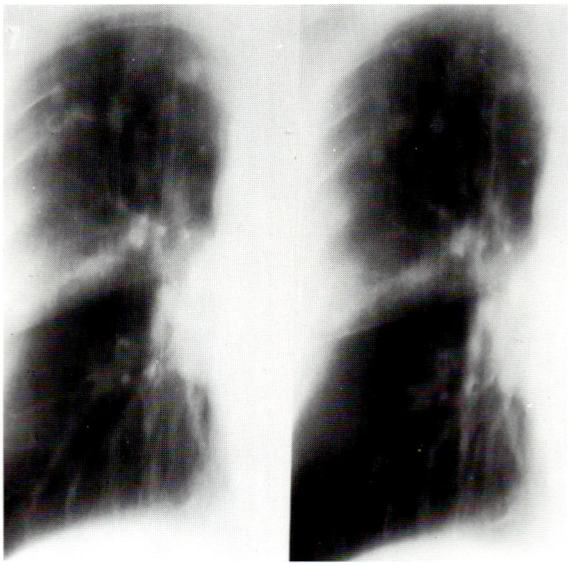

57.2 Right chest tomograms (right: 6 cm from the back, left: 7 cm from the back). A mass shadow is visible in the hilum, atelectasis of S^3a, and small cavity changes in the upper field.

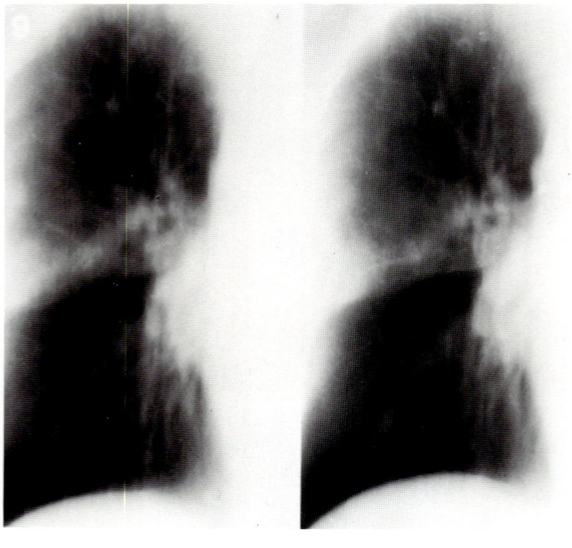

57.3 Right chest tomograms (right: 8 cm from the back, left: 9 cm from the back). In addition to the described changes, irregularity of the wall of the truncus intermedius is visible.

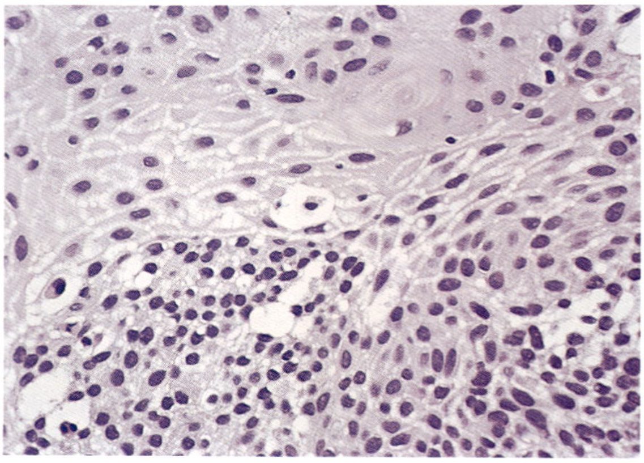

57.4 Pathological findings of the biopsied lung. Note well-differentiated epidermoid carcinoma. Tumour cells are sufficiently differentiated to form such structures as stratum lucidum and stratum corneum. Intercellular bridges are prominent.

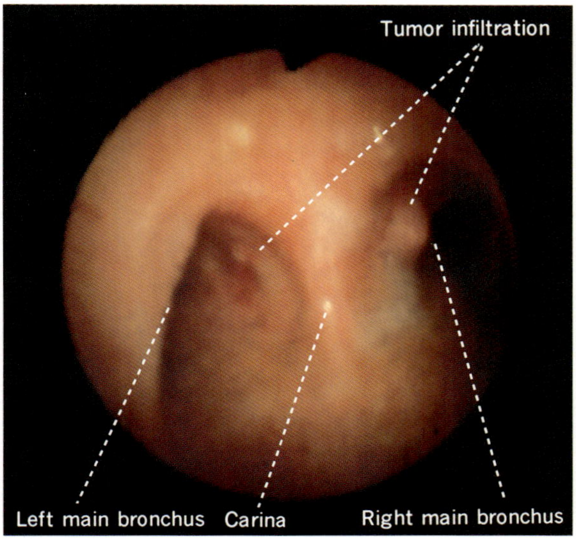

57.5 Bronchoscopic findings at the carina. The tumour invaded the anterolateral part of the bifurcation, which as a result is oedematous and widened.

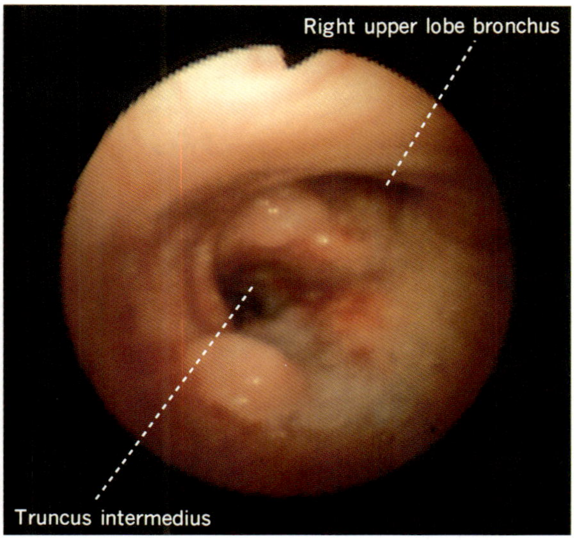

57.6 Bronchoscopic findings in the RUL bronchus and truncus intermedius. The yellow nodular mass is located on the membranous portion of the main bronchus. Bifurcation into the RUL bronchus and truncus intermedius is widened because of tumour invasion.

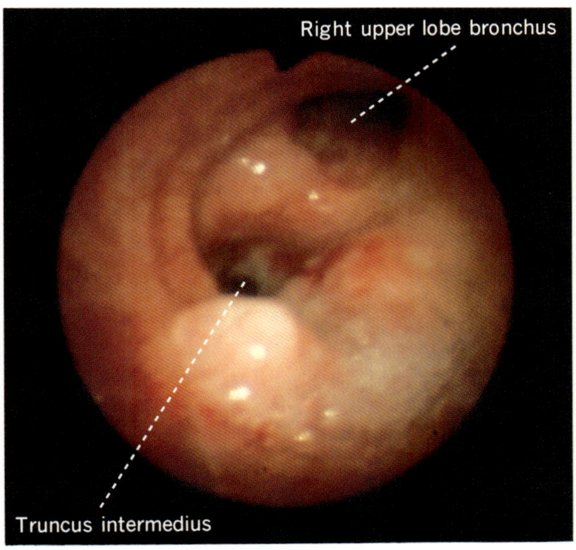

57.7 Close-up of **57.6**. The tumour invades the membranous portion as well. The mucosa is generally reddened.

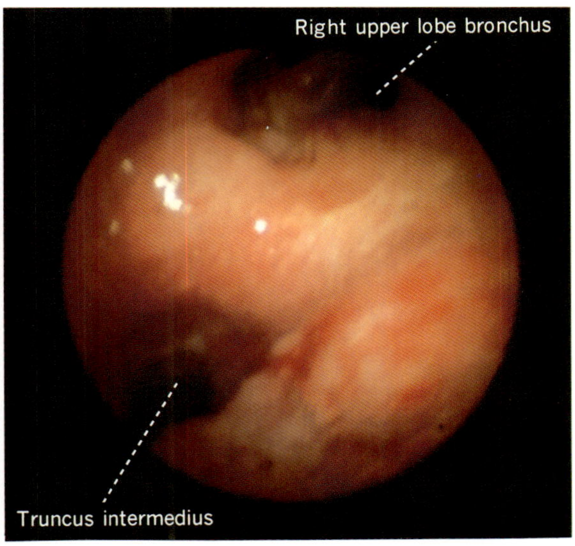

57.8 Close-up of **57.7**. The tumour invasion is strikingly seen, involving the membranous portion, the bifurcation, and the orifice of the RUL bronchus. Normal mucosa is almost replaced by tumour invasion. Biopsy confirmed a definite diagnosis of epidermoid carcinoma.

Case 58: Epidermoid carcinoma in a 68-year-old male.

The patient, who complained of a non-productive cough, was proved to have an epidermoid carcinoma of the lung, originating from right S^6.

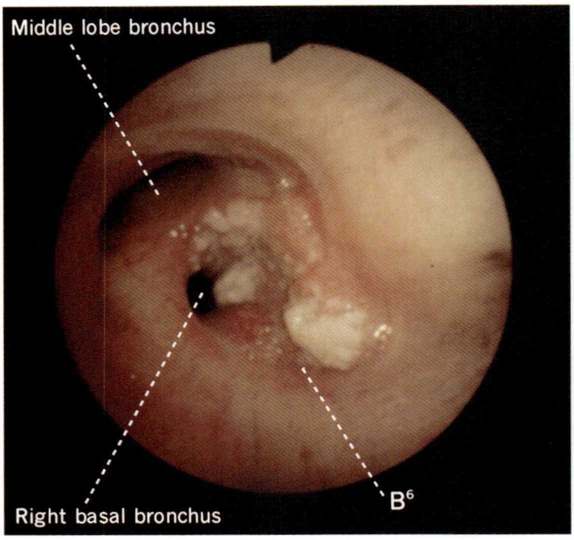

58.1 Bronchoscopic findings in the RML and RLL bronchi. The orifice of B^6 is occluded by a white tumour, which has also invaded the orifice of the RLL bronchus as well as the bifurcation into the RML bronchus.

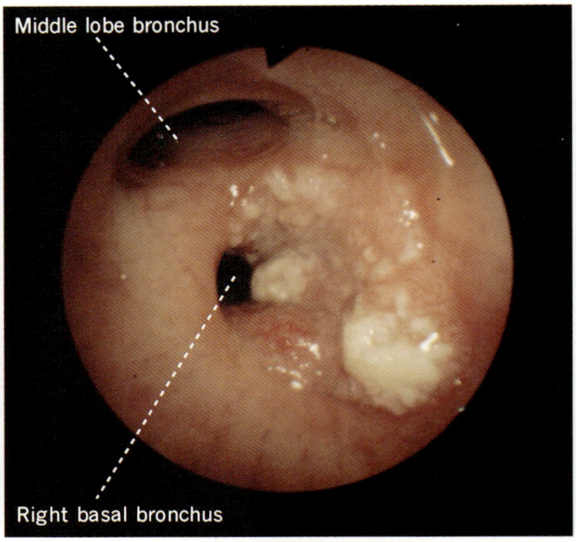

58.2 Close-up of **58.1**. All bifurcations are oedematous and widened and the white tumour is located over the orifices of B^6 and the RLL bronchus.

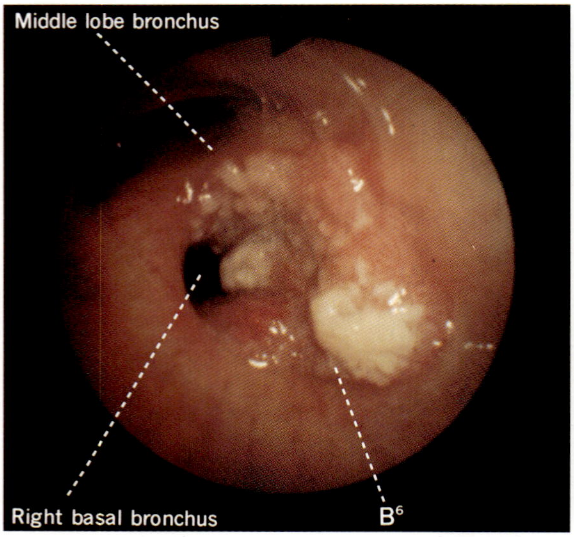

58.3 Close-up of **58.2**. Vascular engorgement on the mucosa of the white tumour is visible.

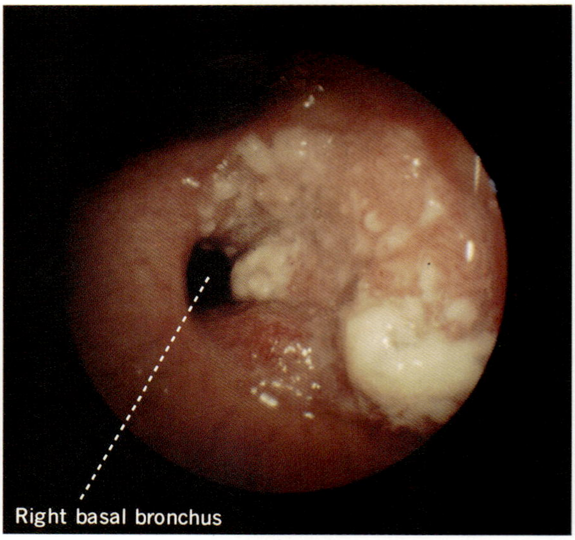

58.4 Close-up of **58.3**. The white tumour is associated with reddened, swollen mucosa and has dilated vessels on it. The orifice of B^6 is extremely stenotic.

Case 59: Epidermoid carcinoma in a 67-year-old male.

This is a patient with epidermoid lung carcinoma of left S^3.

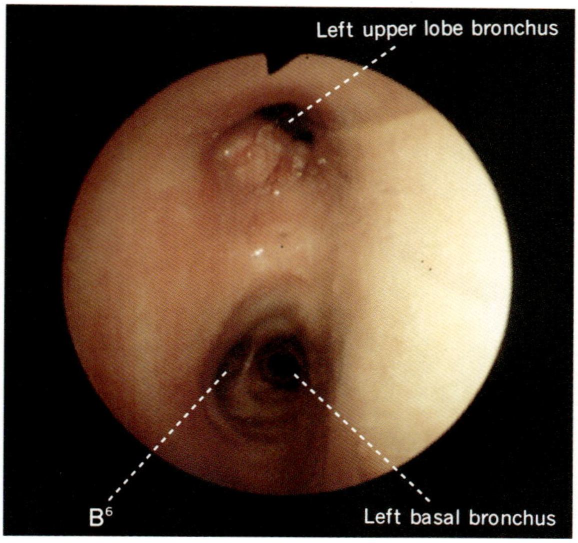

59.1 Bronchoscopic findings in the LUL and LLL bronchi. Bifurcation is oedematous and widened and a tumour with an irregular surface is located at the orifice of the LUL bronchus.

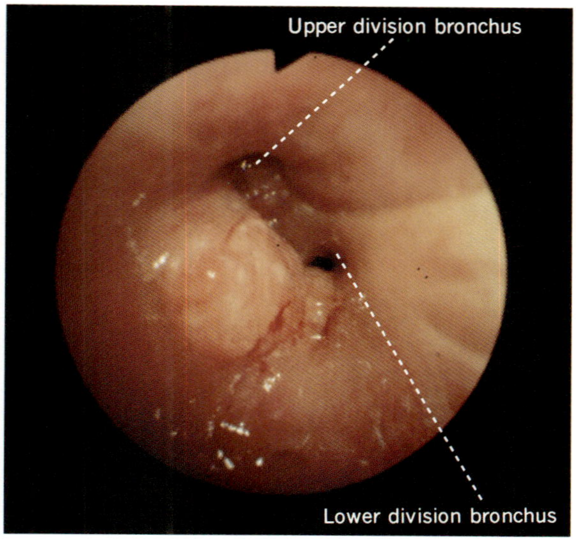

59.2 Bronchoscopic findings in the LUL bronchus. The white tumour accompanying the dilated vessels has occluded the orifice. The orifice of the upper division bronchus is patent although narrowed, while that of the lower division bronchus is almost totally obstructed.

Case 60: Epidermoid carcinoma in a 70-year-old male.

This is a patient with early epidermoid carcinoma of the lung.

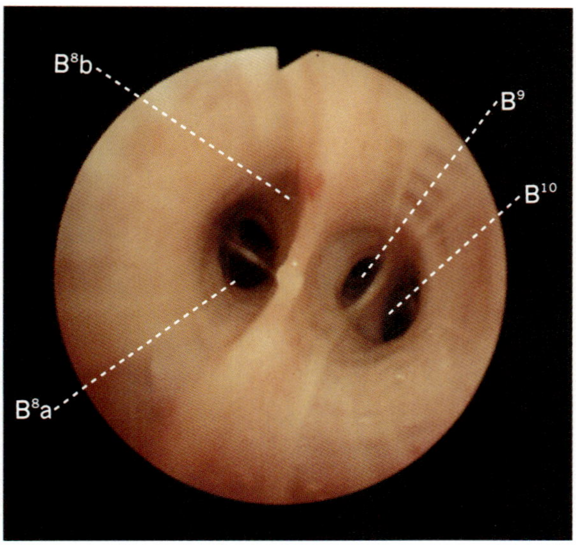

60.1 Bronchoscopic findings in the right basal bronchus. This is a nodule on the bifurcation into B^8 and $B^9 + B^{10}$. Apart from these no abnormalities were visible.

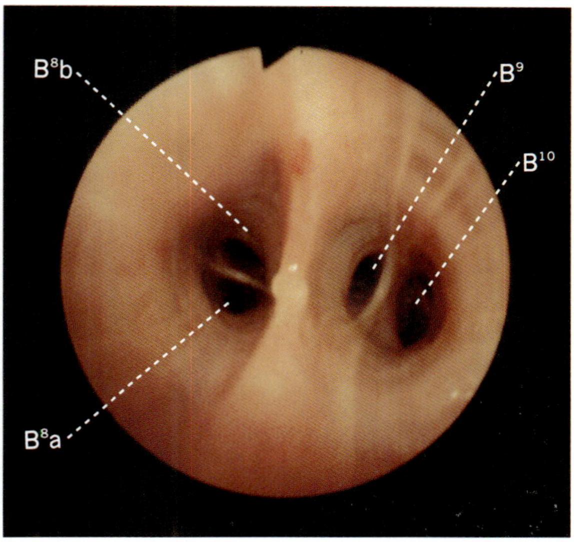

60.2 Close-up of **60.1**. The nodule at the middle of the bifurcation was found to be an epidermoid carcinoma at biopsy.

Case 61: Epidermoid carcinoma in a 55-year-old male.

This is a patient with epidermoid carcinoma of the lung protruding from the left upper lobe.

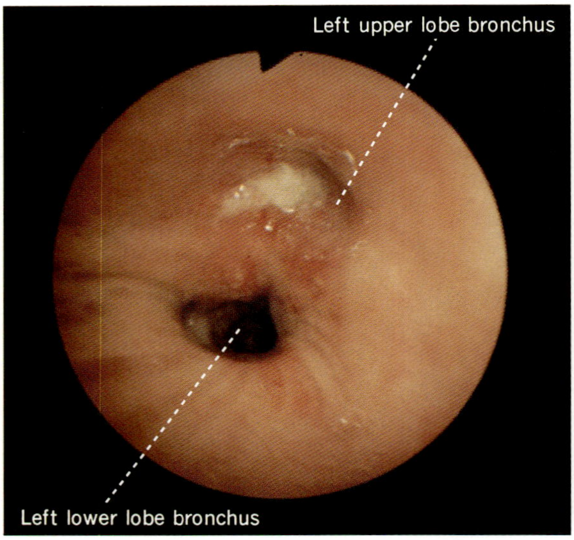

61.1 Bronchoscopic findings in the LUL and LLL bronchi. The bifurcation into the LUL and LLL bronchi is markedly swollen because of tumour invasion. The orifice of the LUL bronchus is occluded by the tumour, which is covered with white necrotic tissue, and the surrounding mucosa is oedematous.

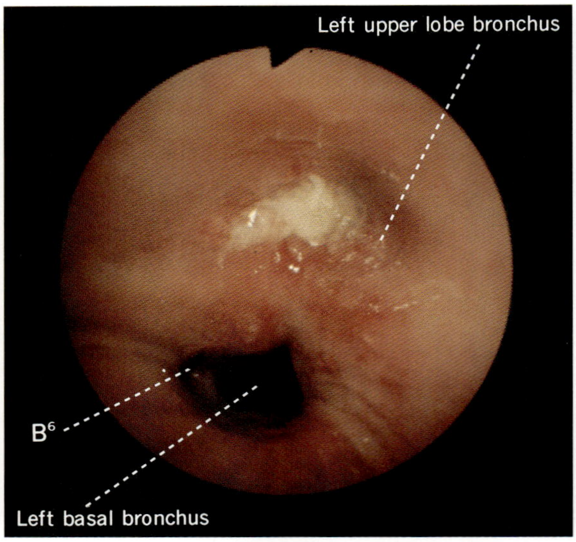

61.2 Close-up of the tumour. The orifice of the LUL bronchus is totally obstructed by the tumour, which has nodular metastases on the bifurcation.

Case 62: Epidermoid carcinoma in a 62-year-old male.

This patient had an epidermoid carcinoma of the lung originating from the LUL bronchus.

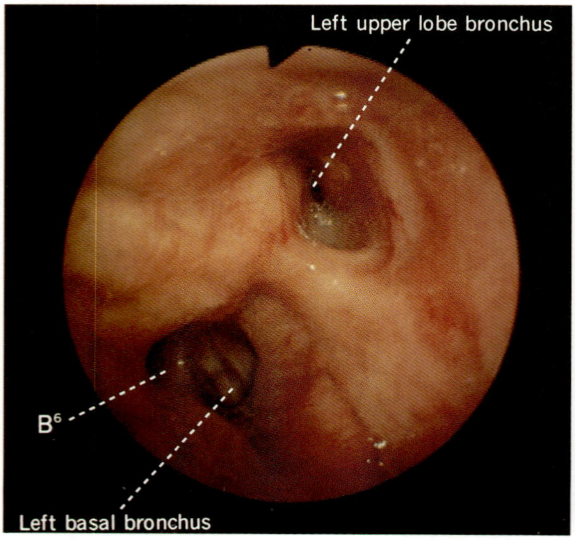

62.1 Bronchoscopic findings in the LUL and LLL bronchi. The bifurcation is widened and the flattened elevation of the mucosa suggests tumour invasion, starting from the lateral part of the bifurcation to the lateral wall of the main bronchus.

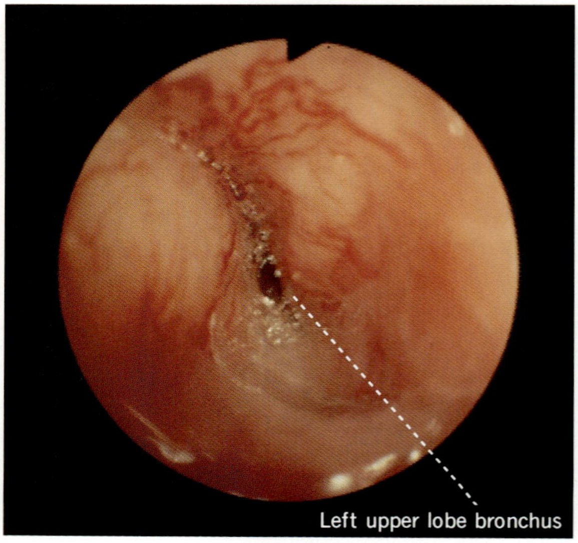

62.2 Close-up of the LUL bronchus. The orifice of the LUL bronchus is almost totally occluded by the tumour; note the air bubbles coming out. The mucosal vessels are prominently engorged.

Case 63: Epidermoid carcinoma in a 54-year-old male.

This patient had an epidermoid carcinoma of the lung originating from the LUL bronchus.

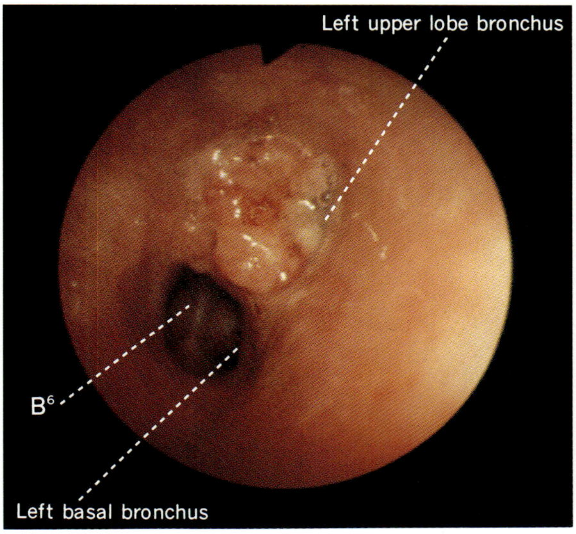

63.1 Bronchoscopic findings in the LUL and LLL bronchi. The bronchial mucosa is generally reddened and oedematous. The nodular mass obstructs the orifice of the LUL bronchus.

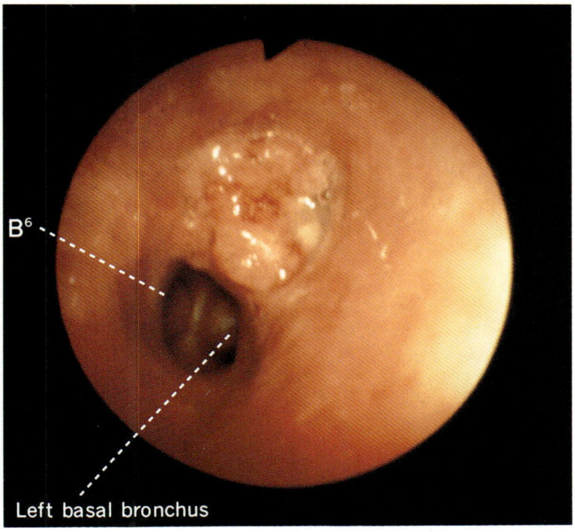

63.2 Close-up of **63.1**. The tumour with an irregular surface spreads from the orifice of the LUL bronchus to that of the LLL bronchus.

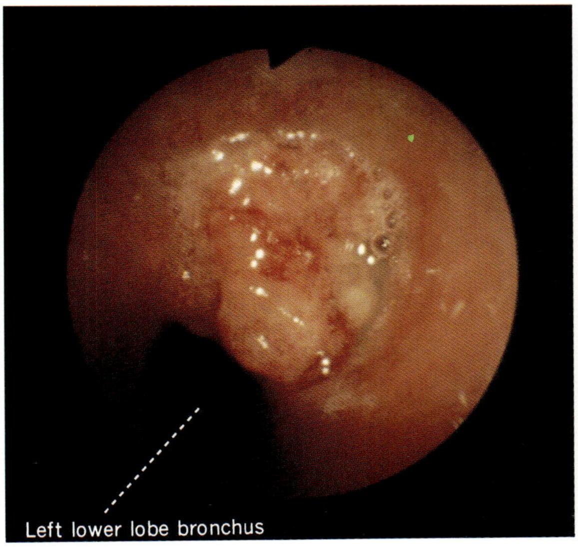

63.3 Close-up of the tumour. It is partly covered with a white coat; the vessels on the tumour and the surrounding mucosa are dilated.

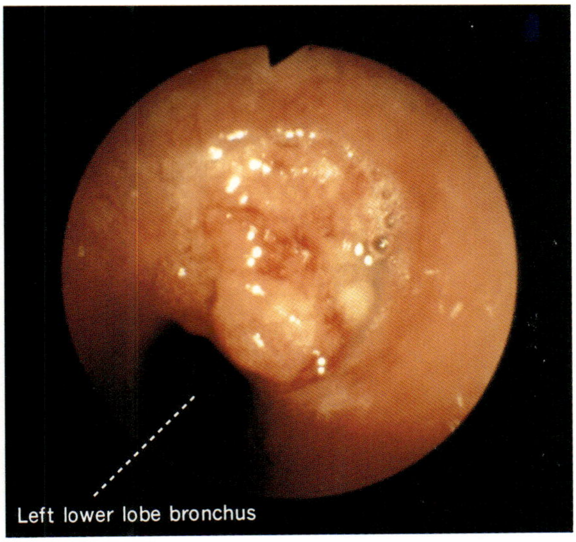

63.4 A further close-up of the tumour. Nodular lesions of varying sizes, covered with white necrotic tissue are visible.

Case 64: Epidermoid carcinoma in a 70-year-old male.

This patient has early epidermoid carcinoma of the lung in left B^3.

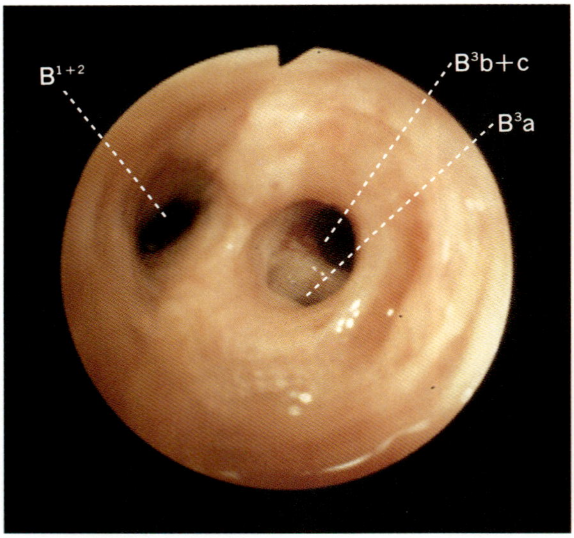

64.1 Bronchoscopic findings in the left upper-division bronchus. The bifurcation between B^3 and B^{1+2} appear almost normal but irregular to a slight degree. A protruding lesion with haemorrhage on the bifurcation of the subsegmental bronchi of B^3 is visible.

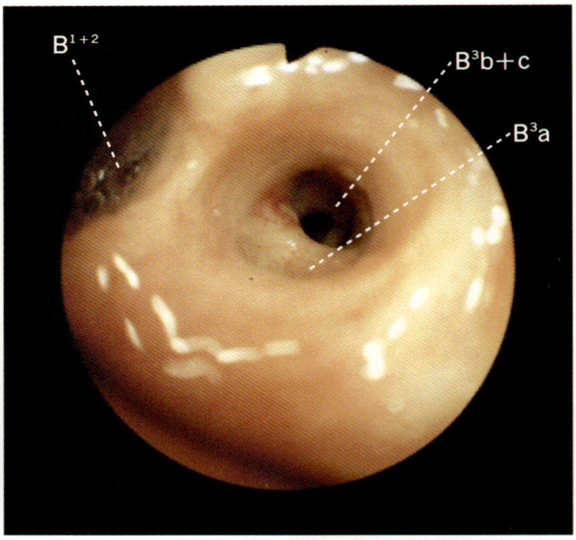

64.2 Bronchoscopic findings in left B^3. On the bifurcation of the subsegmental bronchi of B^3, there is a small protruding lesion with haemorrhage, which at biopsy was proved to be an epidermoid carcinoma.

Case 65: Epidermoid carcinoma in a 49-year-old male.

This patient had an epidermoid carcinoma arising from left B^9.

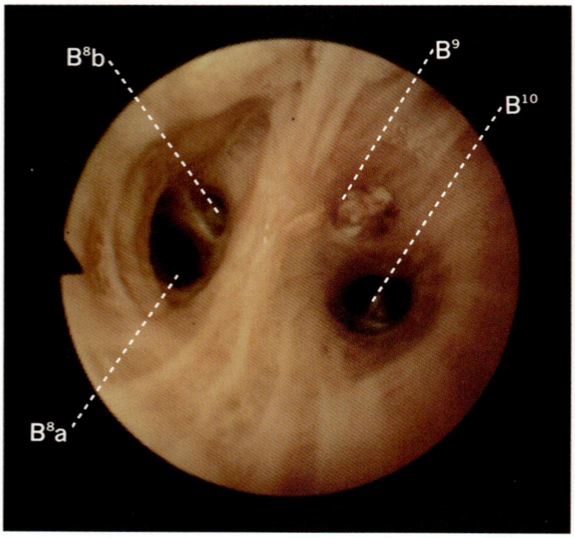

65.1 Bronchoscopic findings in left B^8, B^9 and B^{10}. Bifurcation between B^8 and B^{9+10} remains intact, although a little widened. The orifice of B^9 is occluded by a white-coated tumour.

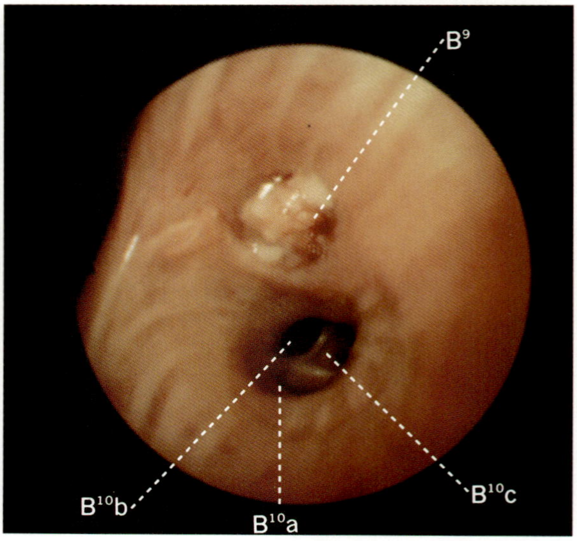

65.2 Bronchoscopic findings in left B^9 and B^{10}. The orifice of B^9 is completely occluded by a white-coated tumour, although the surrounding mucosa remains unchanged.

Case 66: Epidermoid carcinoma in a 59-year-old male.

The patient complained of a cough. Chest radiograph showed bilateral hilar lymphadenopathy as well as linear shadows radiating from the hilum.

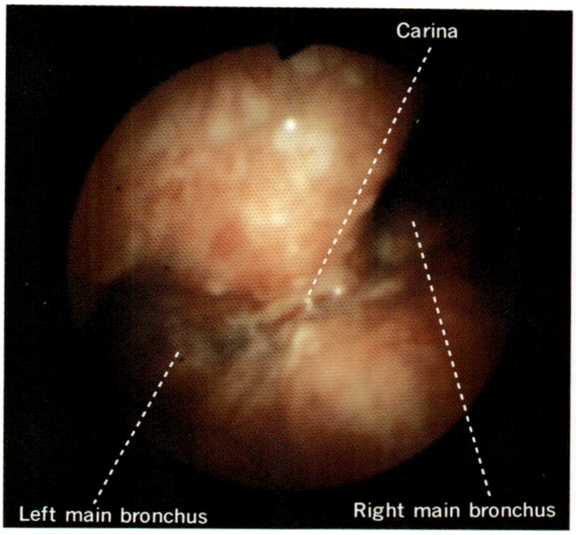

66.1 Bronchoscopic findings of the carina. The bifurcation is prominently widened as well as reddened and swollen, suggesting that the submucosa has been invaded by the tumour.

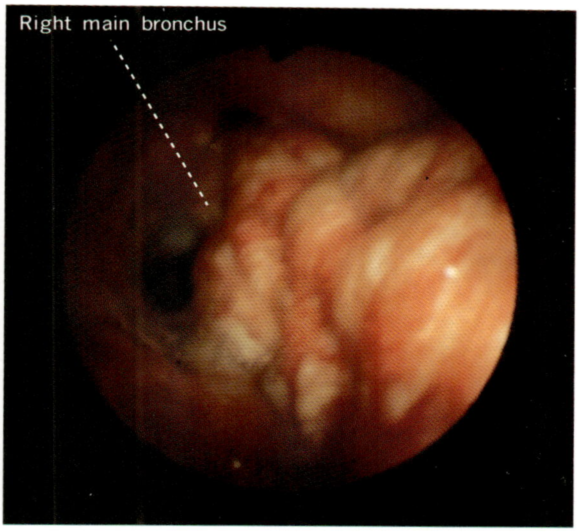

66.2 Bronchoscopic findings in the right main bronchus. The membranous portion is covered with a nodular mass, with vascular dilatation and partial white coatings.

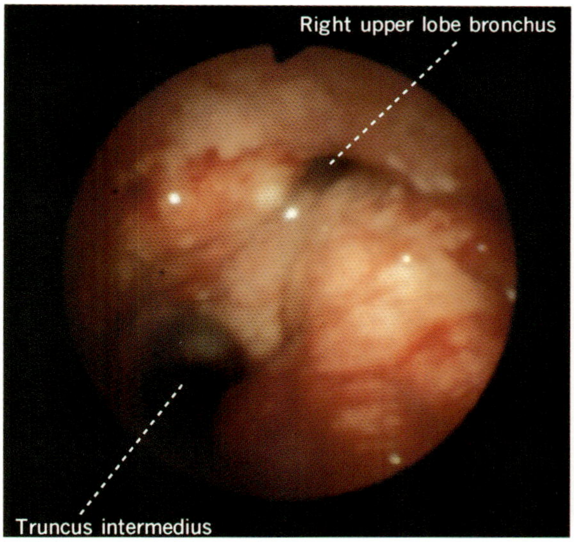

66.3 Bronchoscopic findings in the RUL bronchus and truncus intermedius. The bifurcation into the RUL is strikingly widened, narrowing its orifice.

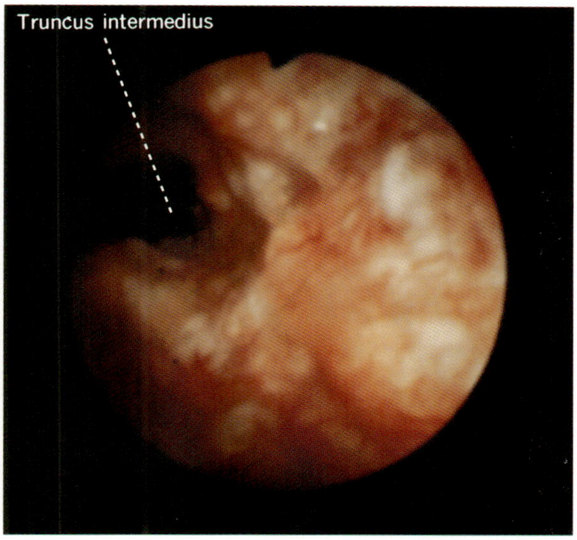

66.4 Bronchoscopic findings of the truncus intermedius. The tumour has invaded the membranous portion and lateral wall, narrowing the lumen diameter to less than half. The mucosal vessels are markedly dilated and white necrotic tissue is visible.

Case 67: Epidermoid carcinoma in a 57-year-old male.

This patient had an epidermoid carcinoma of the lung, forming a spherical mass with smooth surface at the orifice of the left upper-division bronchus.

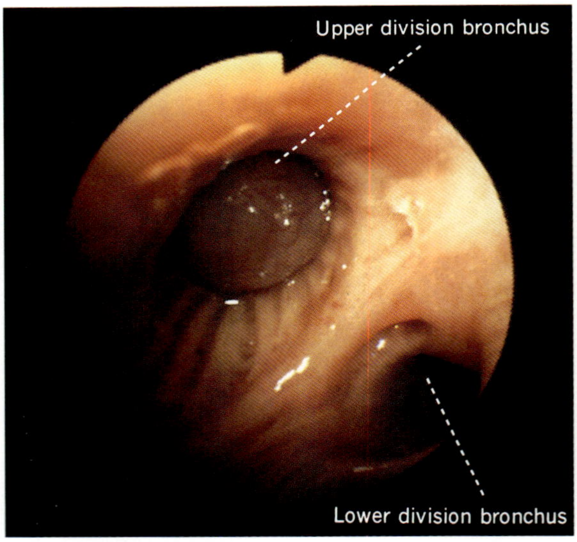

67.1 Bronchoscopic findings in the LUL bronchus. A purple spherical mass with a network of vessels on its surface was located in the upper-division bronchus.

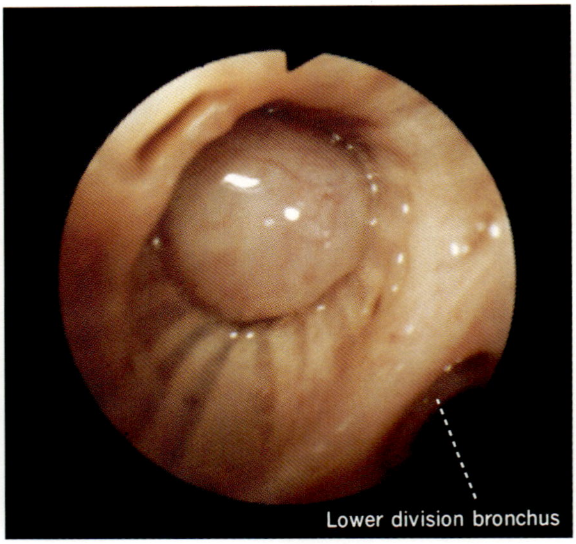

67.2 Bronchoscopic findings in the upper-division bronchus. The tumour has a smooth surface, within which the vessels are visible. The bifurcation into the lower-division bronchus is rather widened.

Case 68: Epidermoid carcinoma in a 72-year-old male.

This patient had an epidermoid carcinoma which originated from left B^5; polymyositis and interstitial pneumonia were also present.

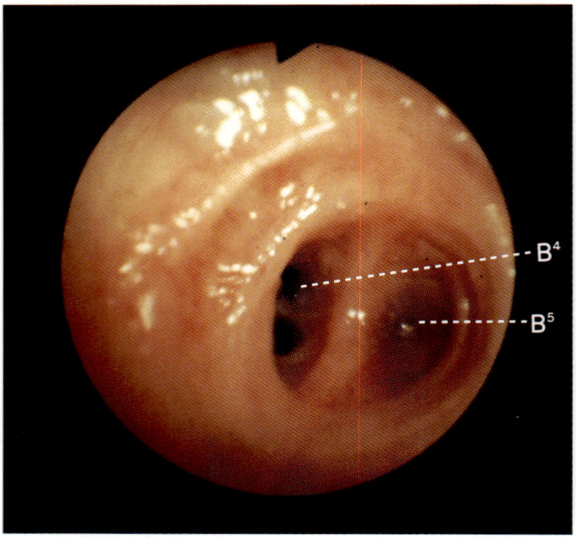

68.1 Bronchoscopic findings in the left lower-division bronchus. The bifurcation between B^4 and B^5 is obviously widened. The orifice of B^5 is obstructed by the tumour, the surface of which contains bloody secretion.

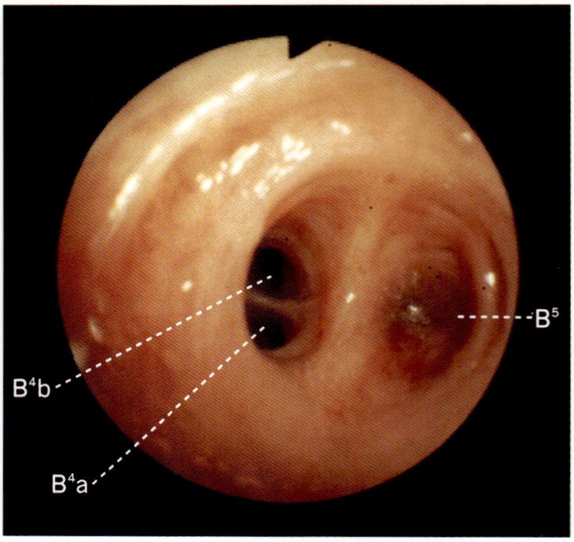

68.2 Close-up of **68.1**. The bifurcation appears oedematous. At the orifice of B^5 is a tumour with dilated vessels on its surface.

Case 69: Epidermoid carcinoma in a 66-year-old male.

This patient had an epidermoid carcinoma of the lung arising from the LUL bronchus. He complained of a non-productive cough.

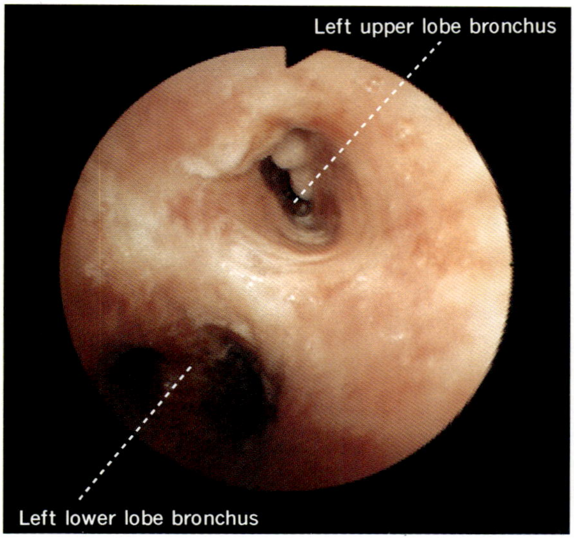

69.1 Bronchoscopic findings in the LUL and LLL bronchi. The bifurcation between the LUL and LLL bronchi is widened and the basal bronchus as well as B^6 are narrowed. A white tumour is situated around the orifice of the LUL bronchus.

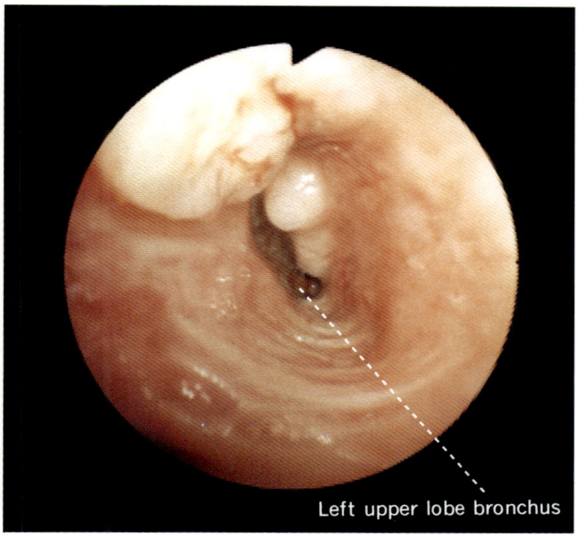

69.2 Bronchoscopic findings in the LUL bronchus. The white tumour has a relatively smooth surface.

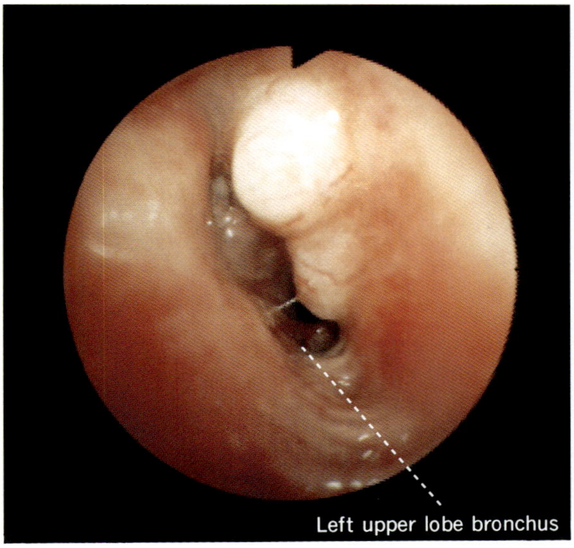

69.3 Close-up of **69.2**. The white tumour with a smooth surface sits on the right side and the mucosa on the other side is also protruding and results from tumour invasion. The small vessels are visible through the surface of the tumour.

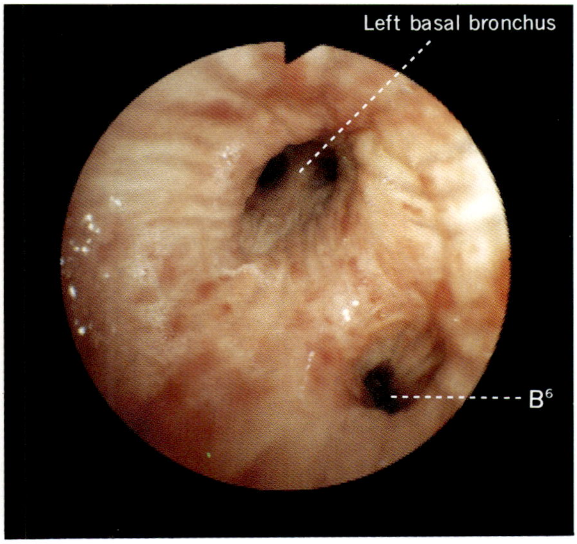

69.4 Bronchoscopic findings in the LLL bronchus. Orifices of both B^6 and the basal bronchus have irregular walls with oedematous mucosal changes. The bifurcation into B^6 is strikingly widened. These findings are compatible with submucosal invasion by the tumour.

Case 70: Epidermoid carcinoma in a 70-year-old male.

This patient had an epidermoid carcinoma of the LUL bronchus showing polypoid growth, initially presumed to be carcinoid based.

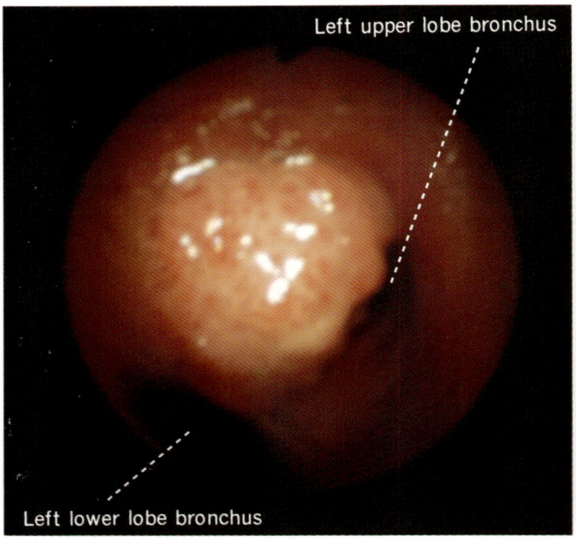

70.1 Bronchoscopic findings in the LUL bronchus. A tumour with a nodular strawberry-like surface. There is a narrow space on the right side.

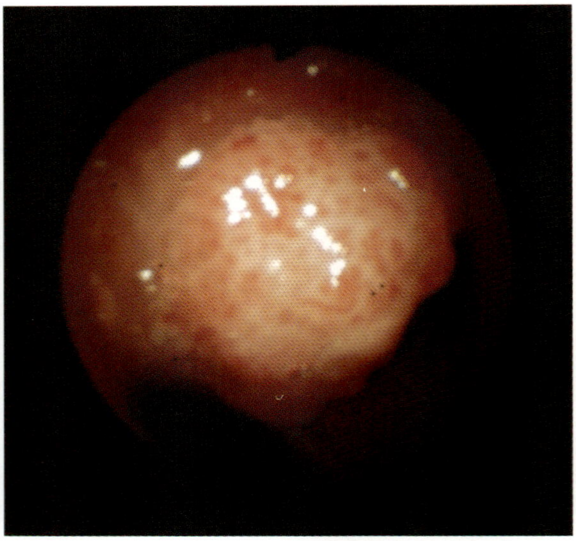

70.2 Close-up of the tumour in **70.1**. The surface has protruding lesions of varying sizes, giving it a strawberry-like appearance.

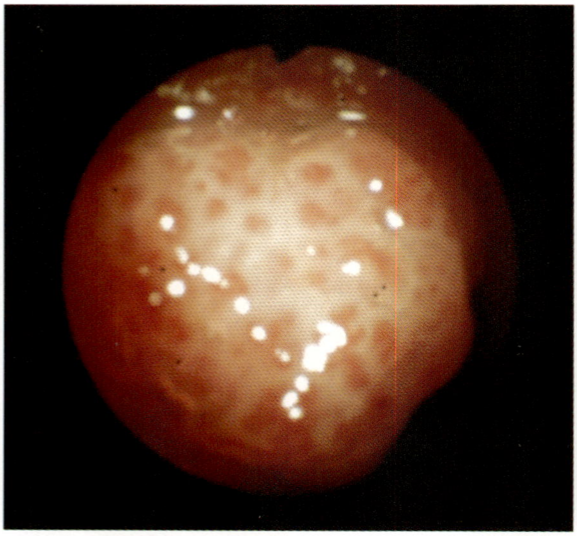

70.3 Further close-up of the tumour. The milky necrotic tissue is dotted with several red nodules. Biopsy confirmed the diagnosis.

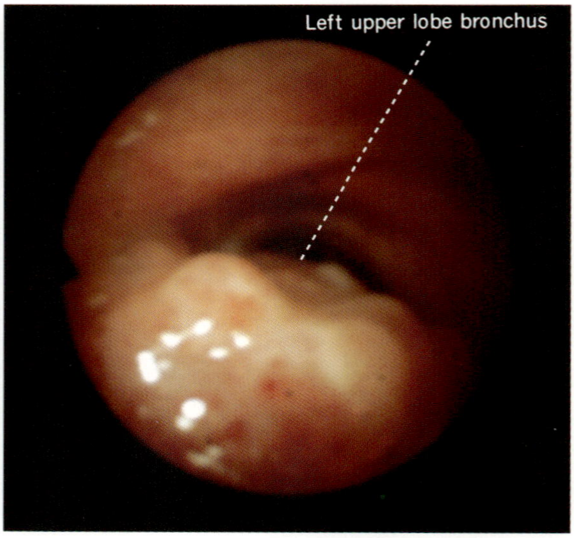

70.4 The space between the tumour and the bronchial wall is visible. Note the tumour continuing distally.

Case 71: Epidermoid carcinoma in a 75-year-old male.

This patient had an epidermoid carcinoma that occluded the orifice of the RUL bronchus. Two courses of chemotherapy, which consisted of cis-platinum and mitomycin C, were prescribed, resulting in necrosis of the bifurcation into the RUL bronchus.

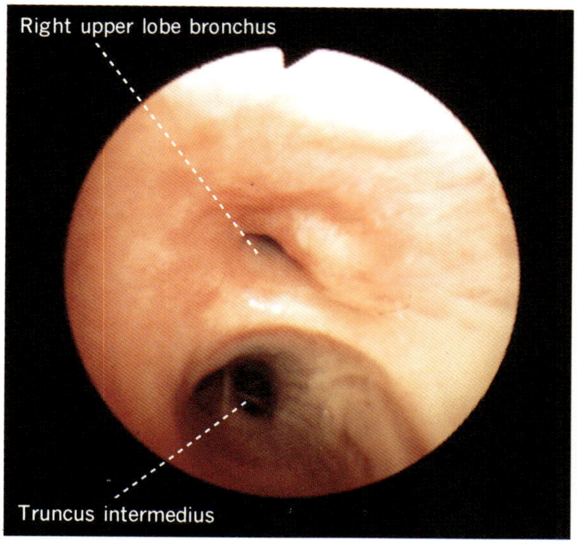

71.1 Bronchoscopic findings in the RUL bronchus and truncus intermedius. The bifurcation is rather widened and the orifice of the RUL bronchus is narrowed.

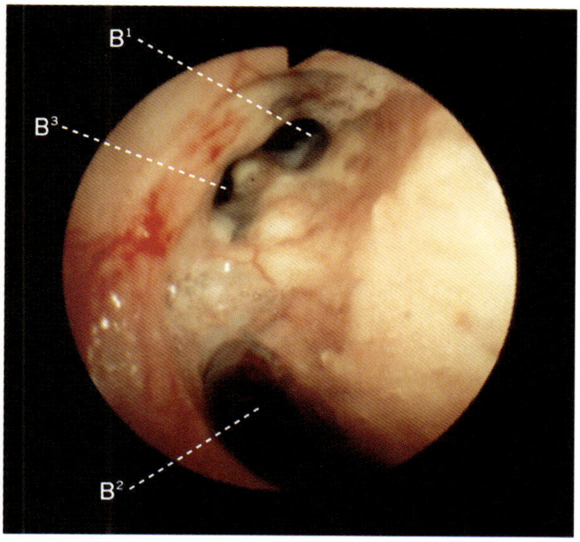

71.2 Bronchoscopic findings at the bifurcation into the RUL bronchus. The bifurcation between B^1 and B^3 is necrotic.

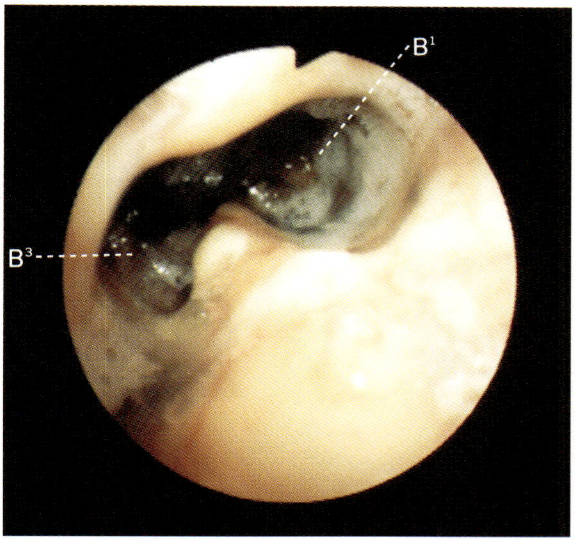

71.3 Bronchoscopic findings in right B^1 and B^3. The bifurcation between them has been replaced by necrotic black tissue.

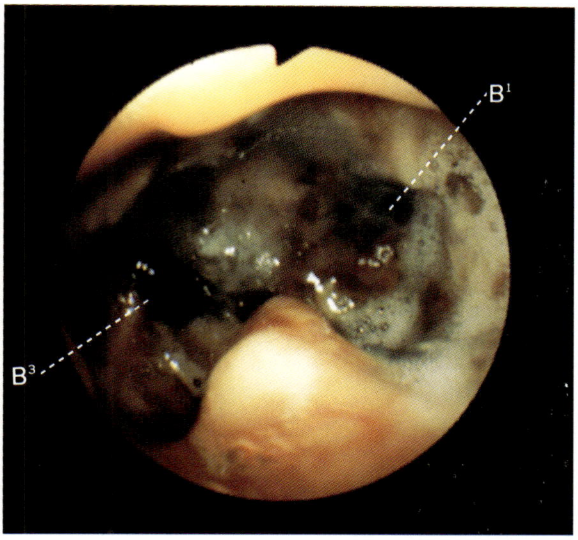

71.4 Close-up of **71.3**. The orifices of B^1 and B^3 are hardly visible through the mucus and necrotic tissue. Massive haemoptysis may occur and should not be ignored.

Case 72: Epidermoid carcinoma (poorly differentiated) in a 61-year-old male.

The patient noticed lympadenopathy of the right side of the neck in October 1979. He visited the clinic with a persistent cough in January 1980. He had experienced haemoptysis since May and dyspnoea on exertion since July. He was hospitalised. He had a history of sinusitis for which he underwent surgery at 24 years of age and of aortic stenosis at 35 years of age. He stated that he smoked 6,000 cigarettes per year.

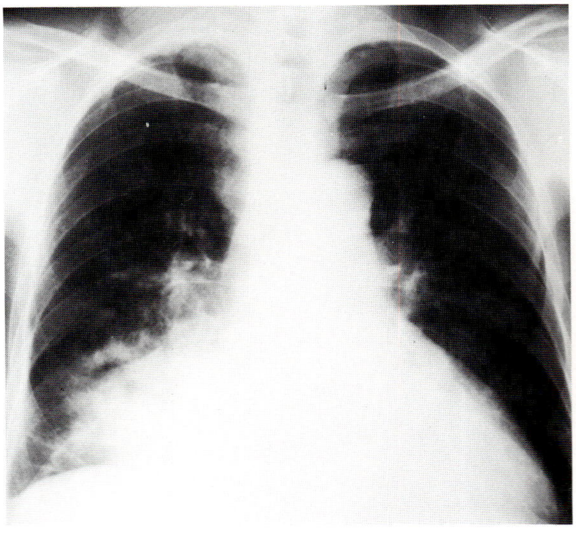

72.1 Posteroanterior chest radiograph. Cardiomegaly and right pleural effusion are present. An enlargement of the right hilum associated with a pneumonic infiltrate in the right lower zone is visible, obliterating the right heart border. Lymphadenopathy of the right side of the neck may be present.

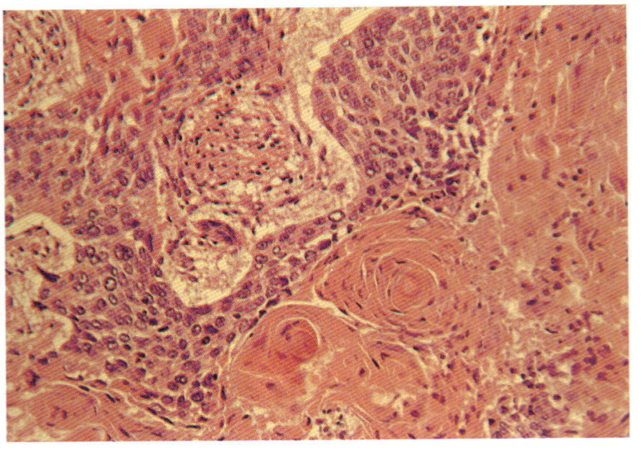

72.2 Histopathology of the transbronchial lung biopsy. The bronchial lumen is packed with epidermoid carcinoma, forming the cancer pearls. The tumour cells look identical, although some cells appear spindle-shaped.

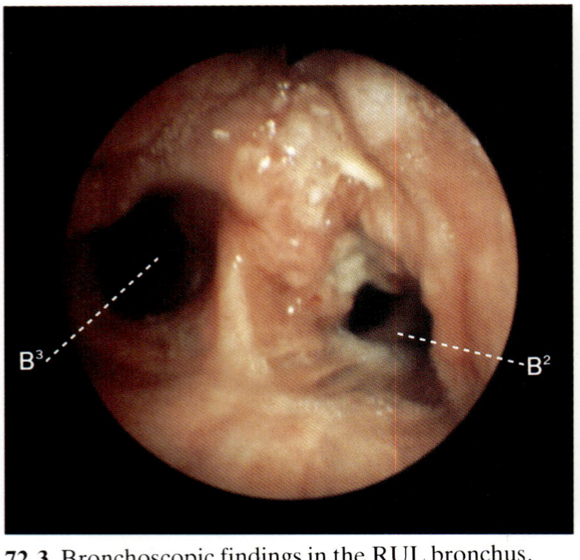

72.3 Bronchoscopic findings in the RUL bronchus. The orifice of B^1 is occluded by the tumour and that of B^2 is stenotic as well.

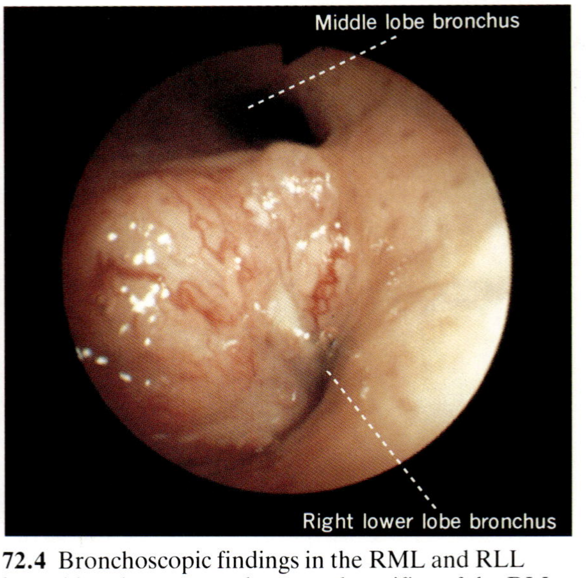

72.4 Bronchoscopic findings in the RML and RLL bronchi. A huge mass obstructs the orifice of the RLL bronchus which is still patent minimally. The tumour has an irregular surface with visible vessels beneath it.

Case 73: Large cell carcinoma of the lung (poorly differentiated) in a 56-year-old female.

The patient, who had been asthmatic for 10 years, presented with haemoptysis once or twice a month since January 1980. Increasing dyspnoea since June and worsening haemoptysis once a week with left-sided chest pain since July prompted her to visit the clinic. She was hospitalised in an orthopnoeic state in September.

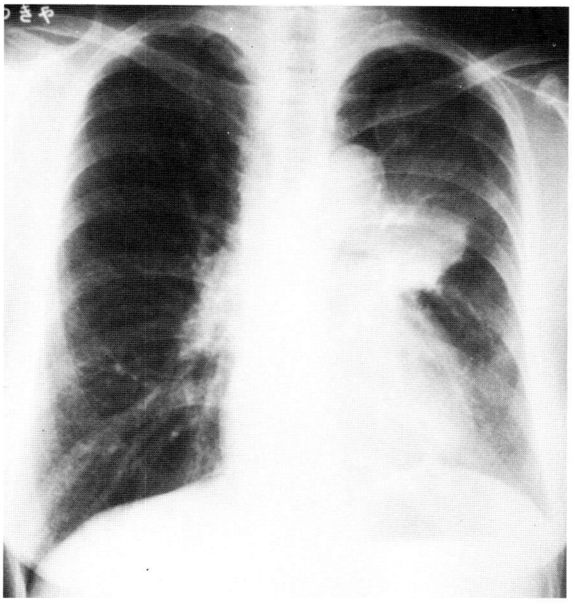

73.1 Posteroanterior chest radiograph. A mass shadow, 4 cm in diameter, is located at the left hilum, with atelectasis of left upper lobe.

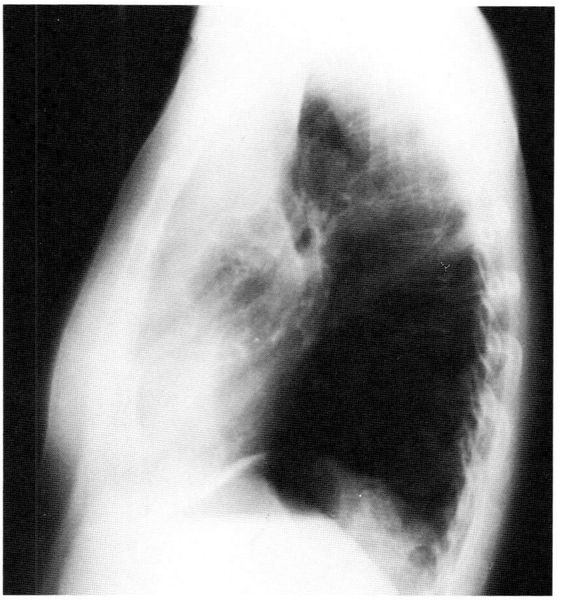

73.2 Lateral chest radiograph. Atelectasis of the left upper lobe is visible.

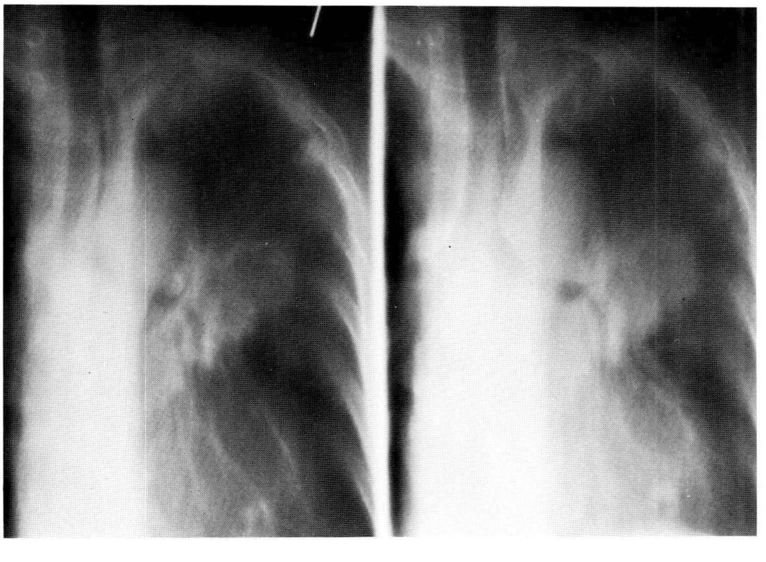

73.3 Chest tomogram (left: 7 cm from the back; right: 8 cm from the back). The LUL bronchus is occluded, while the LLL bronchus is partly patent.

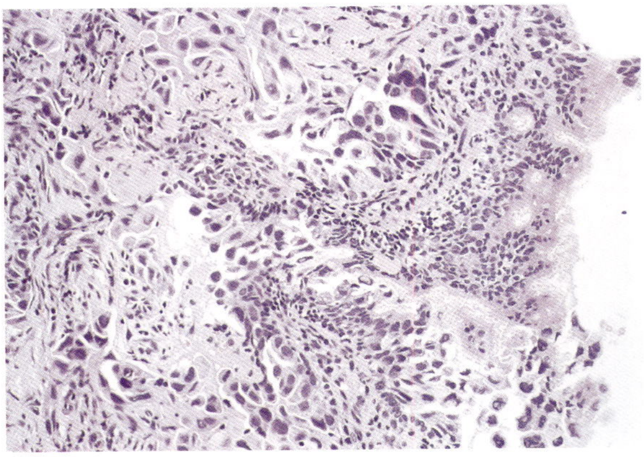

73.4 Histopathology of the biopsied lung. The cluster of tumour cells infiltrates the fibrous tissue. They have pleomorphic nuclei and abundant cytoplasm. The intercellular bridges are not recognised.

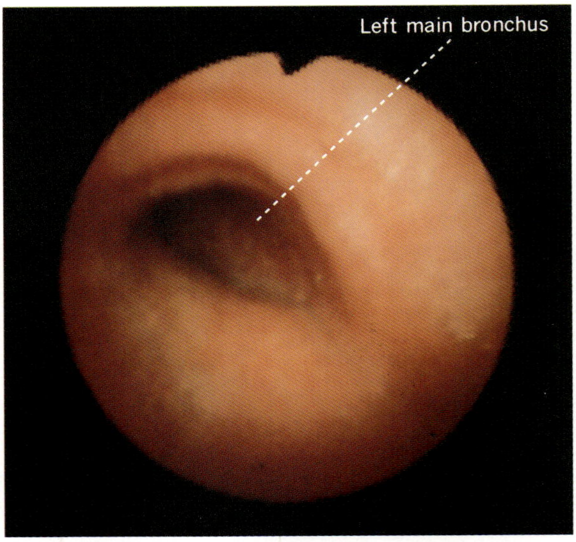

73.5 Bronchoscopic findings of the left main bronchus. The mucosa is reddened and swollen, narrowing the lumen of the bronchus.

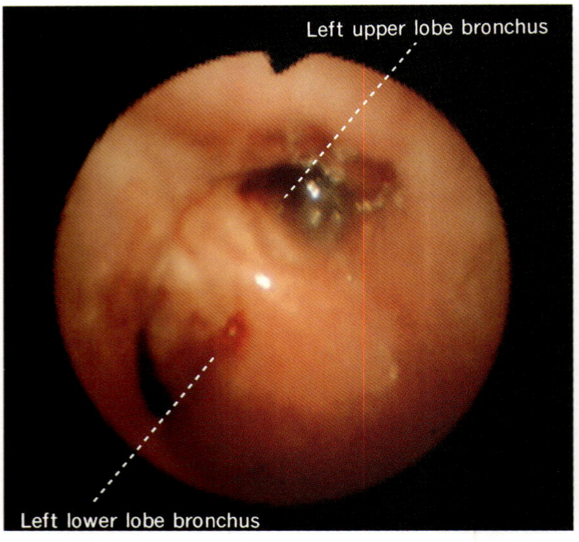

73.6 Bronchoscopic findings in the LUL and LLL bronchi. The bifurcation is strikingly widened and the mucosa is generally reddened and swollen. Air bubbles are coming out from the orifice of the LUL bronchus, suggesting its minimal patency. The orifice of the LLL bronchus is narrowed.

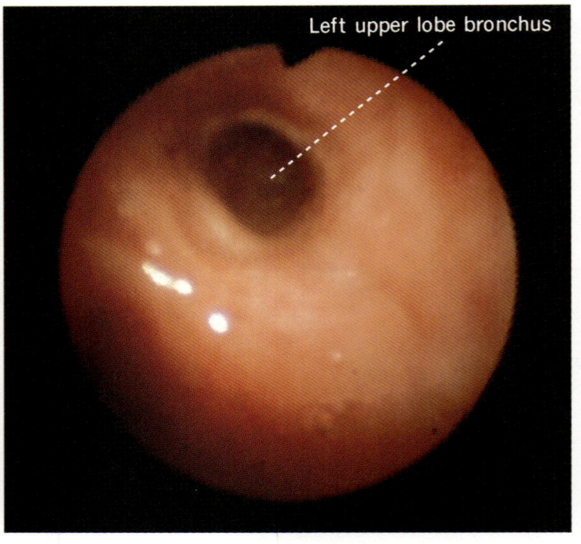

73.7 Bronchoscopic findings in the LUL bronchus. The bifurcation as well as the surrounding mucosa is oedematous, associated with the stenotic orifice. Biopsy of this lesion revealed large-cell anaplastic carcinoma.

Case 74: Large-cell carcinoma in a 75-year-old male.

This patient had a large-cell carcinoma arising from right S^2. He complained of a non-productive cough.

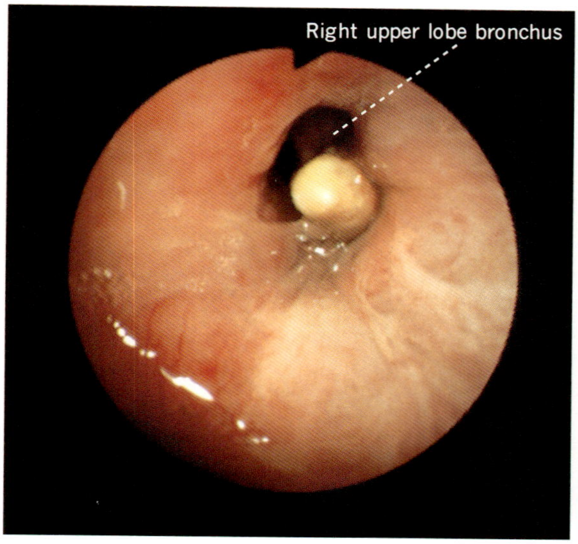

74.1 Bronchoscopic findings in the RUL bronchus. A yellow polypoid tumour protrudes from the orifice. The surrounding mucosa appears irregular and oedematous, with vascular engorgement.

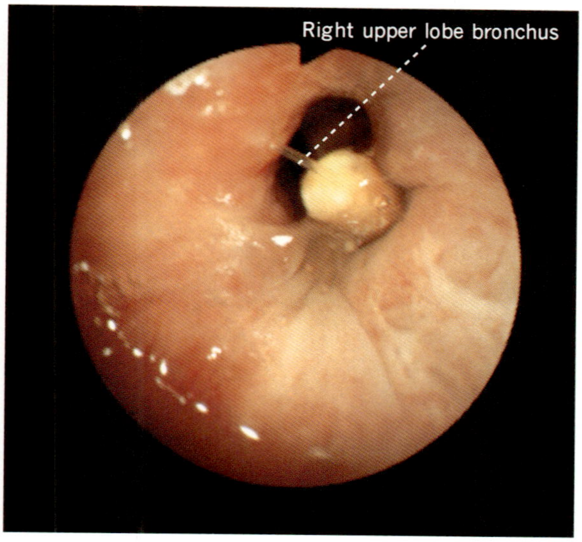

74.2 Close-up of **74.1**. Oedema and tumour invasion have involved the surrounding mucosa. The RUL bronchus is markedly narrowed at the bifurcation.

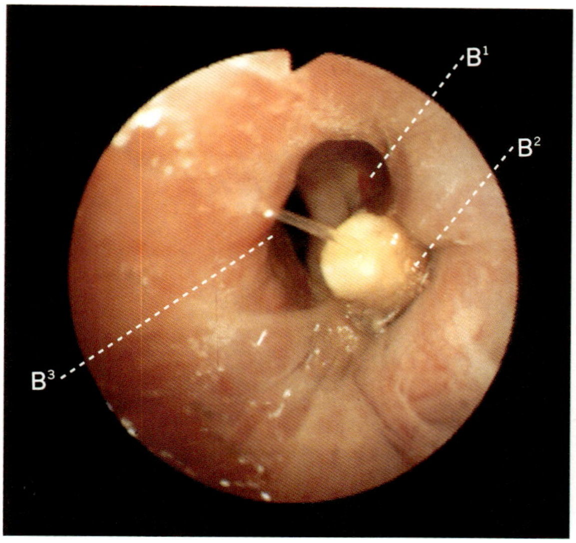

74.3 Further close-up of **74.2**. Mucous secretion has attached itself to the tumour.

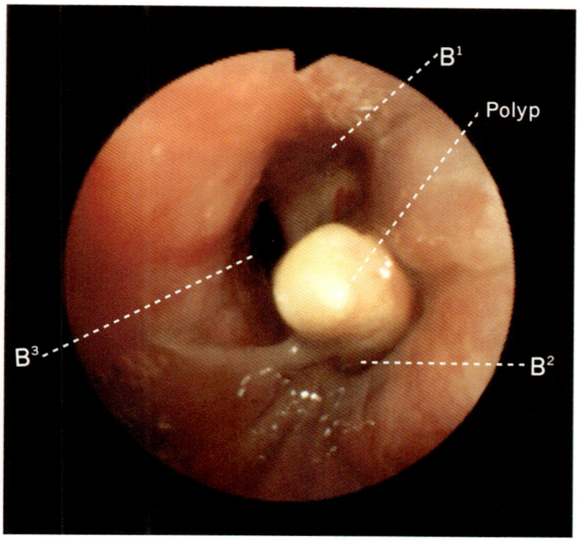

74.4 Further close-up of **74.3**. The yellow necrotic tissue covers the surface of the tumour, beyond which the orifice of B^3 is visible.

Case 75: Large-cell carcinoma in a 62-year-old male.

This patient had a large-cell lung carcinoma of right B^6.

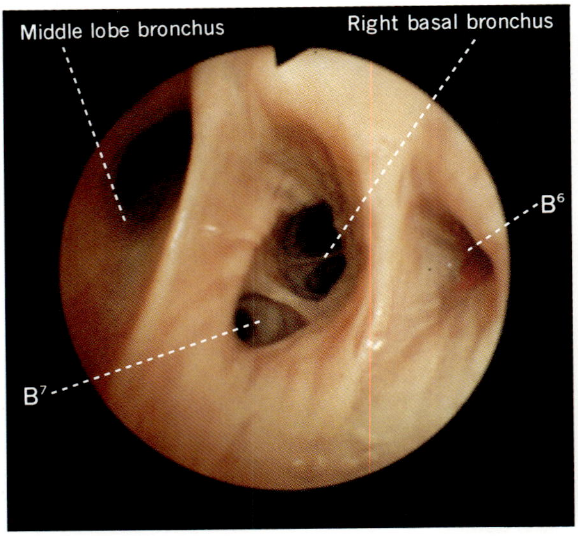

75.1 Bronchoscopic findings in the RLL bronchus. The bifurcation into B^6 is rather widened, despite leaving the surrounding mucosa intact. A red tumour is visible in B^6.

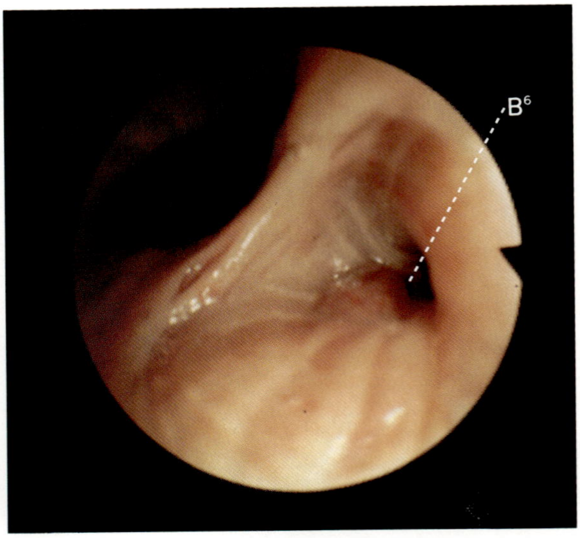

75.2 Bronchoscopic findings in B^6. There is a tumour with abundant vessels, which at biopsy was proved to be a large-cell carcinoma.

Case 76: Large-cell carcinoma in a 60-year-old male.

This patient had a large-cell lung carcinoma which arose from the right main bronchus and truncus intermedius.

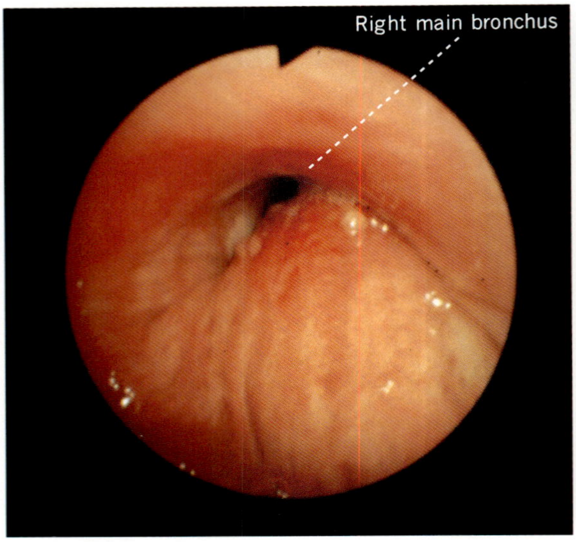

76.1 Bronchoscopic findings in the right main bronchus. The main bronchus is grossly narrowed by protrusion of the membranous portion proximally from the bifurcation into the RUL bronchus. The surface of the tumour appears nodular and is covered with the white necrotic tissue.

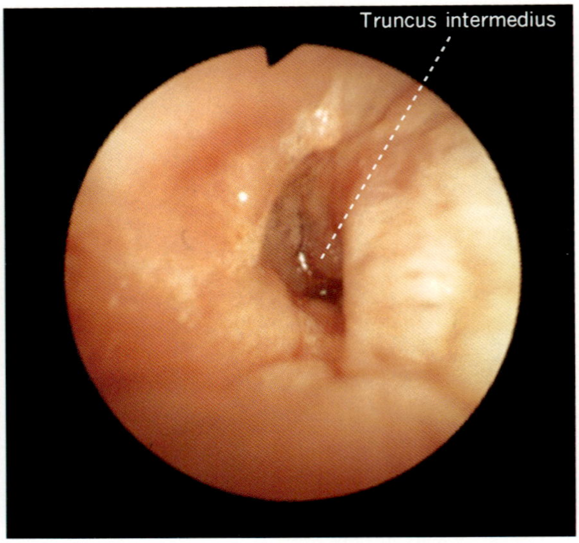

76.2 Bronchoscopic findings in the truncus intermedius after two courses of chemotherapy. Whereas the tumour previously located at the orifice of the right main bronchus has disappeared, the truncus intermedius is occluded by the nodular tumour.

9 Primary lung cancer (adenocarcinoma)

Case 77: Adenocarcinoma in a 50-year-old male.

This patient, with a history of smoking 6,000 cigarettes per year, had been well until April 1980, when he presented with a non-productive cough, which came on when he took a deep breath.

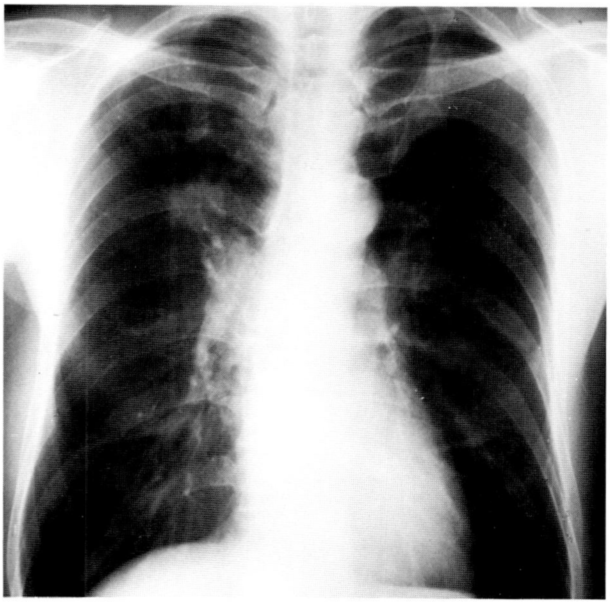

77.1 Posteroanterior chest radiograph. The lungs appear hyperinflated, suggesting the presence of pulmonary emphysema. A tumour shadow, 2.5-3 cm in diameter is visible around the base of the RUL bronchus.

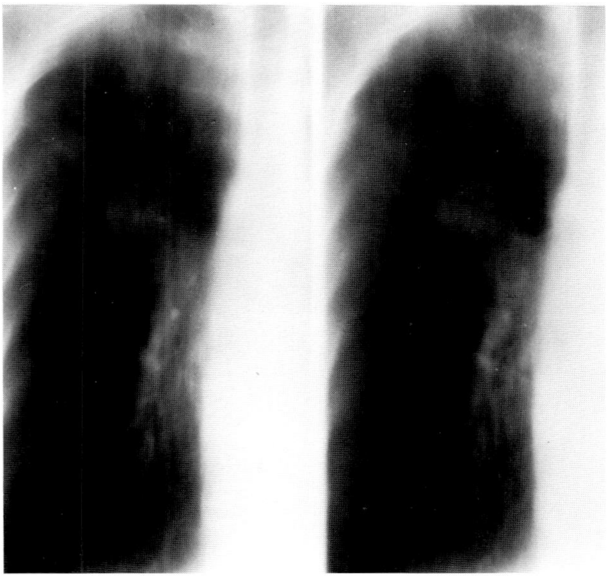

77.2 Chest tomogram (left: 7 cm from the back; right: 8 cm from the back). Note the radiological triad of carcinoma: spicular radiation, notch sign and inhomogeneity.

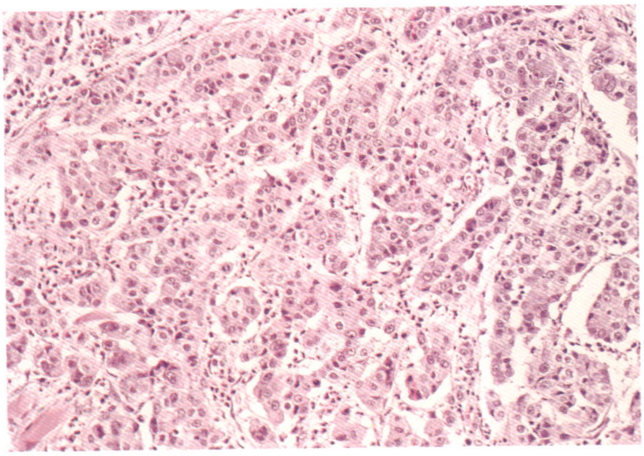

77.3 Pathological findings showing the papillary type of moderately differentiated adenocarcinoma.

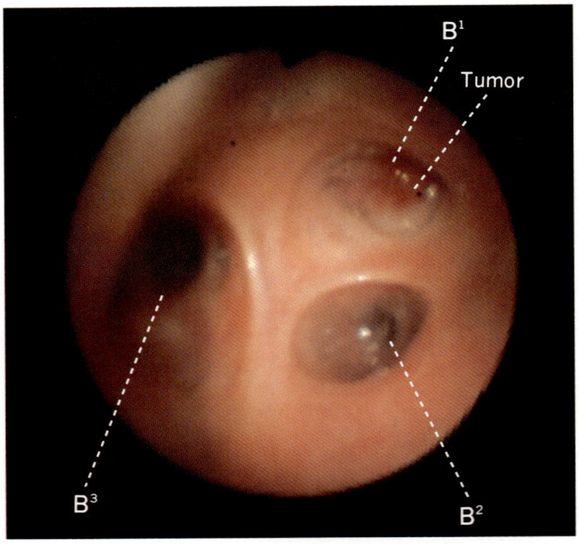

77.4 Bronchoscopic findings in the RUL bronchus. A tumour is visible at the orifice of B^1.

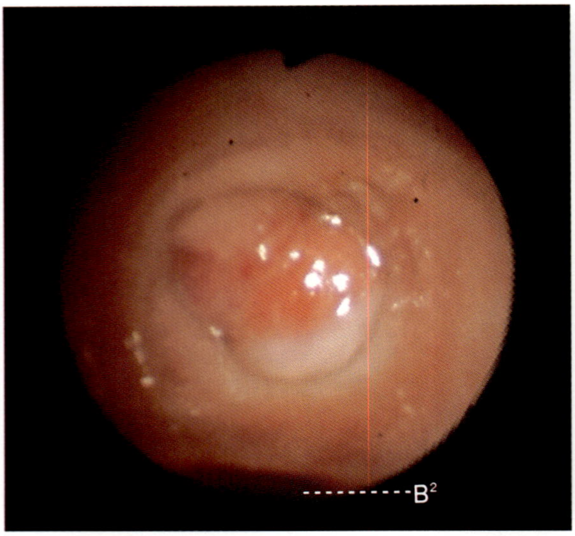

77.5 Bronchoscopic findings in B^1. The orifice of B^1 is totally occluded by a tumour with a relatively smooth surface.

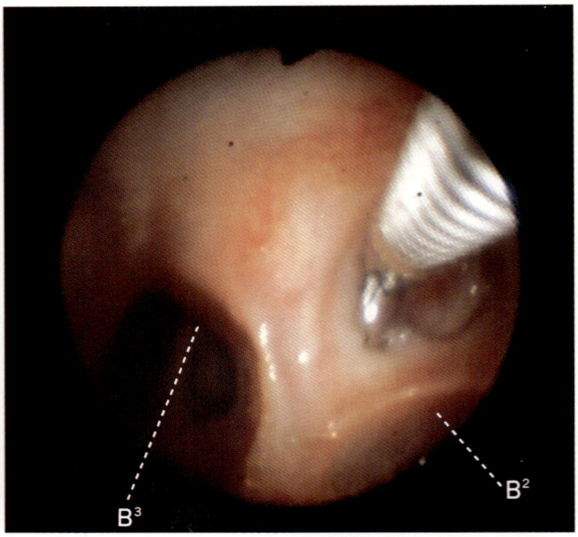

77.6 Biopsy being carried out on the tumour, which was diagnosed as an adenocarcinoma.

Case 78: Adenocarcinoma in a 65-year-old male.

The patient had been well until several years ago when he started to present with a productive cough probably as a result of chronic bronchitis. He had a history of smoking 8,000 cigarettes per year. Since Februrary 1981 he has complained of facial oedema, which suggested superior vena cava syndrome and led to his hospitalisation.

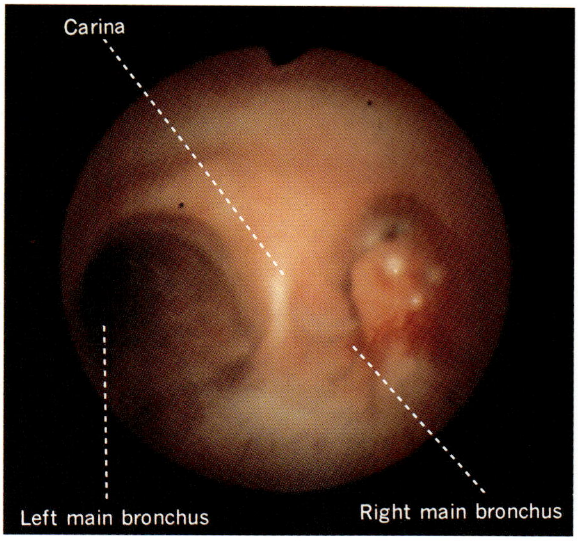

78.1 Bronchoscopic findings at the carina. At the orifice of the RUL bronchus, a tumour arising on the posterolateral side of the bronchial wall is visible.

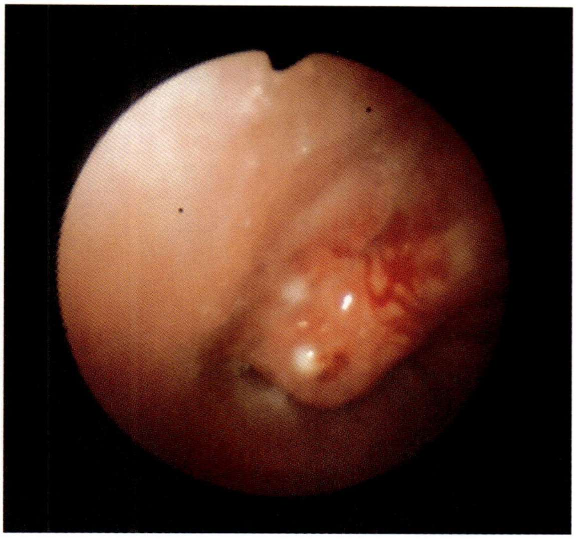

78.2 Bronchoscopic appearance of the tumour. It is rich in blood vessels and partly covered with a white coat.

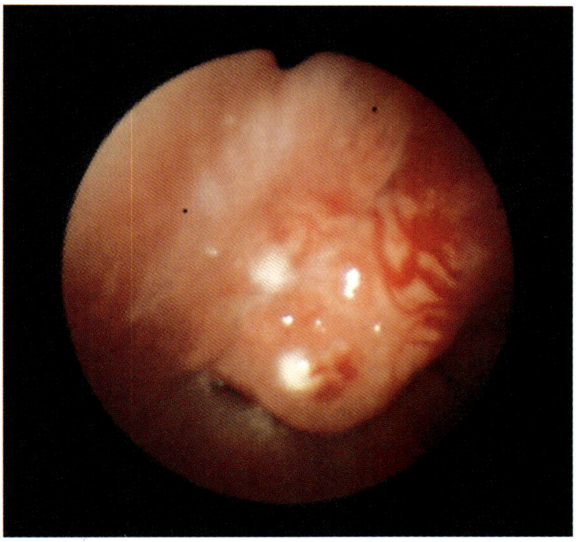

78.3 Close-up of the tumour. The white surface has multiple nodules with vascular dilatation.

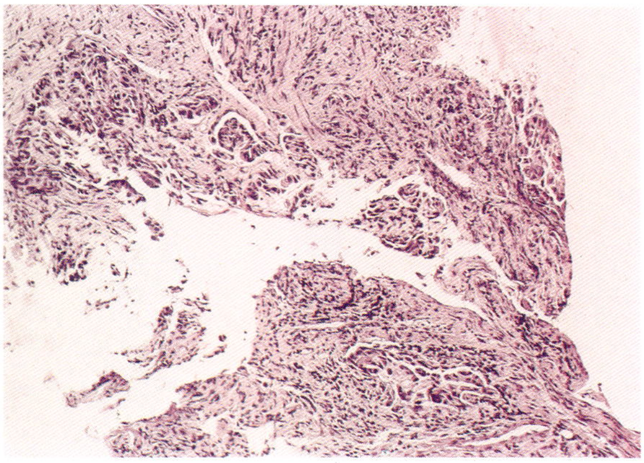

78.4 Histopathology shows adenocarcinoma.

Case 79: Adenocarcinoma in a 64-year-old female.

This patient had a polypoid adenocarcinoma of the truncus intermedius, which caused atelectasis of the RML and RLL.

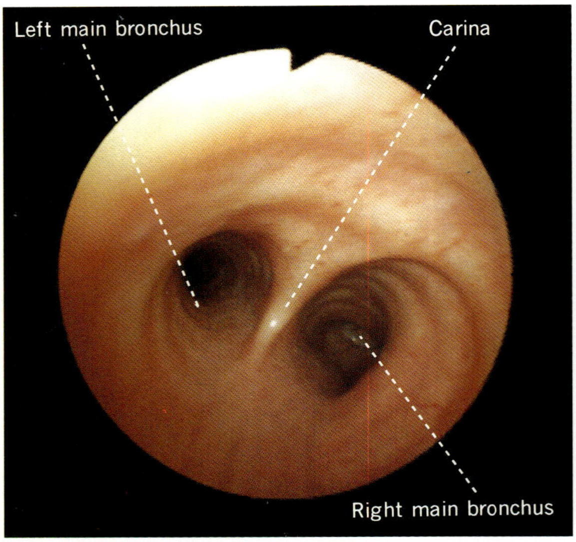

79.1 Bronchoscopic findings at the carina. The bifurcation is rather widened.

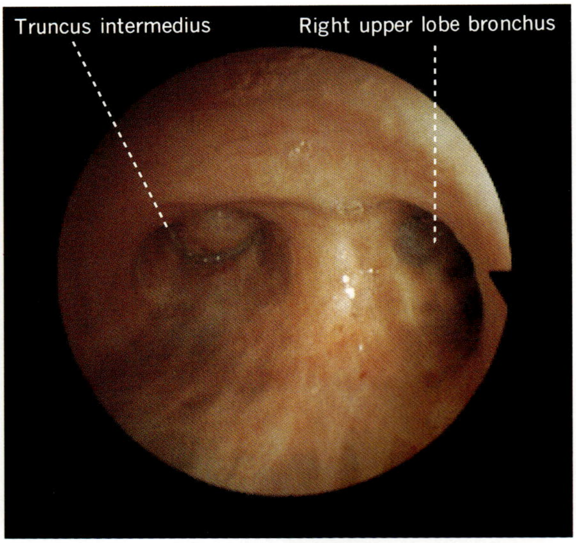

79.2 Bronchoscopic findings in the RUL bronchus and truncus intermedius. The bifurcation is oedematous and widened and a tumour occludes the truncus intermedius.

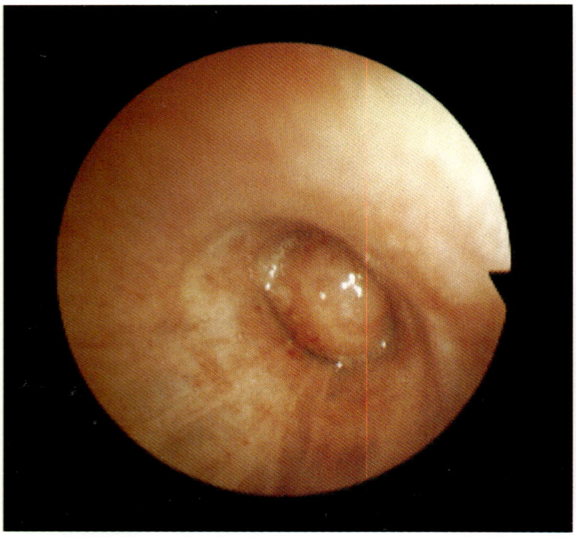

79.3 Bronchoscopic findings in the truncus intermedius. The tumour is covered with a thin layer of necrotic tissue. The longitudinal corrugations of the membranous portion remain almost intact.

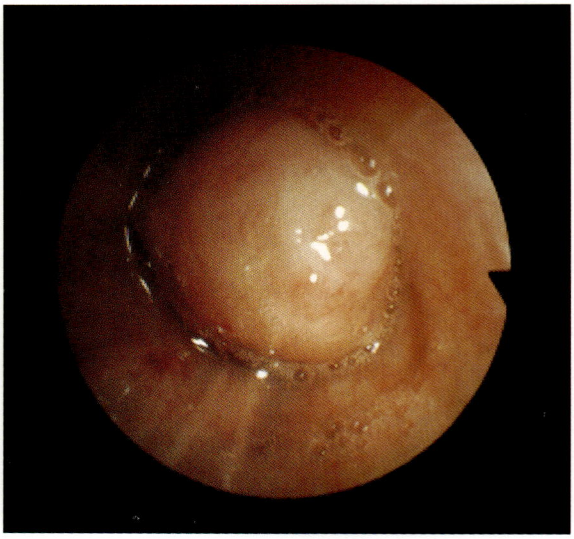

79.4 Close-up of the tumour. The relatively smooth-surfaced tumour is surrounded by air bubbles, which suggests that patency is minimal. Biopsy of the tissue confirmed the diagnosis.

Case 80: Adenocarcinoma in an 80-year-old male.

This patient's adenocarcinoma originated from the right basal bronchus, and was complicated by fluid in the right pleura. Cytology confirmed the diagnosis.

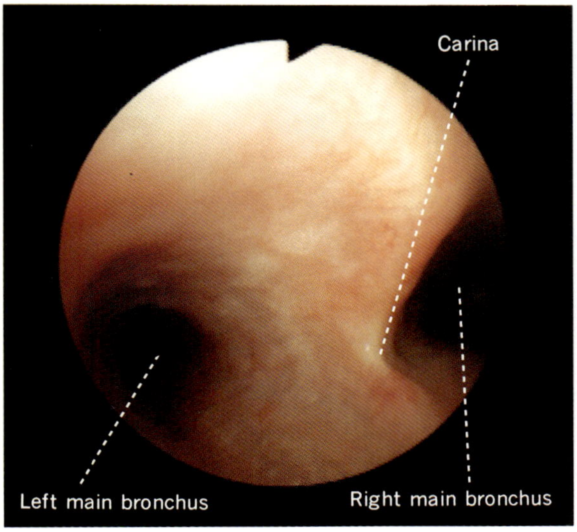

80.1 Bronchoscopic findings at the carina. The bifurcation is slightly widened and the mucosa around the orifice of the left main bronchus appears irregular. The mucosal vessels are dilated.

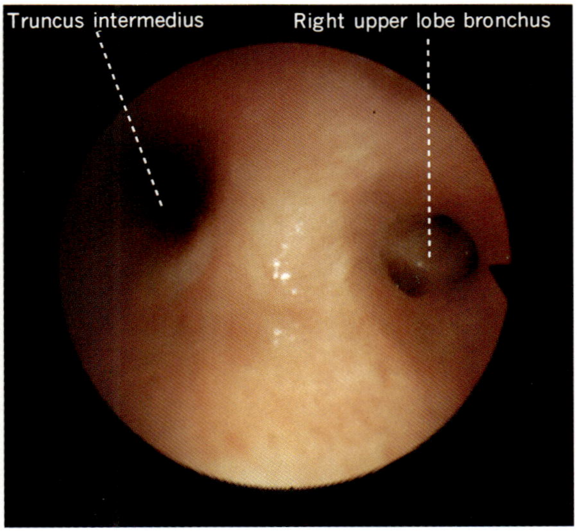

80.2 Bronchoscopic findings in the RUL bronchus and truncus intermedius. The bifurcation is strikingly widened as well as oedematous.

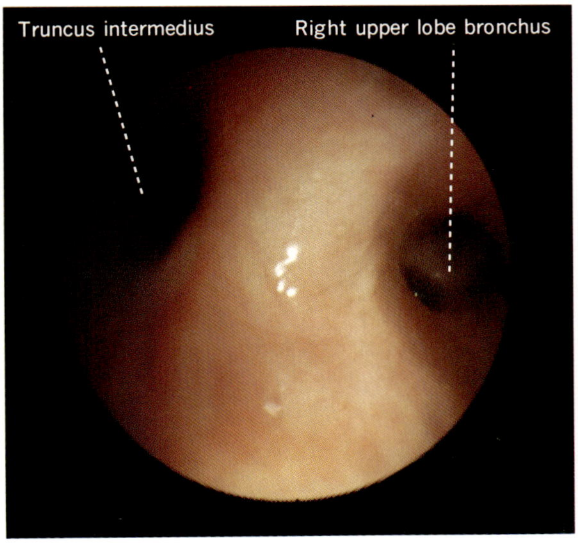

80.3 Close-up of **80.2**. The bifurcation is oedematous. Small vessels are visible beneath the mucosa.

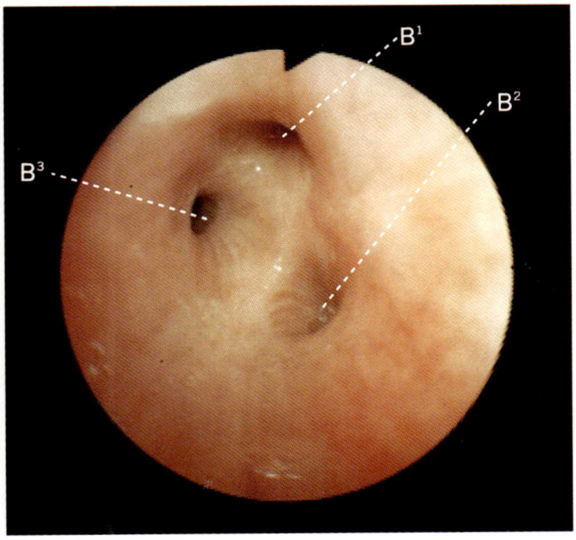

80.4 Bronchoscopic findings in the RUL bronchus. Each bifurcation is oedematous and widened, thus narrowing the lumen of each segmental bronchus. The surrounding mucosa also appears oedematous.

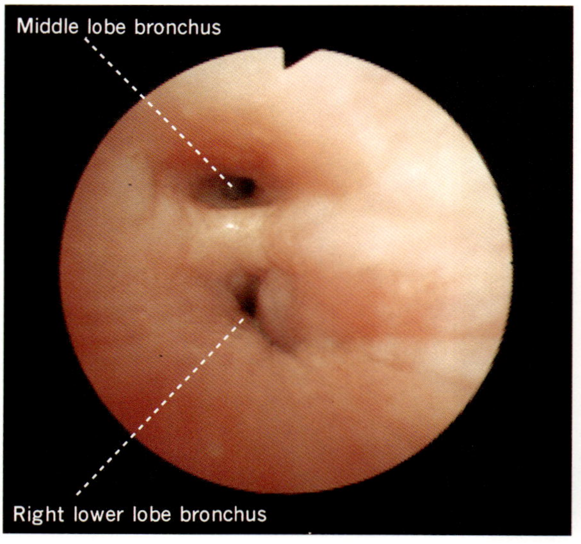

80.5 Bronchoscopic findings in the RML and RLL bronchi. The bifurcation into the RML and RLL bronchi is oedematous and widened, narrowing both bronchial orifices. The surrounding mucosa is oedematous and irregular, suggesting submucosal invasion by the tumour.

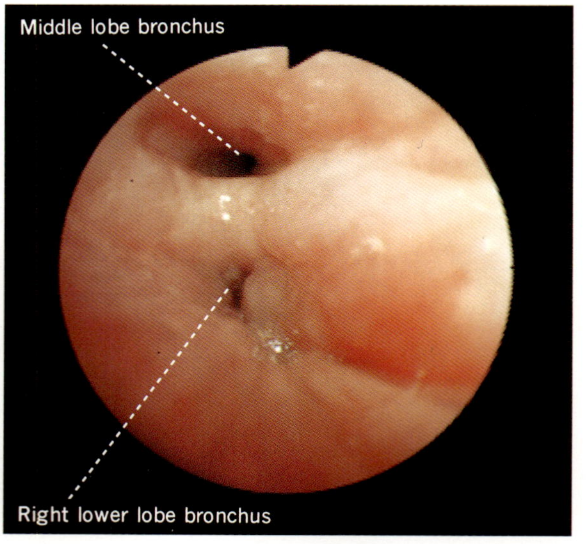

80.6 Close-up of **80.5**. The bifurcation into the RML bronchus appears oedematous as well as irregular, narrowing the orifice of the RLL bronchus.

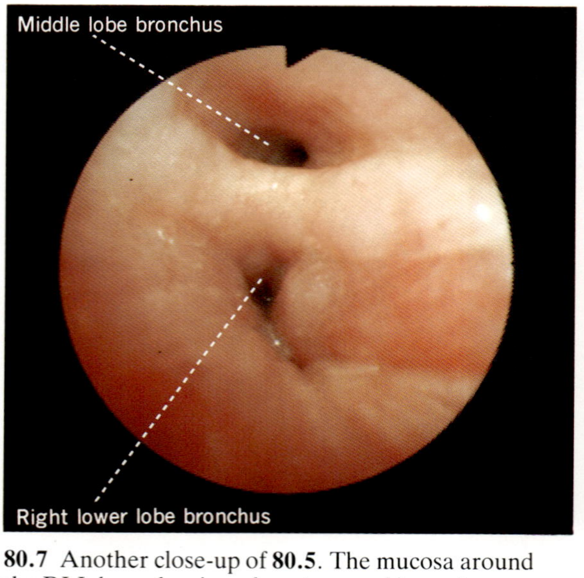

80.7 Another close-up of **80.5**. The mucosa around the RLL bronchus is oedematous and irregular.

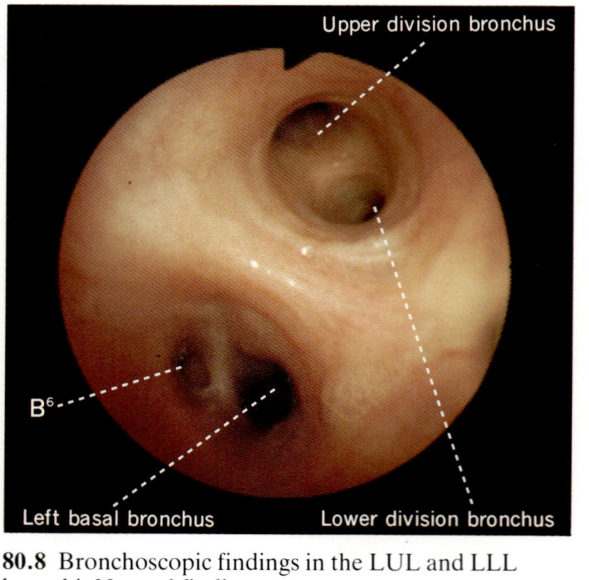

80.8 Bronchoscopic findings in the LUL and LLL bronchi. Normal findings.

Case 81: Adenocarcinoma in a 68-year-old male.

This patient had adenocarcinoma and complained of haemoptysis. The adenocarcinoma originated from the LUL bronchus, and there was metastasis to the right basal bronchus.

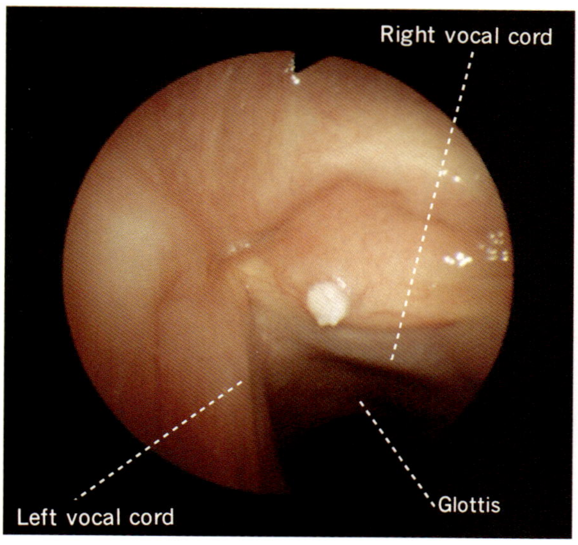

81.1 Bronchoscopic findings at the glottis. There is a white nodule on the right vocal cord.

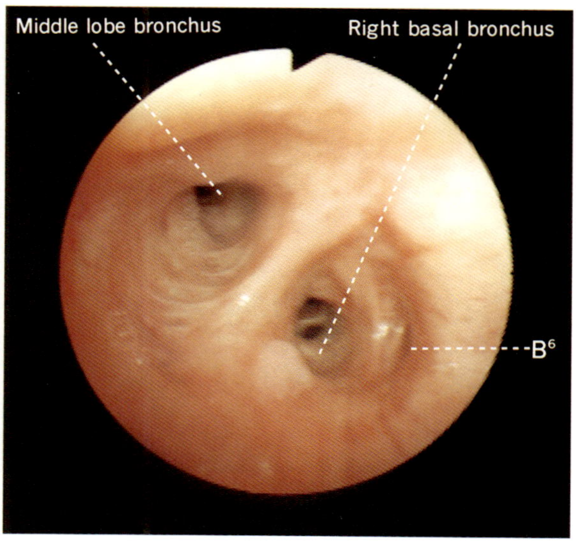

81.2 Bronchoscopic findings in the RML and RLL bronchi. Bifurcation into the RML bronchus is rather widened. A tumour a different colour from the surrounding mucosa of the LUL bronchus is visible at the orifice of the RLL bronchus.

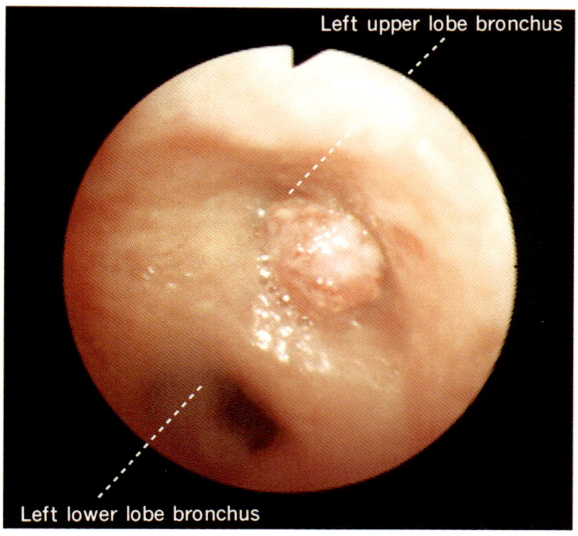

81.3 Bronchoscopic findings in the LUL bronchus. The tumour with an irregular surface occludes the orifice of the LUL bronchus; note the widened bifurcation.

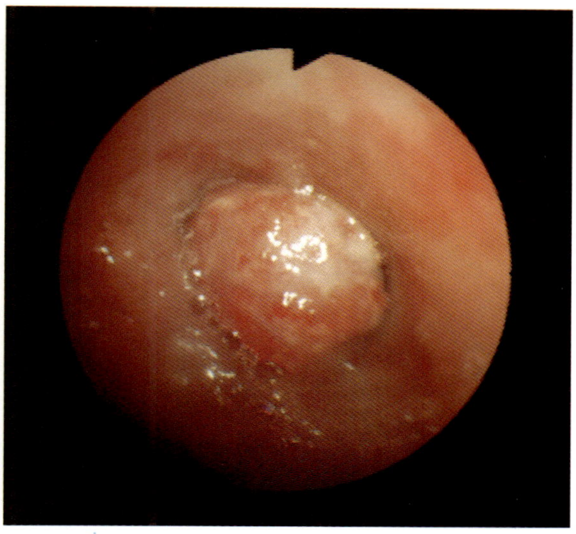

81.4 Close-up of the tumour. The irregular-surfaced tumour is covered with white necrotic tissue.

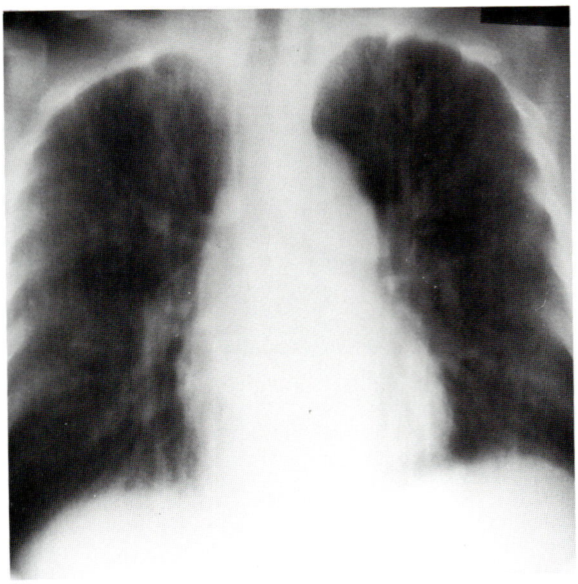

84.3 Chest tomogram (7 cm from the back). The same findings as **84.1** are again demonstrated.

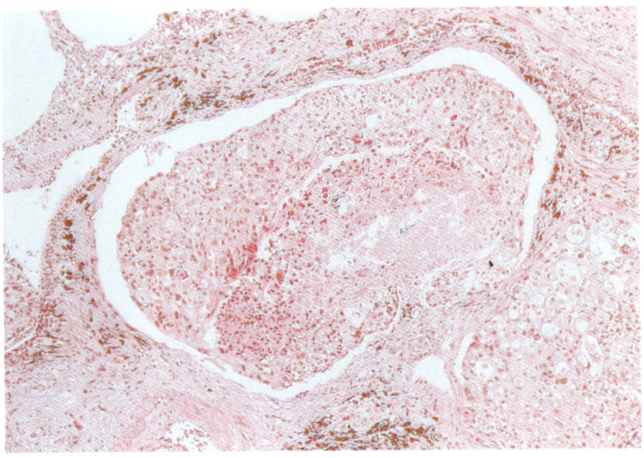

84.4 Histopathology of the biopsied lung. Among fibrous tissue, there is a nest of tumour cells. Glandular structures are formed by the tumour cells in the lymphatics. The cells are rich in cytoplasm.

Case 82: Adenocarcinoma in a 50-year-old male.

This patient had adenocarcinoma of the left upper-division bronchus. He complained of haemoptysis.

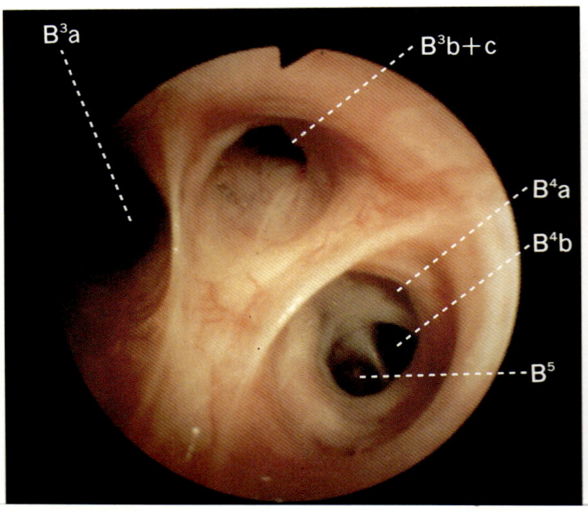

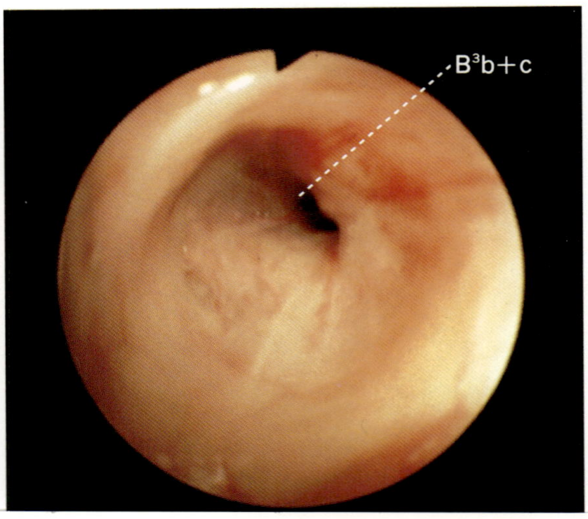

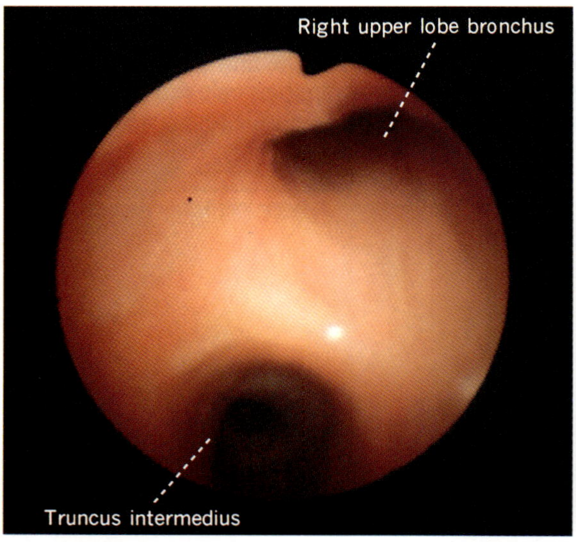

84.5 Bronchoscopic findings in the RUL bronchus and truncus intermedius. The bifurcation is oedematous and widened and the longitudinal corrugations into the RUL bronchus have almost disappeared.

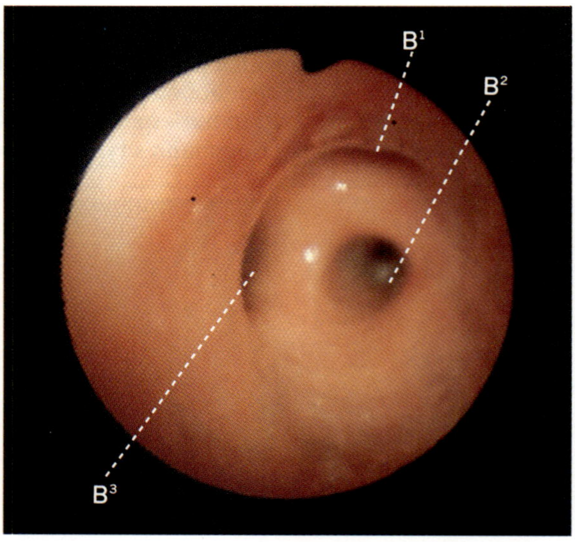

84.6 Bronchoscopic findings in the RUL bronchus. Each bifurcation is grossly widened and the mucosa is oedematous.

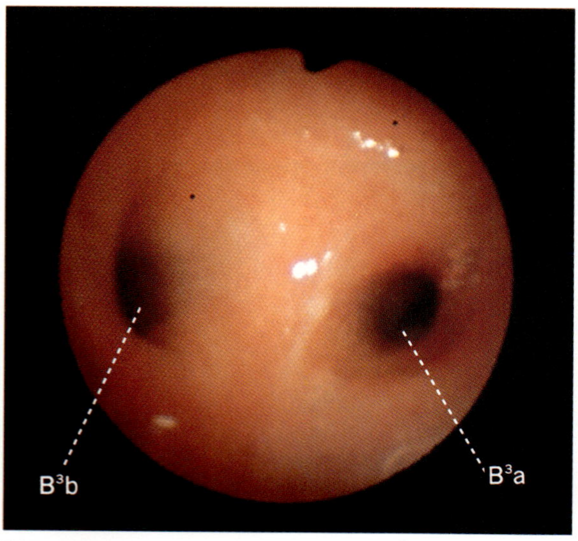

84.7 Bronchoscopic findings in right B^3. The mucosa is markedly reddened and oedematous as a result of impaired lymphatic drainage of the lungs.

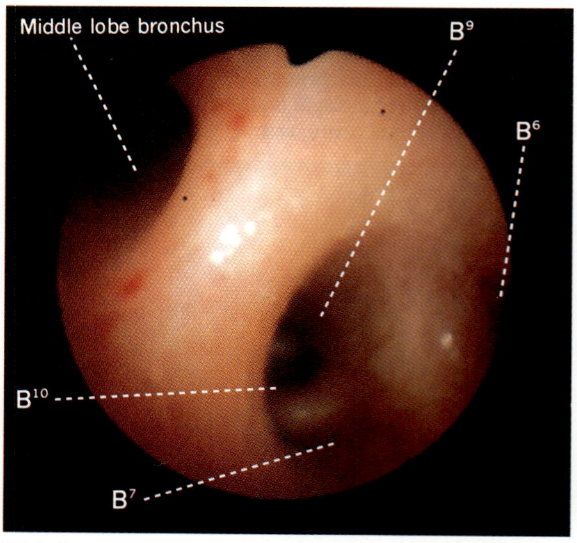

84.8 Bronchoscopic findings in the RML and RLL bronchi. Not only the bifurcation into the RML bronchus but those into B^9 and the subsegmental bronchus of B^{10} appear strikingly oedematous.

Case 85: Metastasis of thyroid cancer in an 81-year-old male.

The patient had been well until 2 months earlier when he complained of a persistent cough. He had also produced a small haemoptysis 10 days previously. He had a history of smoking 10,000 cigarettes per year.

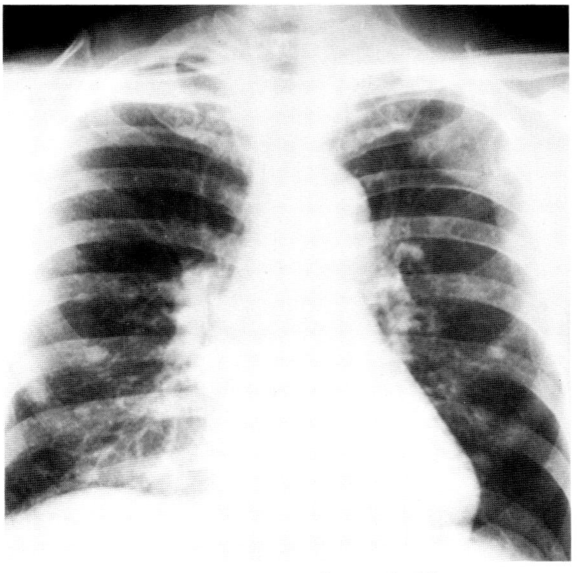

85.1 Posteroanterior chest radiograph. There are scattered round shadows, each 1 cm in diameter, throughout the lungs. A round shadow, 3 cm across, is also seen inferior to the right hilum.

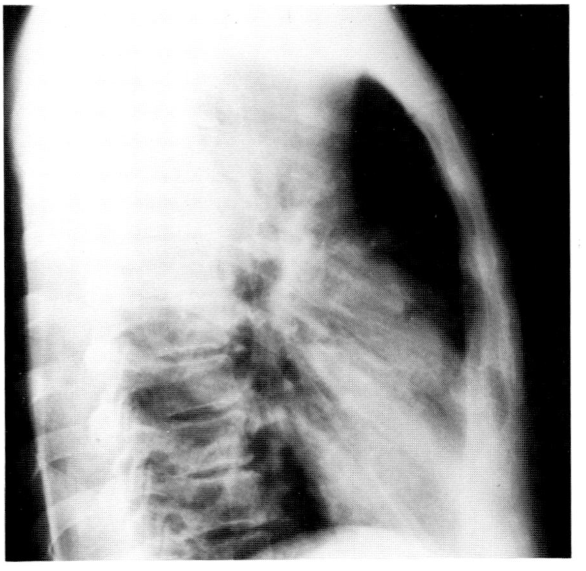

85.2 Lateral chest radiograph. Multiple round shadows are visible in the upper lung zone and over the cardiac shadow.

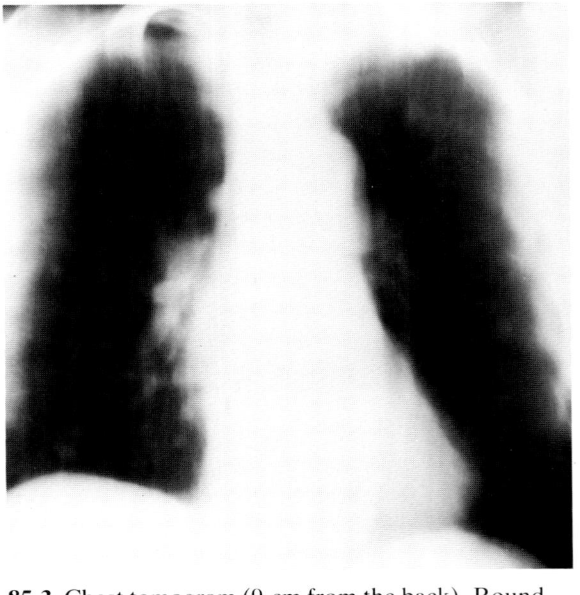

85.3 Chest tomogram (9 cm from the back). Round shadows, 0.5-1 cm in diameter, are scattered throughout the lungs.

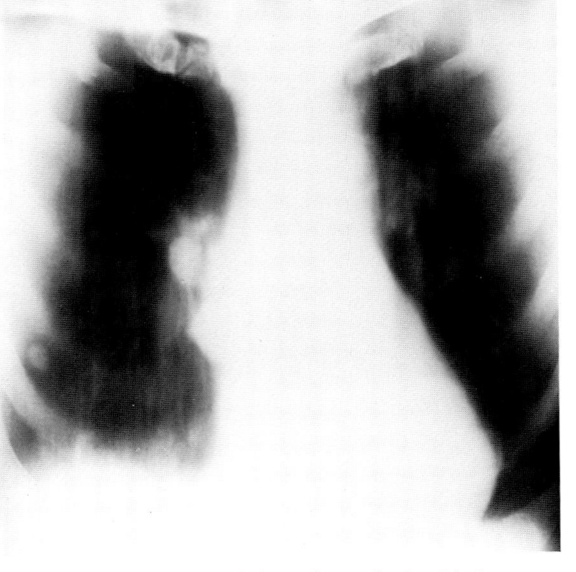

85.4 Chest tomogram (14 cm from the back). In addition to the round shadows, shadows suggesting lymphadenopathy are visible in the right hilum.

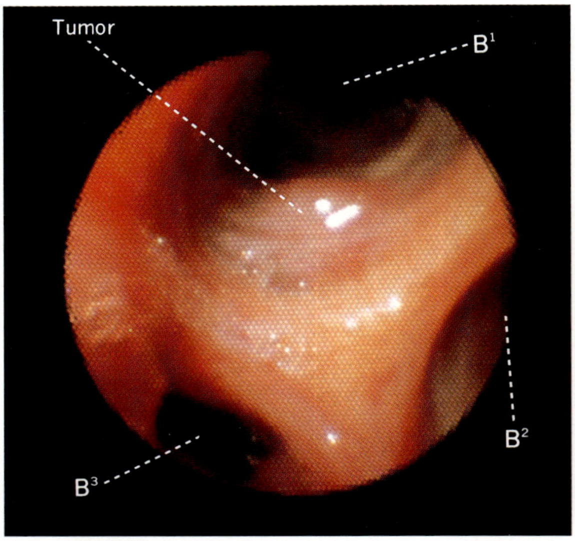

85.5 Bronchoscopic findings in the RUL bronchus. The mucosa is reddened and swollen. At the orifice of B^1 there is a nodule suggesting metastasis via bronchial circulation.

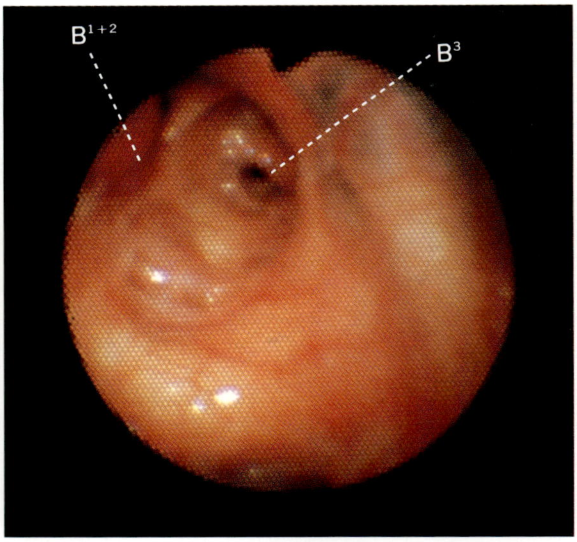

85.6 Bronchoscopic findings in the left upper-division bronchus. There are several pits caused by atrophy of the bronchial glands. The mucosa is reddened and vascular dilatation and anthracosis are clearly evident.

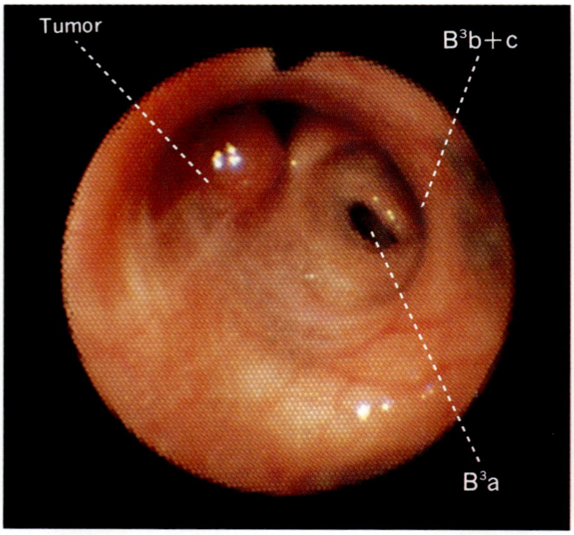

85.7 Close-up of **85.6**. A red tumour protrudes from B^{1+2}.

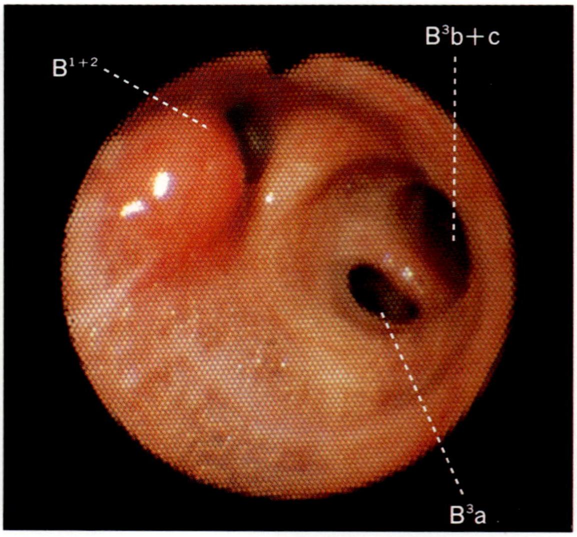

85.8 Further close-up of **85.7**. The red tumour with visible vessels on its surface occludes B^{1+2}. It is suggested that the proliferating tumour is derived from the bronchial circulation.

Case 86: Metastasis of renal cell carcinoma (Grawitz's tumour) in a 75-year-old male.

This patient had renal cell carcinoma, which postoperatively metastatised to the brain, pulmonary parenchyma and endobronchi.

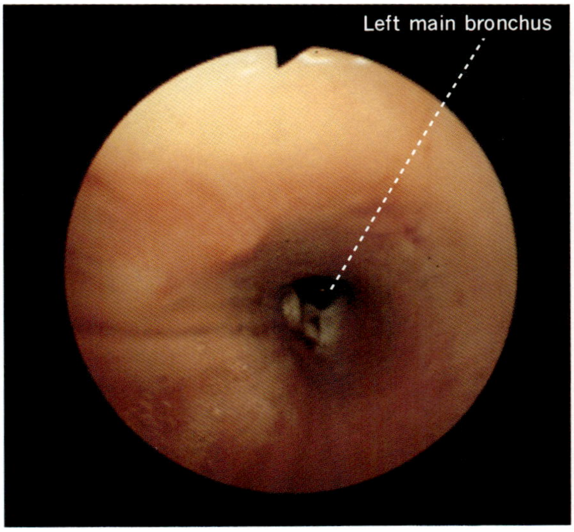

86.1 Bronchoscopic findings in the left main bronchus. On the upper wall a protruding lesion is visible as well as a white tumour beyond it, both of which were metastases.

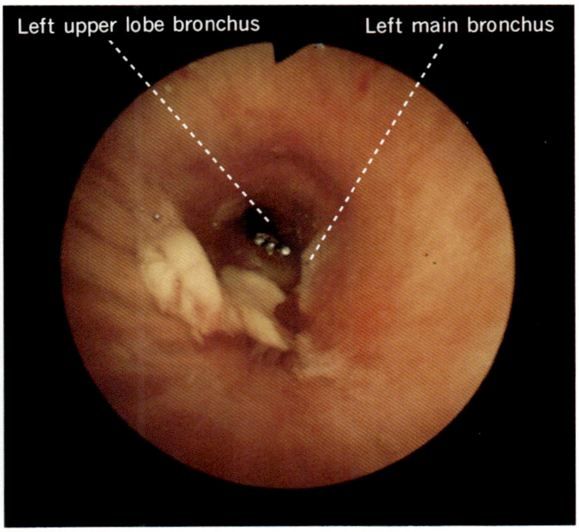

86.2 Further distal view of the left main bronchus. The white tumour is located over the mediastinal side and adheres to the membranous portion of the bronchial wall.

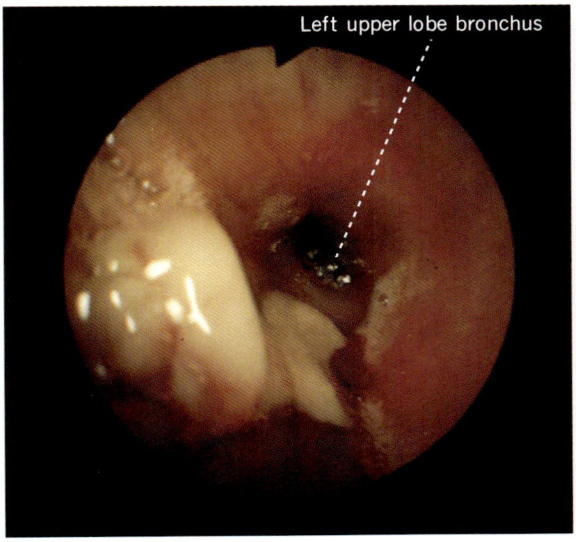

86.3 Close-up of the tumour. It is covered with a thickened white layer, with reddened and swollen mucosa on the opposite side.

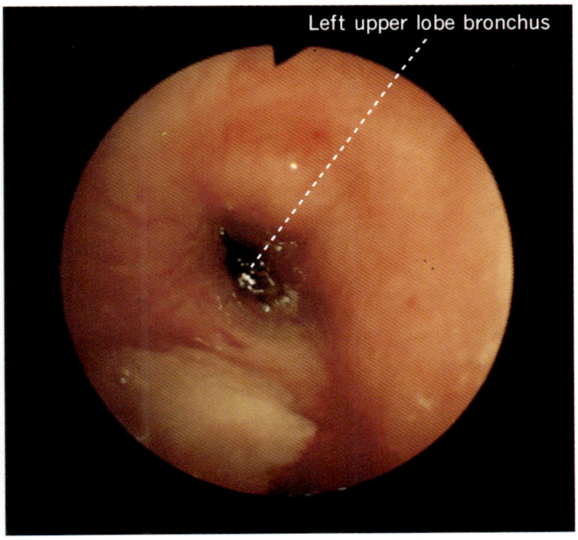

86.4 Bronchoscopic findings beyond the tumour. The membranous portion is covered with the white layer which bleeds easily. The orifice of the LUL bronchus is narrowed and the tumour, proliferating beneath the mucosa, protrudes into it.

Case 87: Metastasis of renal cell carcinoma (Grawitz's tumour) in a 62-year-old male.

The patient presented with haemoptysis, associated with atelectasis of the RML and RLL. A renal cell carcinoma was found later in the left kidney.

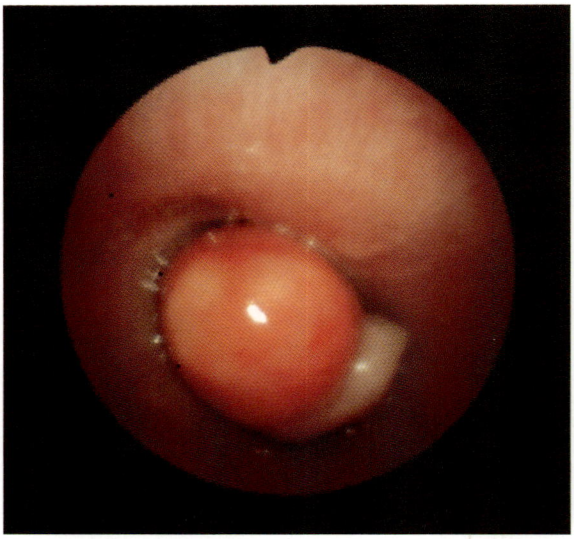

87.1 Bronchoscopic findings in the truncus intermedius. A polypoid tumour with a smooth surface is present at the lower portion of the truncus intermedius. A yellow-white necrotic area is visible on the right.

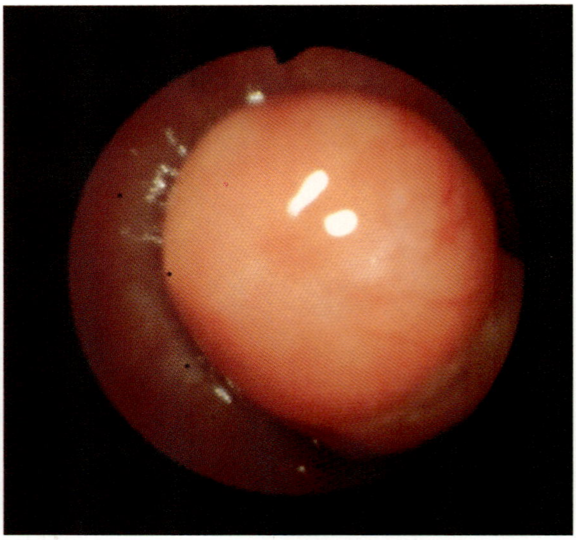

87.2 Bronchoscopic appearance of the tumour. It looks like a tomato. The surface is smooth and a network of vessels is visible.

Case 88: Metastasis of renal cell carcinoma (Grawitz's tumour) in a 72-year-old male.

This patient had a renal cell carcinoma which metastatised to the lungs and bronchi postoperatively.

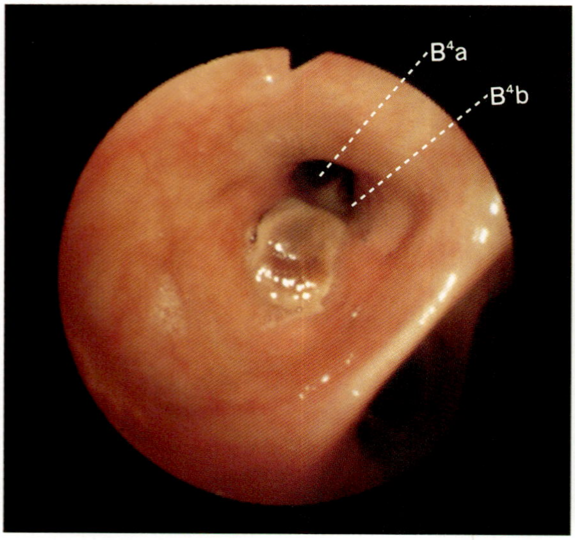

88.1 Bronchoscopic findings in the RML bronchus. While the orifice of B^4 is visible, that of B^5 is obstructed by a red tumour covered with white material.

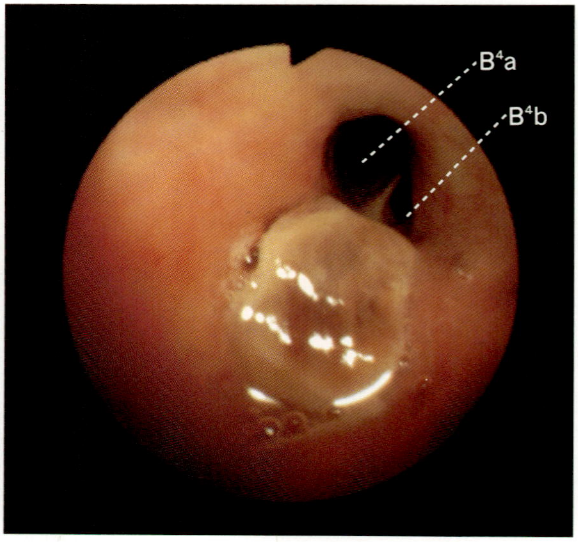

88.2 Close-up of the tumour. While B^4 can be observed down to the subsegmental bronchus, B^5 is completely occluded by the tumour, which was revealed to be a metastasis from the renal cell carcinoma.

Case 89: Metastasis of breast cancer in a 56-year-old female.

This patient had breast cancer metastatising to the lungs and bronchi after the operation.

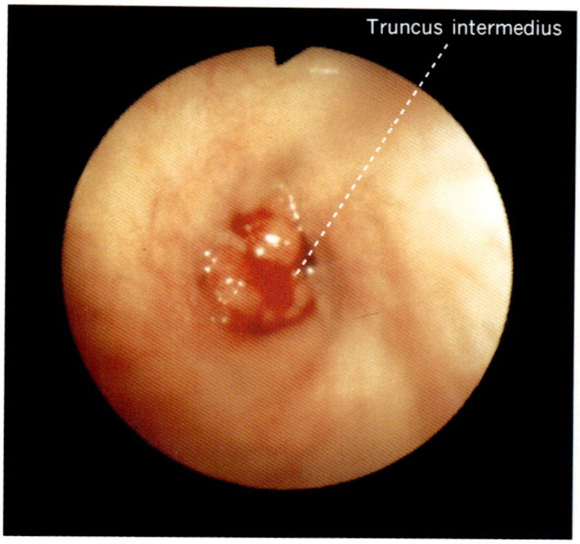

89.1 Bronchoscopic findings in the truncus intermedius. It is occluded by multiple nodules of various sizes.

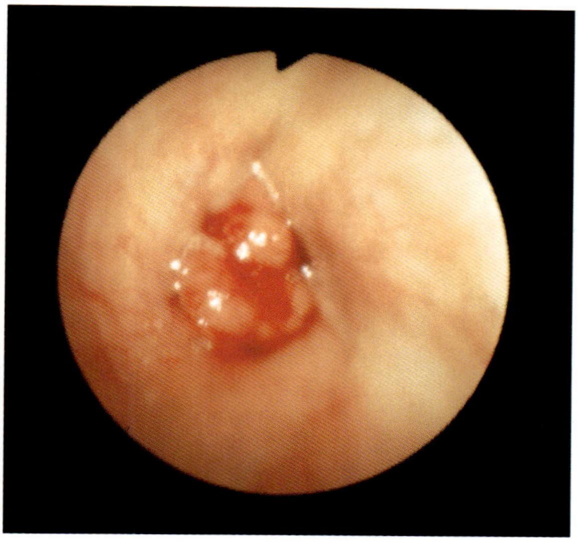

89.2 Close-up of **89.1**. The smooth-surfaced nodules of various sizes occlude the truncus intermedius. Bleeding occurs readily. Dilatation of the small vessels on the surrounding mucosa is present.

Case 90: Metastasis of colon cancer in a 53-year-old female.

This patient had cancer of the colon which metastatised to the lungs and bronchi postoperatively, resulting in atelectasis of the RML and RLL.

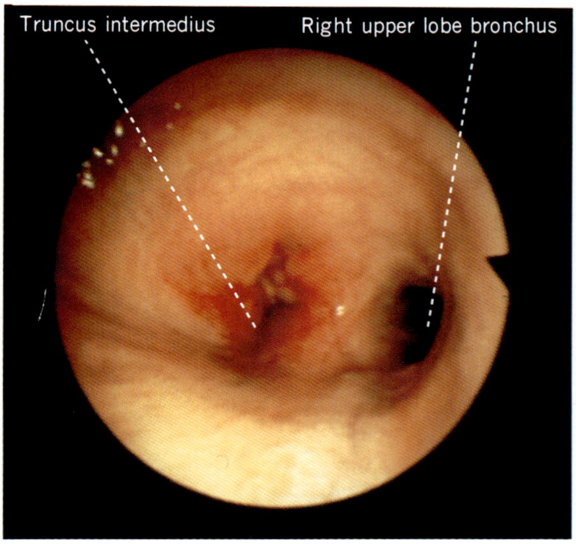

90.1 Bronchoscopic findings in the RUL bronchus and truncus intermedius. The bifurcation is widened and the truncus intermedius is obstructed below it.

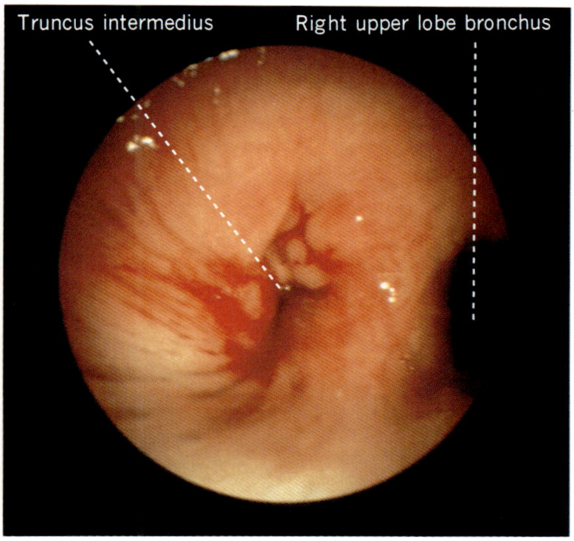

90.2 Close-up of **90.1**. The truncus intermedius is occluded by the nodular tumour which bleeds easily.

Case 91: Metastasis of colon cancer in a 51-year-old male.
This patient had cancer of the colon which metastatised to the lungs and bronchi postoperatively.

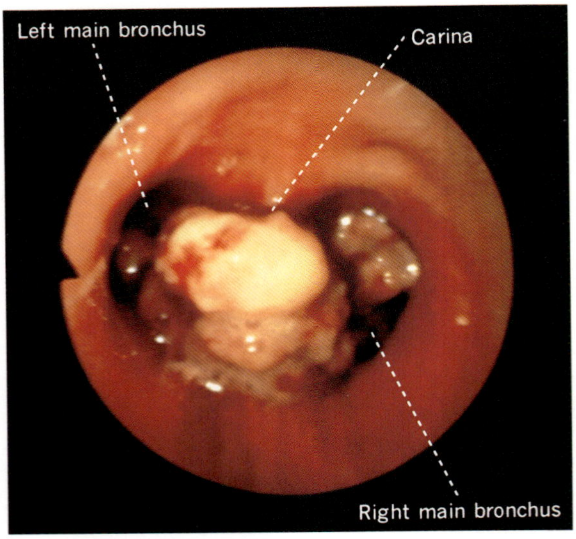

91.1 Bronchoscopic findings at the carina. The bifurcation as well as both main bronchi are partly occluded by the tumour which is covered with yellow-white necrotic tissue. The surrounding mucosa is markedly reddened and swollen. The patient complained of severe dyspnoea.

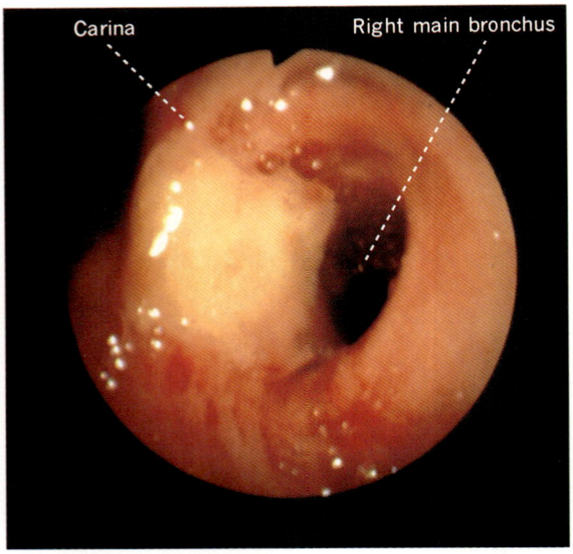

91.2 Bronchoscopic findings at the carina after irradiation. The tumour has reduced in size as a result of radiation therapy which has restored patency to both main bronchi, although the tumour which is covered with thickened, yellow-white necrotic tissue still remains on the bifurcation. The patient's dyspnoea has subsided completely.

Case 92: Metastasis of a melanoma in a 65-year-old female.

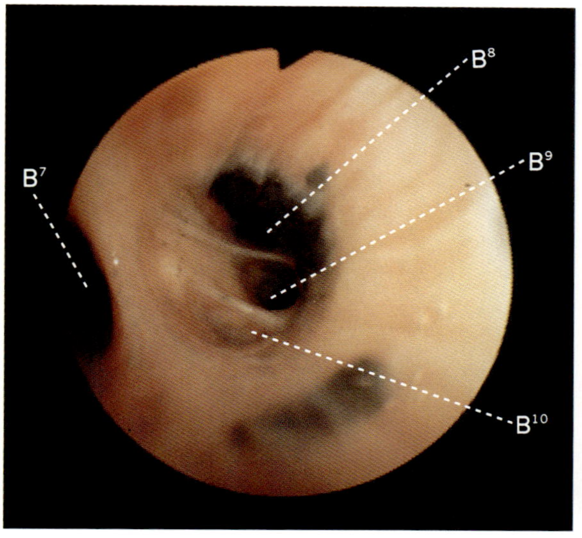

92.1 Bronchoscopic findings in the right basal bronchus. Metastatic lesions of the melanoma can be observed on the mucosa around the orifices of the basal bronchus, B^8, and B^9.

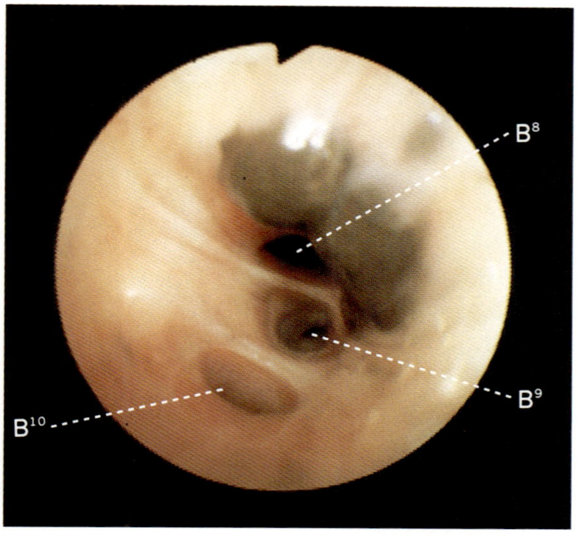

92.2 Close-up of **92.1**. The black tumour protrudes into the orifice of B^8.

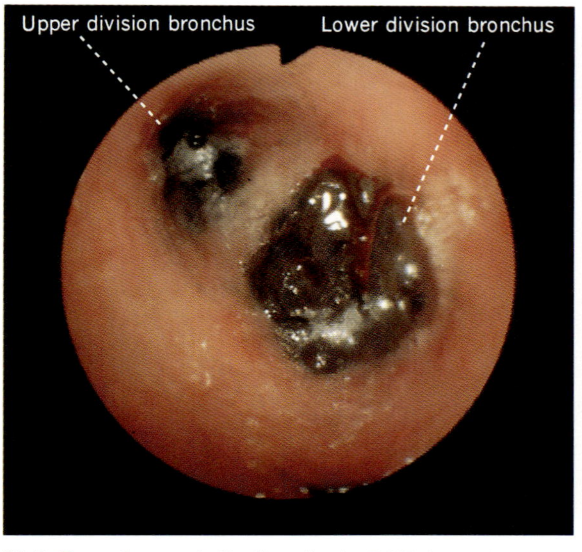

92.3 Bronchoscopic findings in the LUL bronchus. A black metastatic lesion of melanoma is visible.

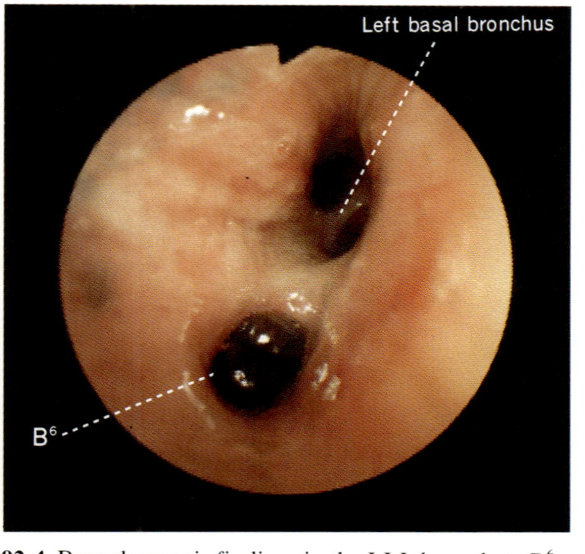

92.4 Bronchoscopic findings in the LLL bronchus. B^6 is totally occluded by the smooth-surfaced black tumour.

11 Tracheobronchial legions from adjacent organs

Case 93: Invasion of the trachea by oesophageal cancer in a 58-year-old male.

The patient, who had oesophageal cancer, presented with cough and haemoptysis.

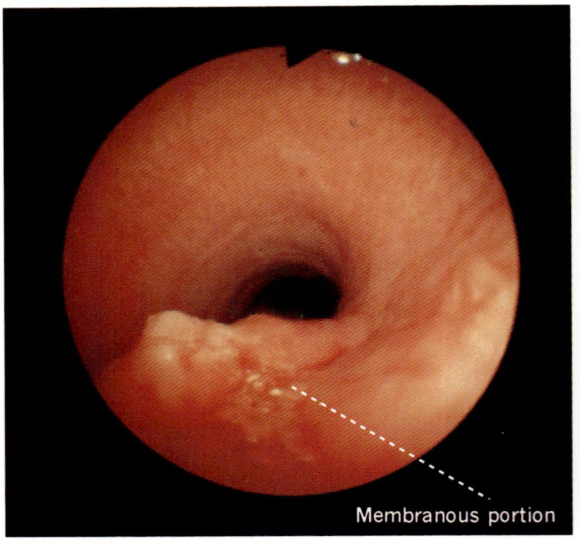

93.1 Bronchoscopic findings in the trachea. A white tumour with an irregular surface is sited mainly on the membranous portion. The trachea appears so oedematous that the tracheal cartilages are obscured. All these findings confirmed direct invasion by oesophageal cancer.

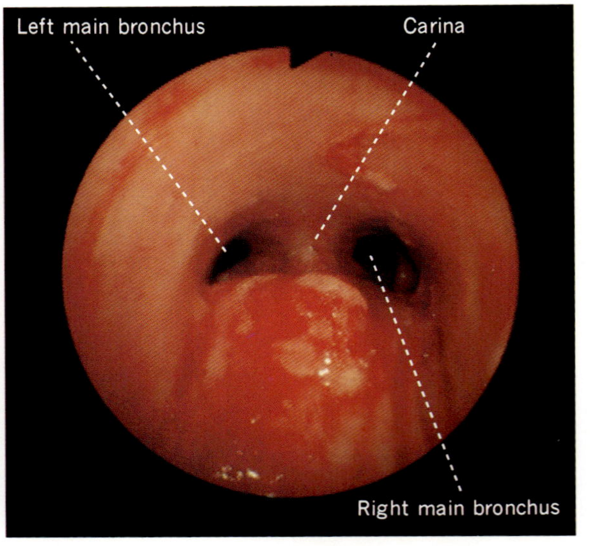

93.2 Bronchoscopic findings at the carina. The white tumour, the mucosa of which bleeds easily, is present on the membranous portion of the bifurcation.

Case 94: Invasion of the trachea by oesophageal cancer in a 58-year-old female.

During the clinical course of the oesophageal cancer, the patient complained of cough and haemoptysis.

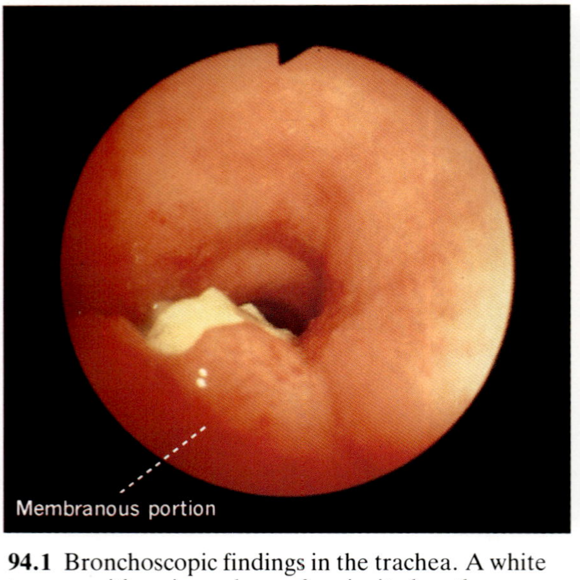

94.1 Bronchoscopic findings in the trachea. A white tumour with an irregular surface is sited on the membranous portion, and the oedematous bronchial wall narrows the lumen. These findings suggest submucosal invasion by the tumour.

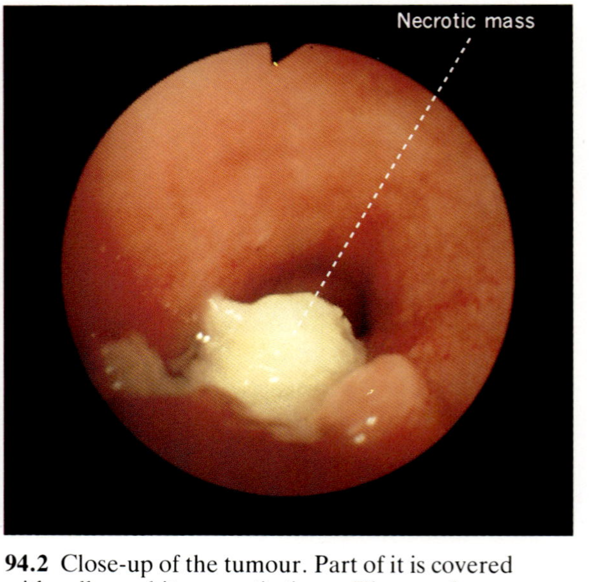

94.2 Close-up of the tumour. Part of it is covered with yellow-white necrotic tissue. The membranous portion appears irregular and the mucosa is so oedematous that it obscures the tracheal cartilages. These observations confirm direct invasion of the trachea by oesophageal cancer.

Case 95: Broncho-oesophageal fistula in a 79-year-old male.

This patient had advanced epidermoid carcinoma of the lung arising from left S^6, with metastasis to the mediastinal lymph nodes. After the patient underwent cancer chemotherapy, he complained of a cough when eating and also had an attack of pneumonia.

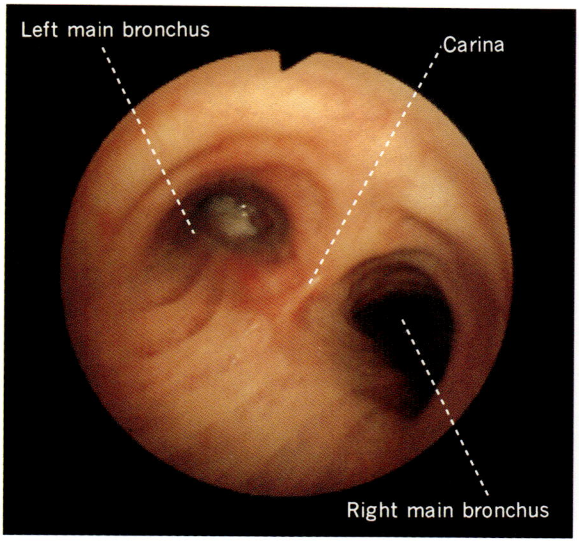

95.1 Bronchoscopic findings at the carina. Although the bifurcation remains unchanged, the mucosa is slightly reddened and swollen at the orifice of the left main bronchus, which is white distally.

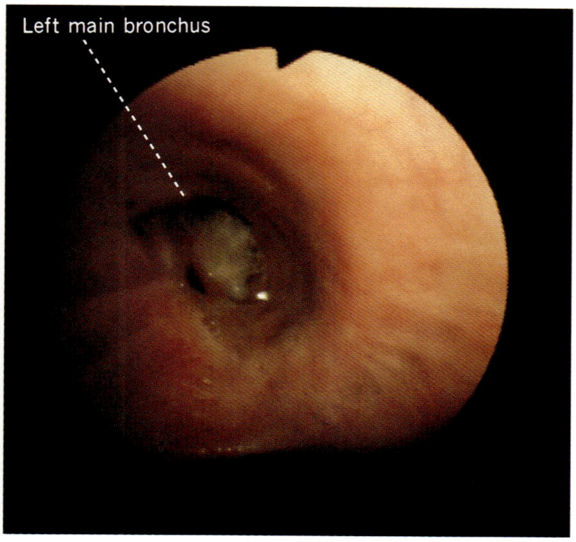

95.2 Bronchoscopic findings in the left main bronchus. While longitudinal corrugations and the rings of cartilage appear almost normal, a yellow-white tumour is visible distally.

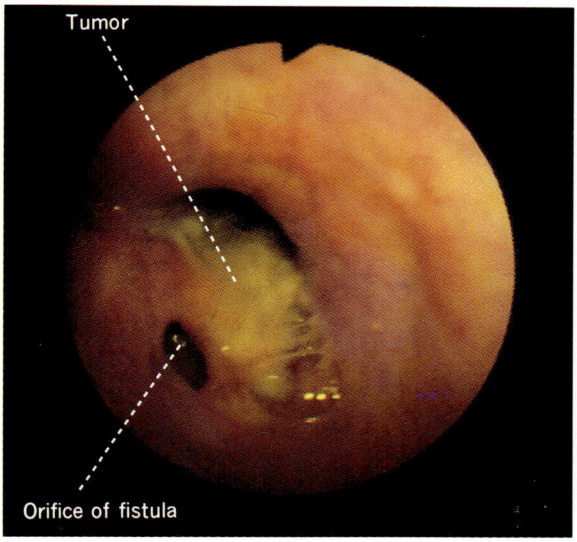

95.3 Close-up of **95.2**. A hole, approximately 5 mm in diameter, is situated behind the white tumour. The surrounding mucosa is oedematous and irregular. The rings of cartilage have been obscured.

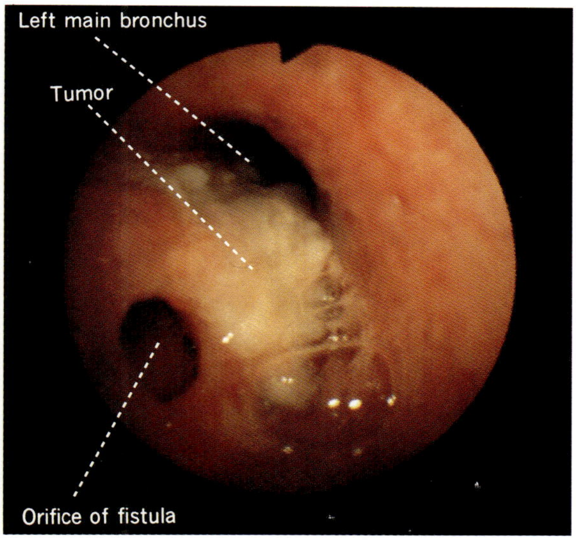

95.4 Close-up of **95.3**. A punched-out hole is sited behind the white tumour. Contrast medium proved it to be a broncho-oesophageal fistula.

Case 96: Malignant lymphoma in a 57-year-old male.

This patient had malignant lymphoma, with marked swelling of the mediastinal lymph nodes.

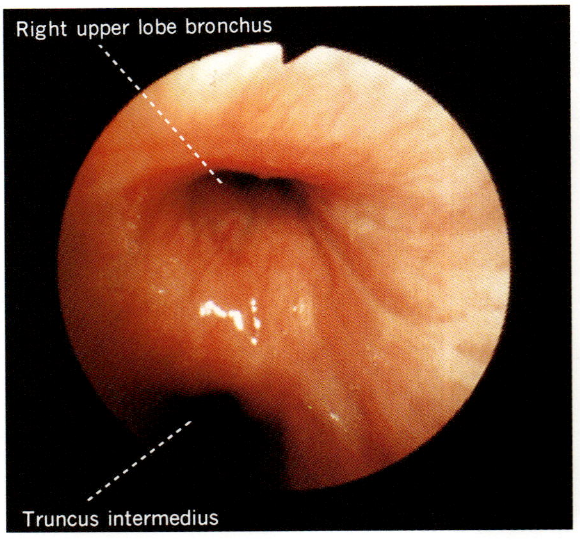

96.1 Bronchoscopic findings in the RUL bronchus. The bifurcation is grossly widened and oedematous, which narrows the orifice of the RUL bronchus.

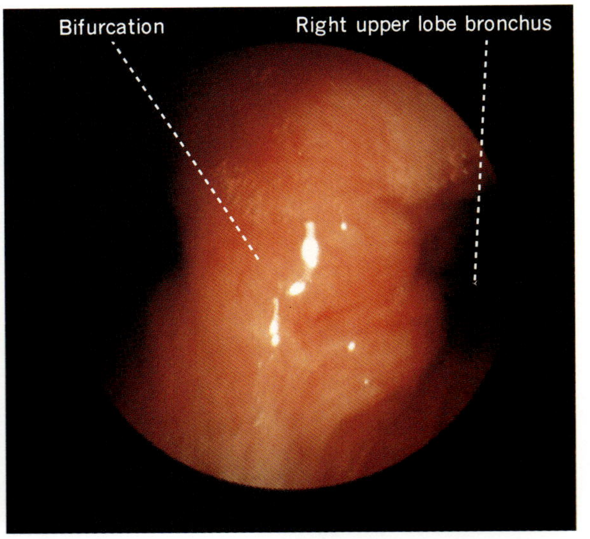

96.2 Close-up of **96.1**. The mucosa is oedematous, reddened and irregular; it is associated with visible dilatation of the vessels. These findings confirm endobronchial invasion by malignant lymphoma.

Case 97: Pseudolymphoma in a 63-year-old female.

The patient had a lung tumour, approximately 5 cm in diameter, in right S^6, for which transbronchial lung biopsy was carried out. It was discovered that the malignant lymphoma primarily originated from the lung. However, a histopathological study of the resected lung confirmed it to be a pseudolymphoma.

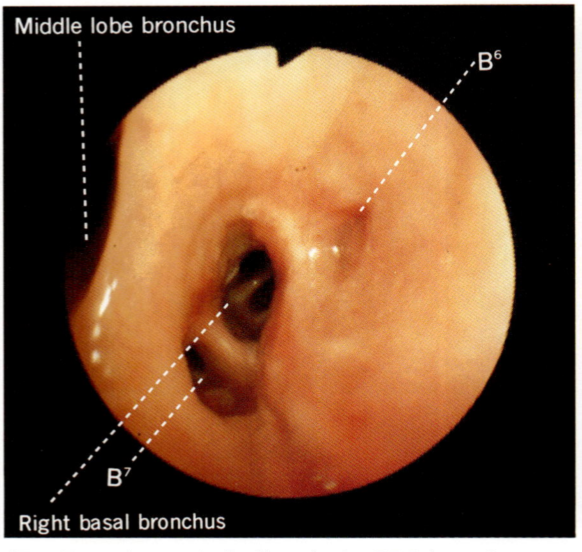

97.1 Bronchoscopic findings in the RLL bronchus. Bifurcation into B^6 is widened and irregular. The orifice of B^6 is rather concave.

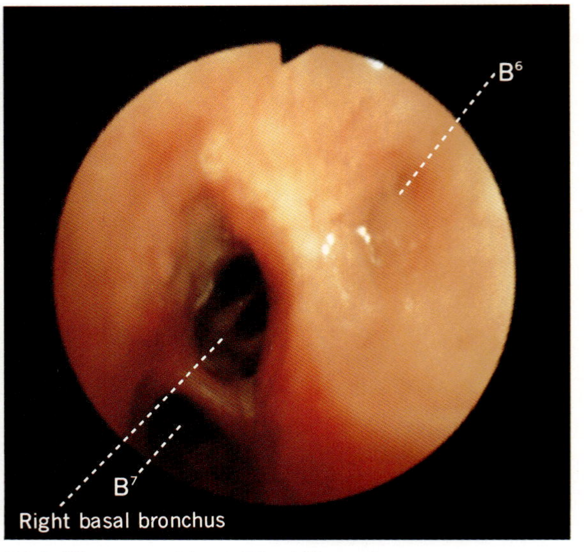

97.2 Close-up of **97.1**. The bifurcation appears widened and irregular. The orifice of B^6 is totally occluded, although not reddened. Biopsy of this lesion suggested malignant lymphoma.

12 Non-malignant bronchial lesions and intrabronchial foreign bodies

Case 98: Endobronchial hamartoma in a 69-year-old male.

This patient had an endobronchial hamartoma, causing atelectasis of right S^3 and a coin lesion.

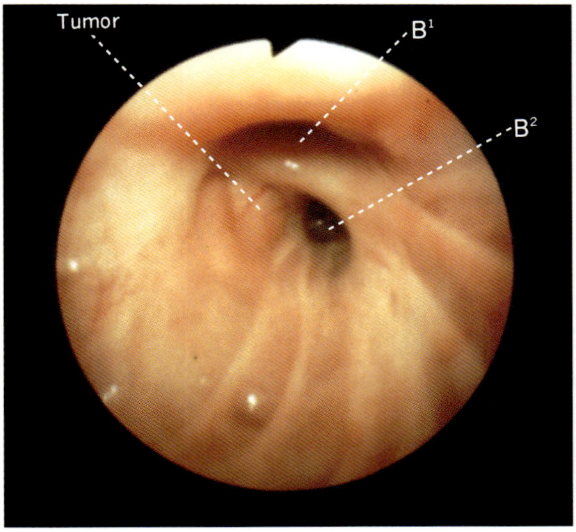

98.1 Bronchoscopic findings in the RUL bronchus. The orifice of B^3 is convex as well as occluded, and there are dilated vessels on the surface. The bifurcation between B^1 and B^2 is oedematous and widened.

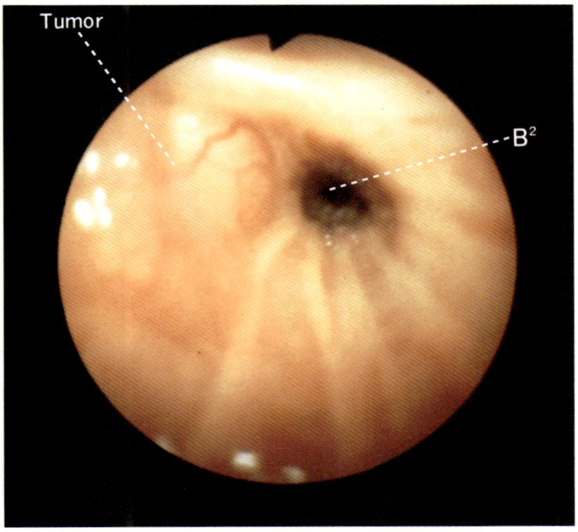

98.2 Bronchoscopic findings in right B^2 and B^3. In addition to the narrowed orifice of B^2, that of B^3 is completely obstructed but convex. Dilated vessels are visible on its surface, although the colour remains normal.

Case 99: Postoperative polyp arising from the bronchial stump in a 61-year-old male.

After this patient underwent left upper lobectomy for lung cancer, he presented with a non-productive cough caused by an inflammatory polyp arising from the bronchial stump.

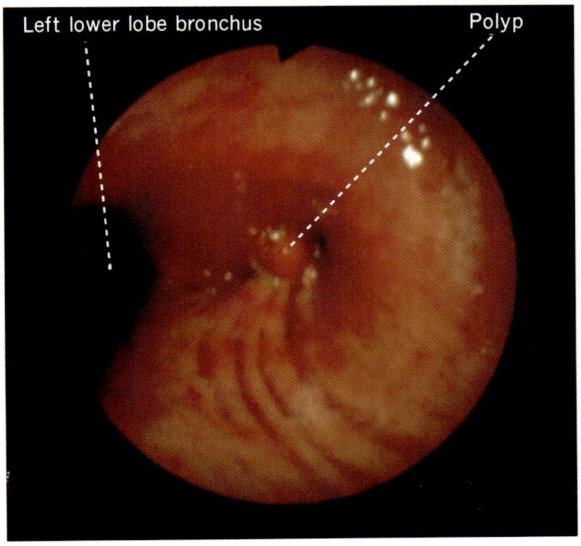

99.1 Bronchoscopic findings in the stump of the LUL bronchus. The stump has a smooth surface. The tumour bled easily. The longitudinal corrugations remained intact.

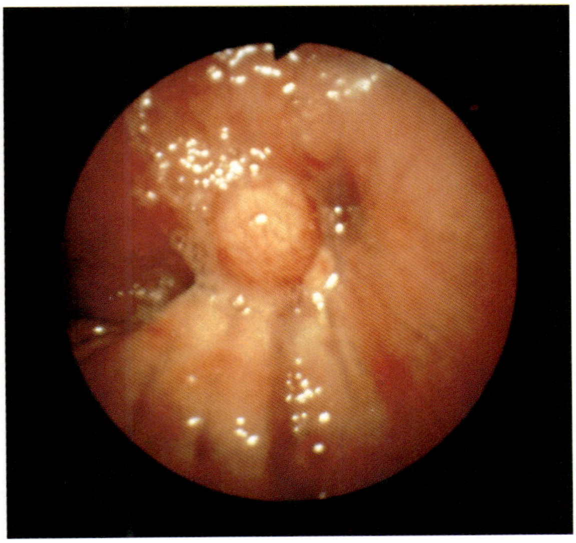

99.2 Close-up of the mass. The spherical tumour has a smooth surface on which the mucosal vessels are visible. The surrounding mucosa is oedematous.

Case 100: Squamous metaplasia in a 60-year-old female.

Because of a persistent non-productive cough, the patient underwent fibreoptic bronchoscopy, which revealed a white mass at the orifice of the right basal bronchus. Severe squamous metaplasia was proved by biopsy, although the bronchoscopic findings suggested the possibility of its being an epidermoid carcinoma. Both the subjective symptoms and the bronchoscopic findings responded to antibiotic (aminobenzylpenicillin) therapy.

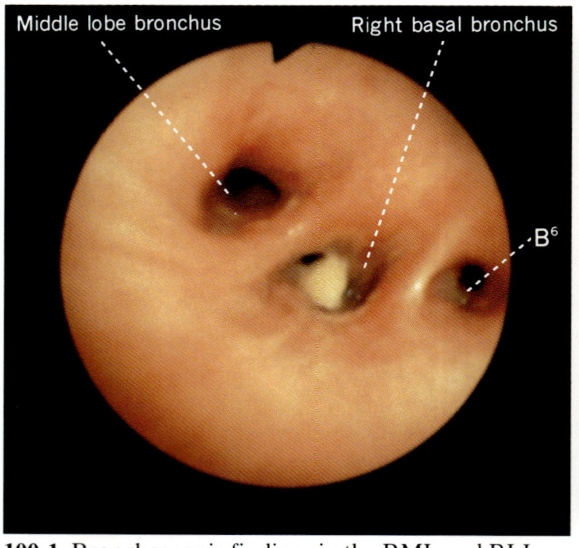

100.1 Bronchoscopic findings in the RML and RLL bronchi. The bifurcation into the RML bronchus is widened and irregular, with a white mass sited at the orifice of the basal bronchus.

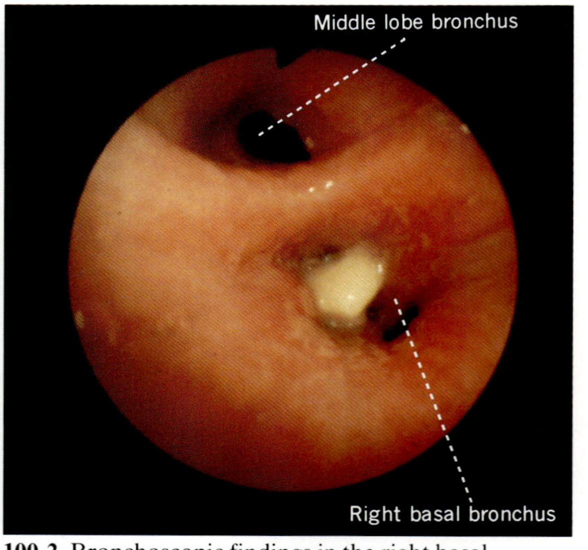

100.2 Bronchoscopic findings in the right basal bronchus. The bifurcation into the RML bronchus is widened and the mucosa is oedematous as well as reddened. Alongside the narrowed orifice of B^6, the orifice of the basal bronchus is occluded by the tumour which is covered with yellow-white necrotic tissue.

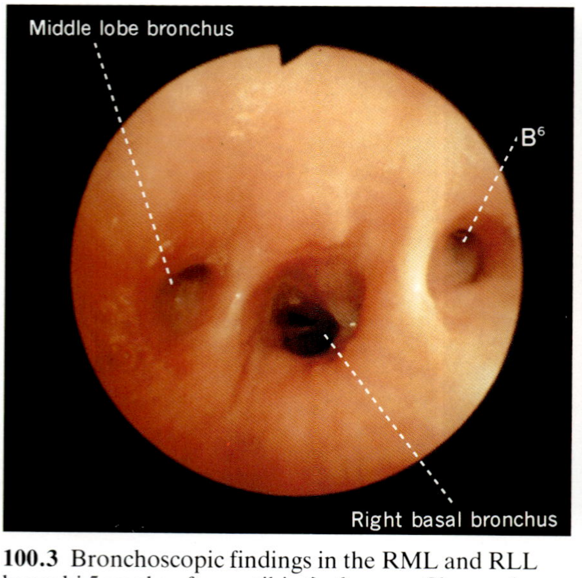

100.3 Bronchoscopic findings in the RML and RLL bronchi 5 weeks after antibiotic therapy. Sharpening of the bifurcation, disappearance of the white necrotic mass, and a normal hue of the surrounding mucosa have been restored.

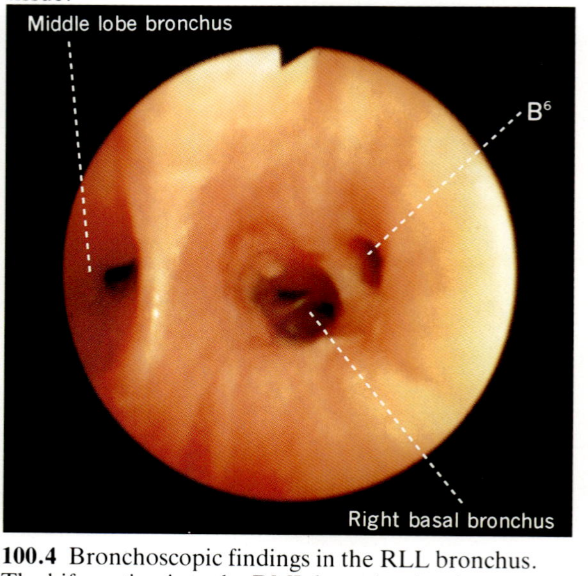

100.4 Bronchoscopic findings in the RLL bronchus. The bifurcation into the RML bronchus has become more sharp-edged, although not completely. The mucosa around the orifice of the basal bronchus still remains reddened to a slight degree; a small protruding lesion is visible on the anterior wall.

Case 101: Bronchial adenoma in a 73-year-old male.

The patient who had pulmonary emphysema underwent fibreoptic bronchoscopy for an occasional cough. Bronchoscopy revealed a bronchial adenoma.

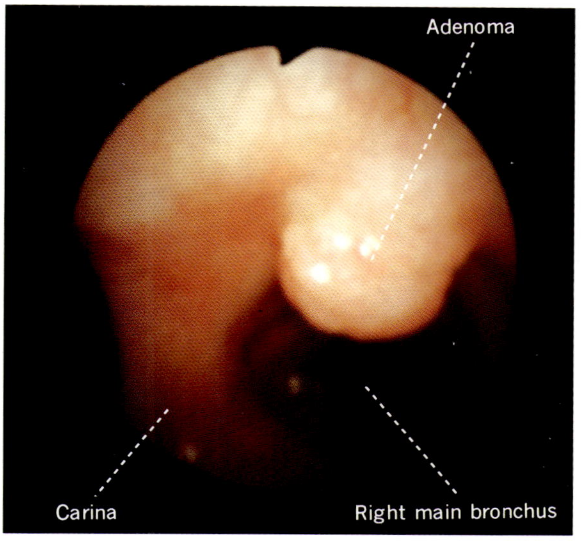

101.1 Bronchoscopic findings in the right main bronchus. On the upper wall a white tumour with an irregular surface is clearly visible.

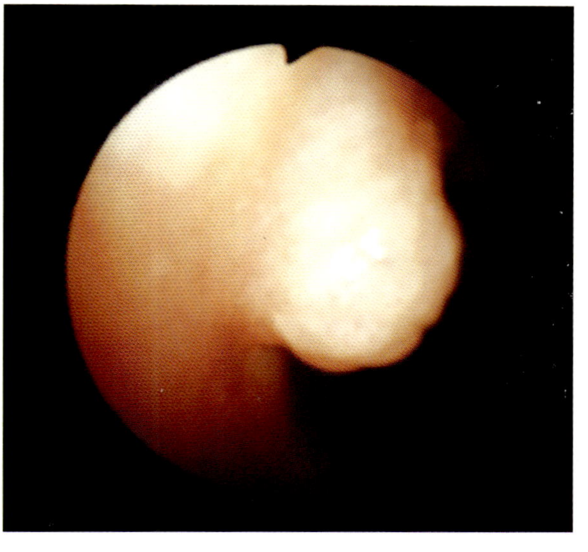

101.2 Close-up of the tumour. Compared with a malignant tumour, there are fewer mucosal vessels on its surface. Biopsy of the tumour confirmed the diagnosis.

Case 102: Foreign bodies in the airway of an 18-year-old male.

The patient presented with increasing cough for several months, although he had no memory of aspiration.

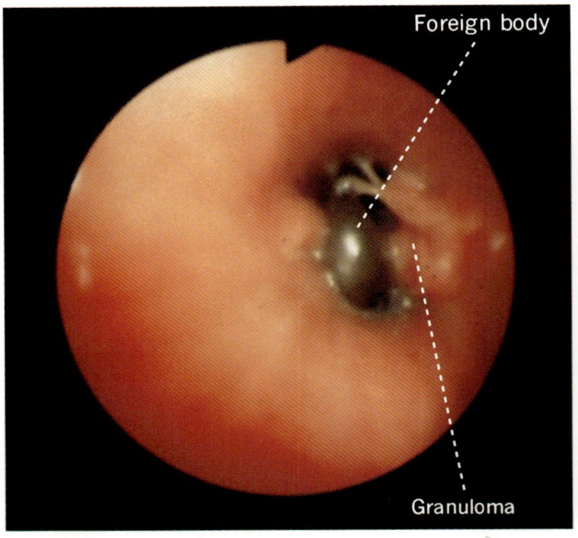

102.1 Bronchoscopic findings in the truncus intermedius. A glossy, black object with a smooth surface, around which granulation tissue proliferates, is visible. The mucosa is reddened and oedematous.

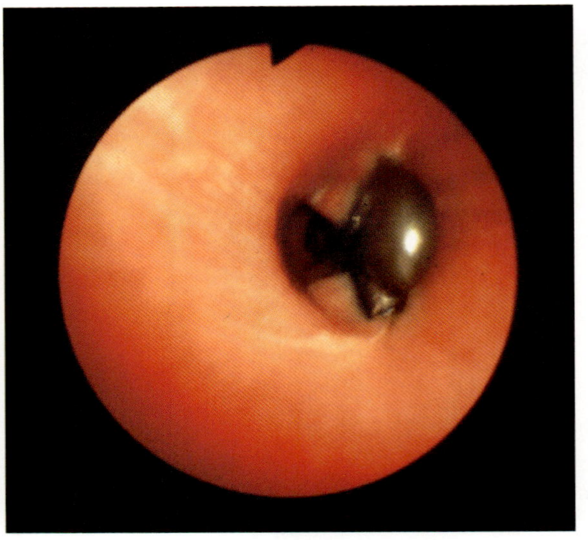

102.2 Examination by forceps revealed that the object was smooth, hard and mobile.

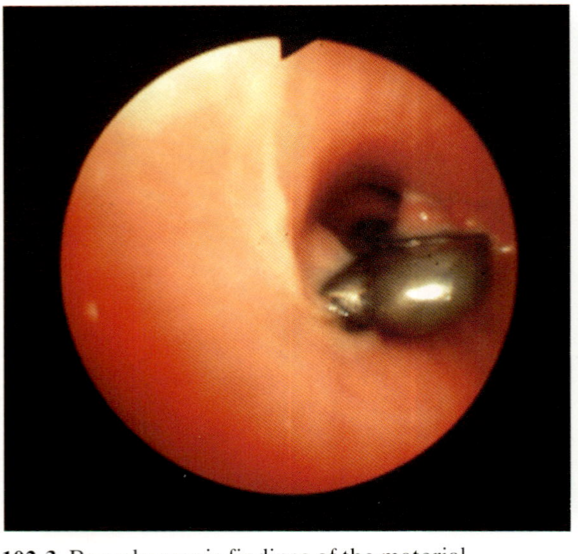

102.3 Bronchoscopic findings of the material retained by the forceps. It was readily removed without haemorrhage.

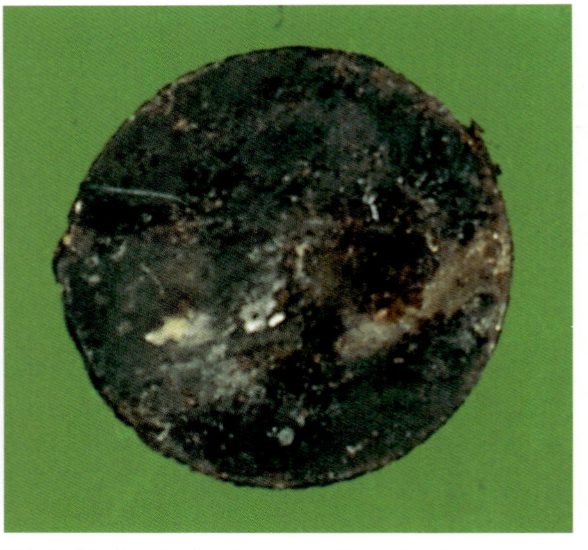

102.4 The foreign body removed by using forceps was found to be the head of a thumbtack.

Case 103: Diffuse cavernous haemangioma of the lung and mediastinum in an 18-year-old male.

The patient was referred to us after a small haemoptysis in winter. It was also pointed out that since 6 years of age a mass shadow involving the mediastinum and both hila was present on his chest radiograph.

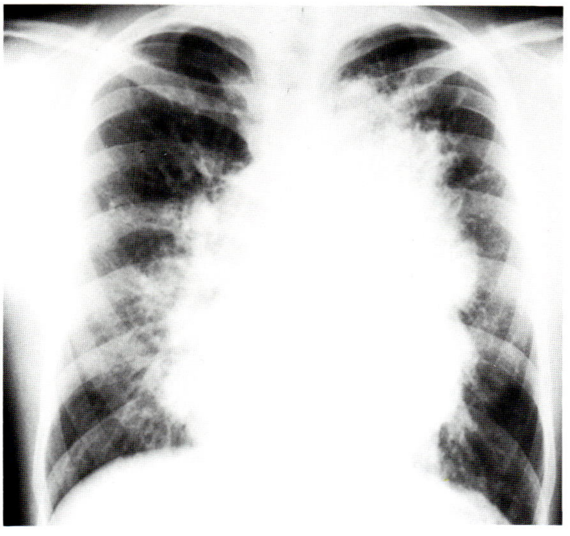

103.1 Posteroanterior chest radiograph. The mediastinum is markedly enlarged, and there are linear and reticular shadows of the blood vessels around it.

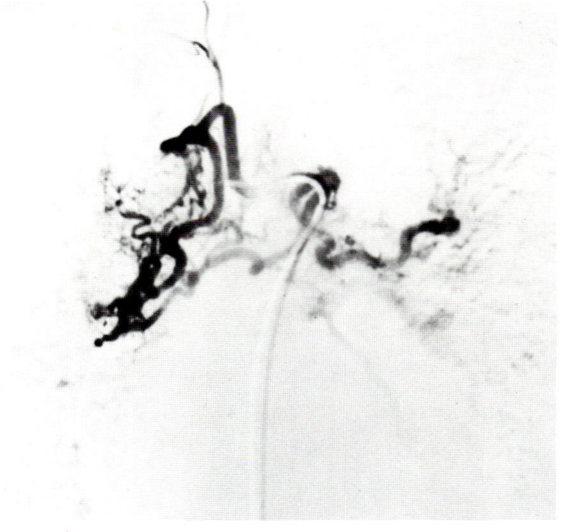

103.2 Bronchial arteriogram. The bilateral bronchial arteries are very tortuous and dilated. The tumour vessels are clearly displayed by a rapid influx of the contrast medium.

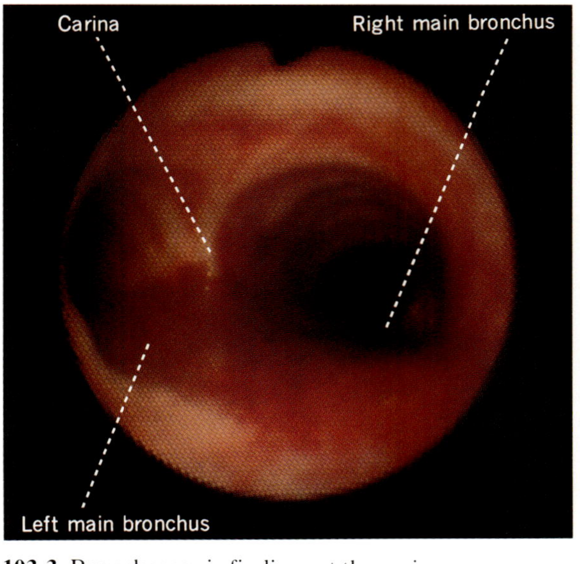

103.3 Bronchoscopic findings at the carina. Dilatation of the vessels and reddening of the mucosa is seen over the membranous portion of the bifurcation.

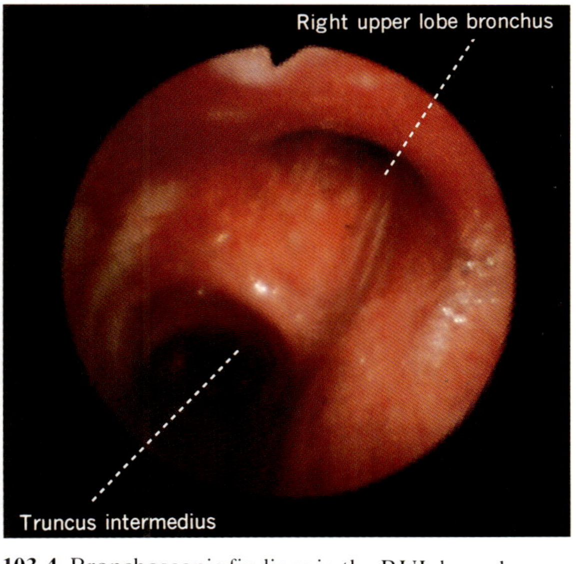

103.4 Bronchoscopic findings in the RUL bronchus. The mucosa is oedematous and dark all over. The condition was diagnosed as a haemangioma.

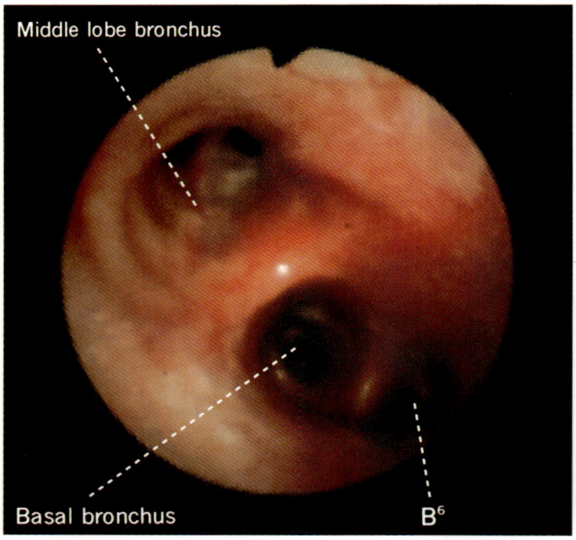

103.5 Bronchoscopic findings in the RML and RLL bronchi. The bifurcation is reddened and swollen becaused of the haemangioma.

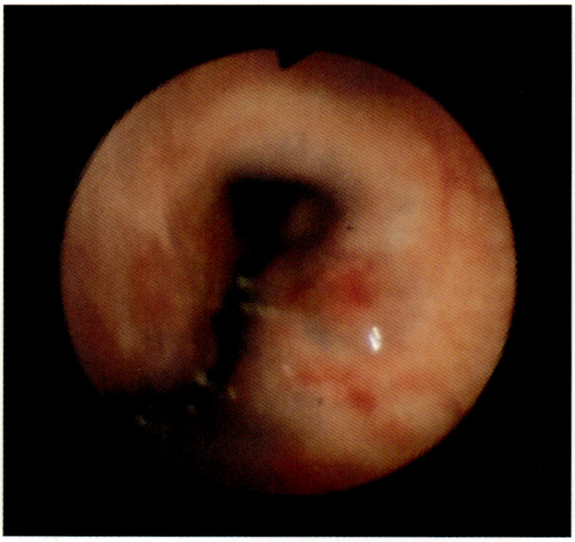

103.6 Bronchoscopic findings in the left main bronchus. The bronchial lumen is narrowed by the protrusion of the haemangioma.

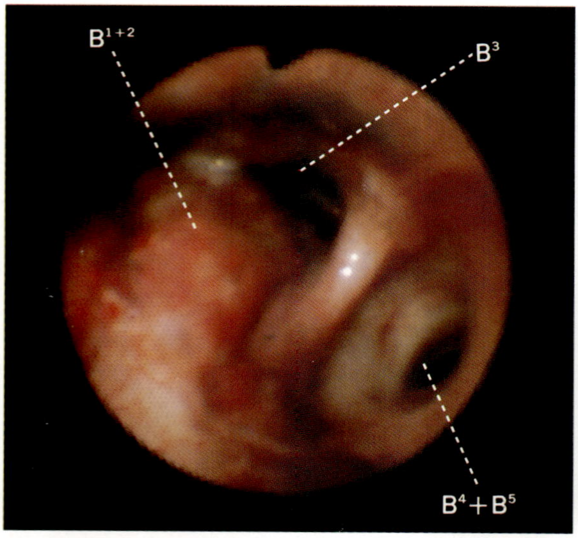

103.7 Bronchoscopic findings in the LUL bronchus. The bifurcation is widened, irregular and dark red in some parts.

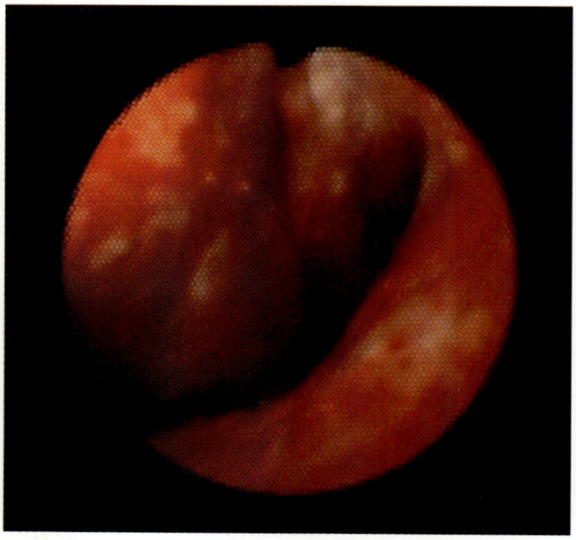

103.8 Bronchoscopic findings in the LLL bronchus. The bronchial wall is strikingly irregular and reddened; again it suggests the presence of a haemangioma.

Case 104: Mitral stenosis in a 46-year-old male.

The patient presented with a history of mild dyspnoea on exertion since he was young. He also complained of a cough with sputum in winter which has lasted for 3 years.

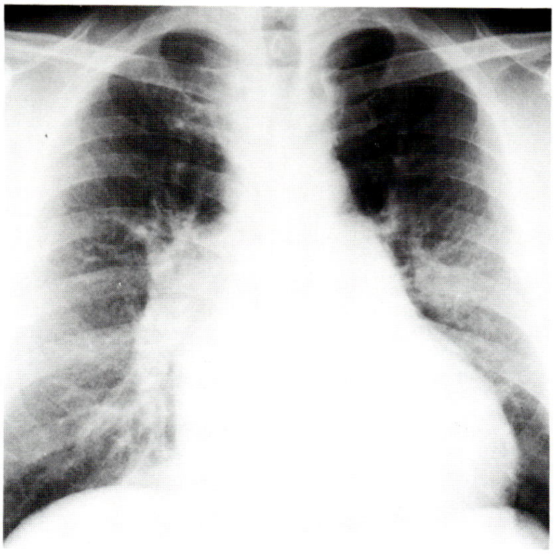

104.1 Posteroanterior chest radiograph. The configuration of the cardiomegaly suggests the presence of mitral stenosis.

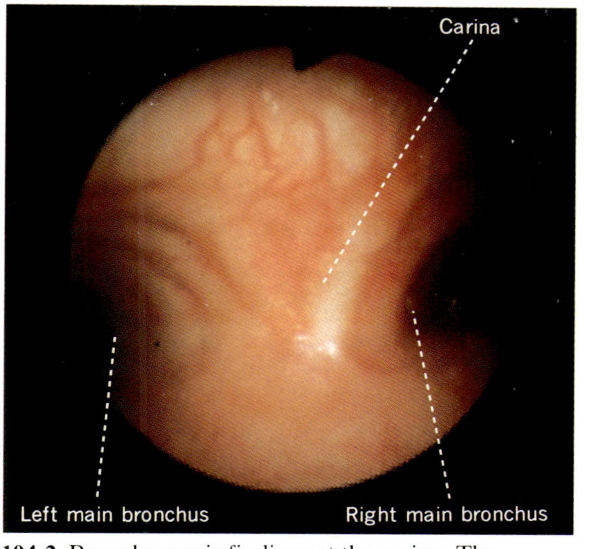

104.2 Bronchoscopic findings at the carina. The mucosal vessels are strikingly engorged and the bifurcation is moderately widened.

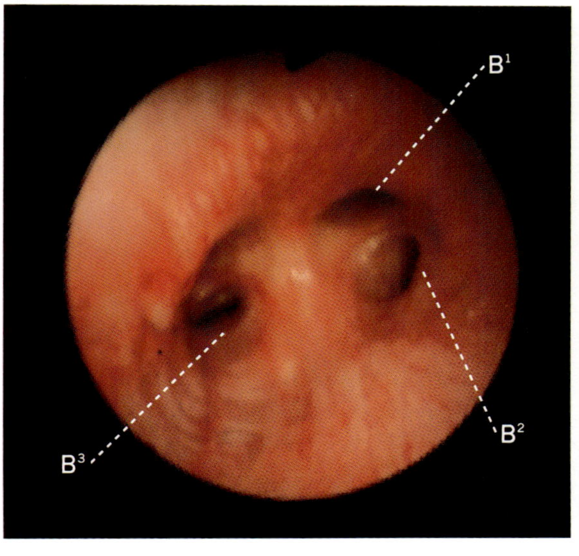

104.3 Bronchoscopic findings in the RUL bronchus. The mucosa appears red and vascular dilatation is present.

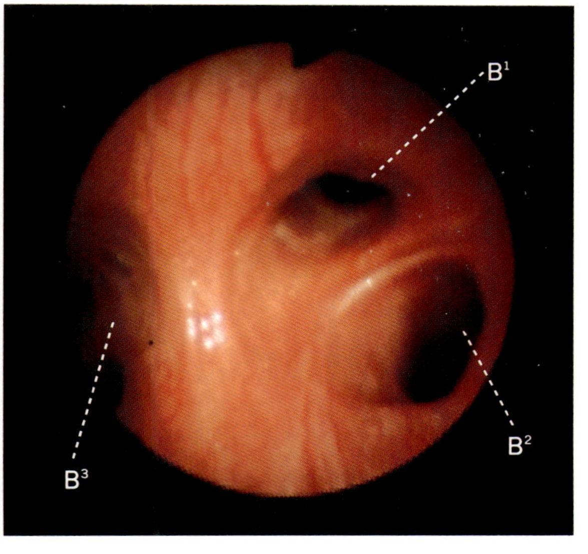

104.4 Close-up of **104.3**. The mucosa is generally red with vascular engorgement.

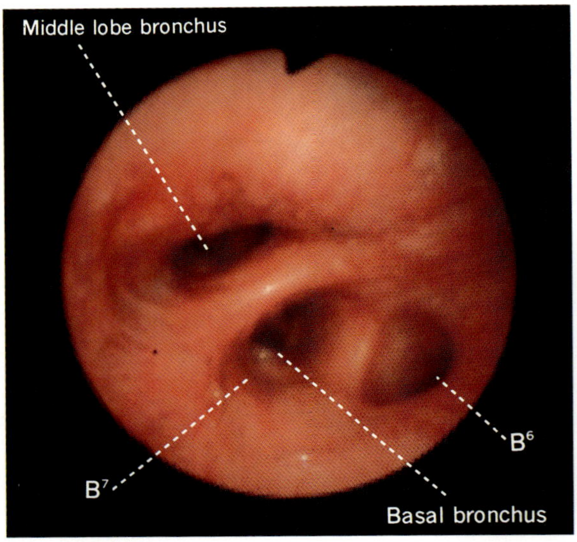

104.5 Bronchoscopic findings in the RML and RLL bronchi. The mucosa is red with vascular dilatation. The bifurcation is slightly widened. Parts of the bronchial walls seem irregular.

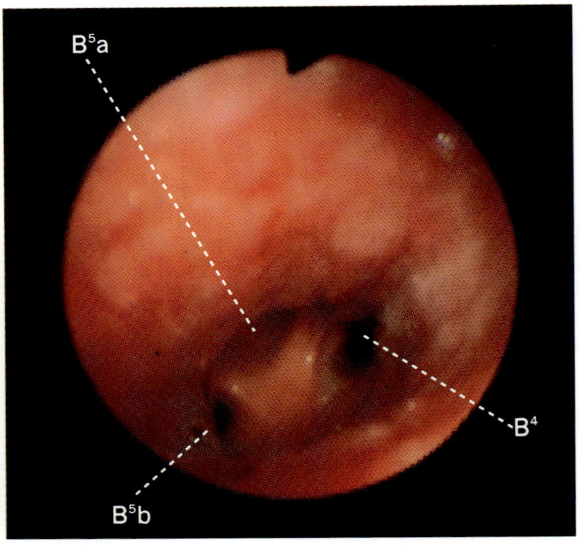

104.6 Bronchoscopic findings in the RML bronchus. The mucosa is generally red and irregular.

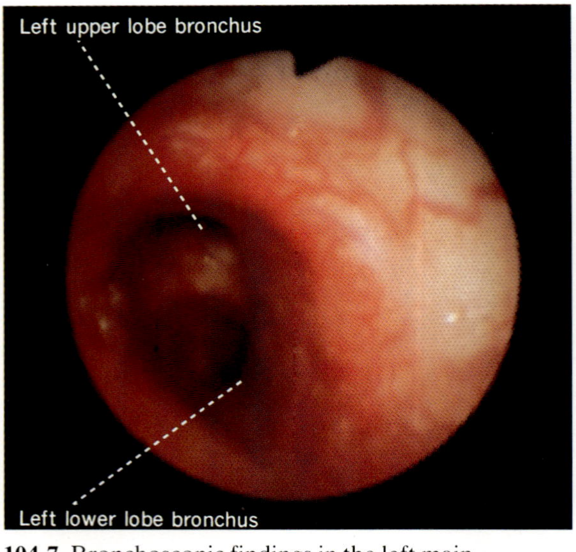

104.7 Bronchoscopic findings in the left main bronchus. Note the tortuous, dilated vessels in the surrounding mucosa.

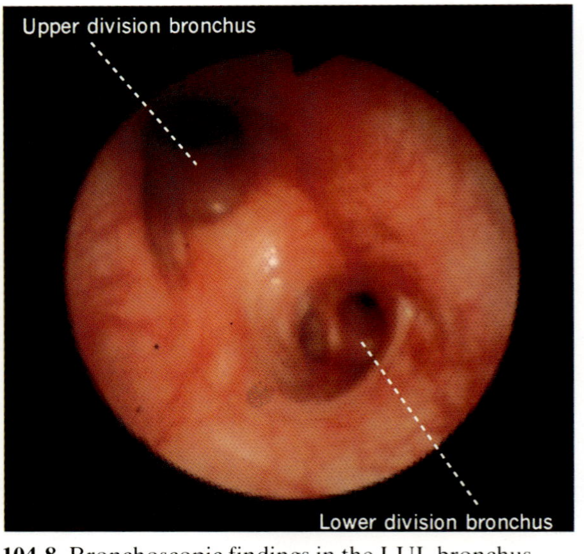

104.8 Bronchoscopic findings in the LUL bronchus. The mucosa is red and the mucosal vessels are strikingly dilated, suggesting the elevation of pulmonary venous pressure and resultant pulmonary congestion of this disease.

Case 105: Cardiomyopathy in a 64-year-old female.

The patient had a history of repeated hospitalisation for cardiomyopathy associated with congestive heart failure or angina pectoris for several years. She was again admitted in December 1981 with congestive heart failure. Her electrocardiogram showed right bundle branch block.

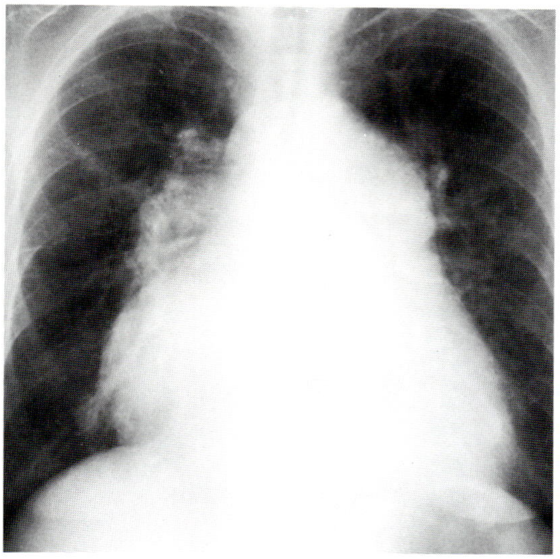

105.1 Posteroanterior chest radiograph. Note marked cardiomegaly (CTR = 63%) and enlargement of the hila, in addition to Kerley B lines.

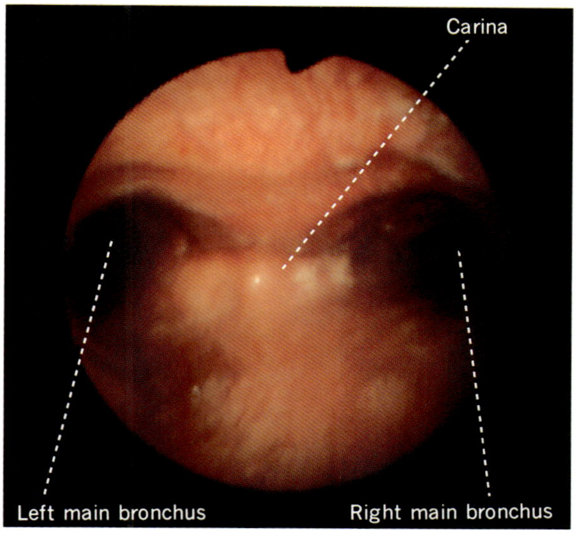

105.2 Bronchoscopic findings at the carina. Note the tortuous, dilated vessels.

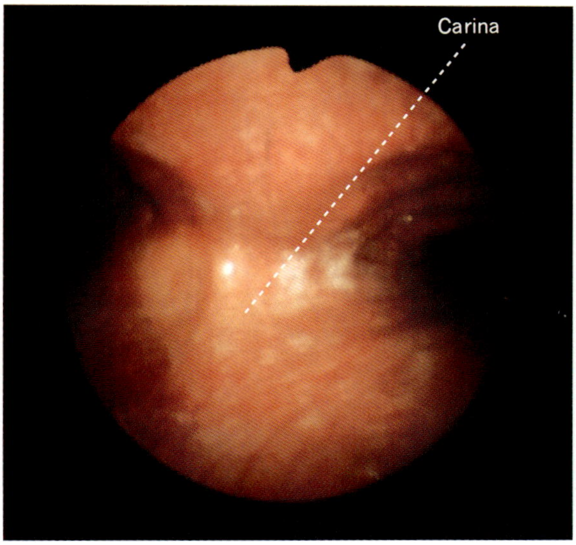

105.3 Close-up of the carina. The mucosa is irregular and reddened, with tortuous vessels.

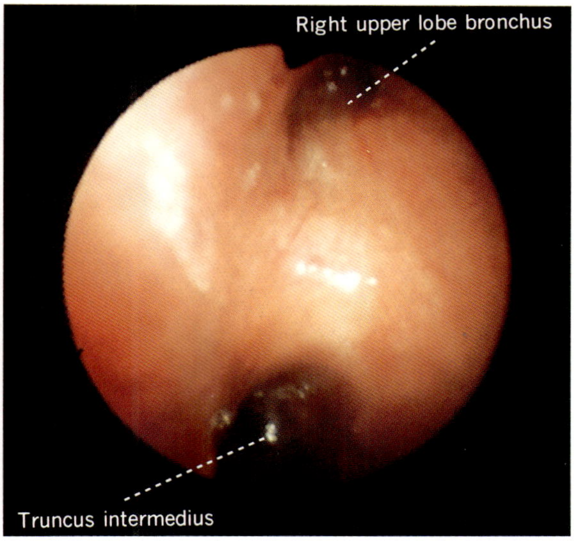

105.4 Bronchoscopic findings in the RUL bronchus. The bifurcation is widened and swollen.

Case 106: Pulmonary oedema in a 42-year-old male.

The patient, an asthmatic since childhood, developed productive cough and dyspnoea at 30 years of age. He also had an additional history of haemoptysis from March 1981. Physical examination revealed clubbing and marked cyanosis.

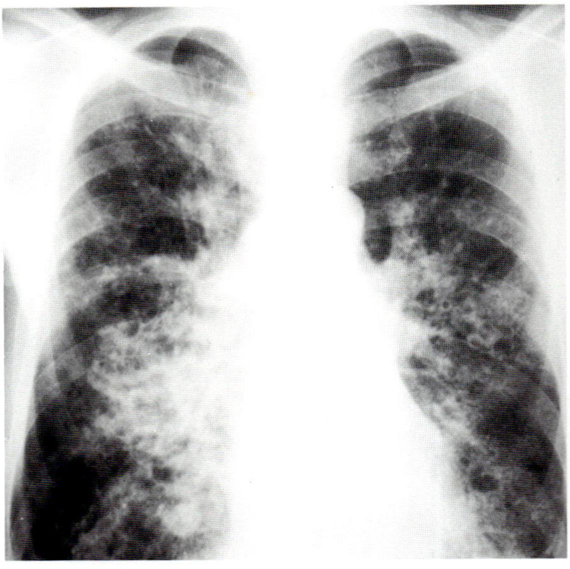

106.1 Posterolateral chest radiograph. The reticular pattern is obvious throughout the lungs; this appearance is referred to as 'honeycomb lung'.

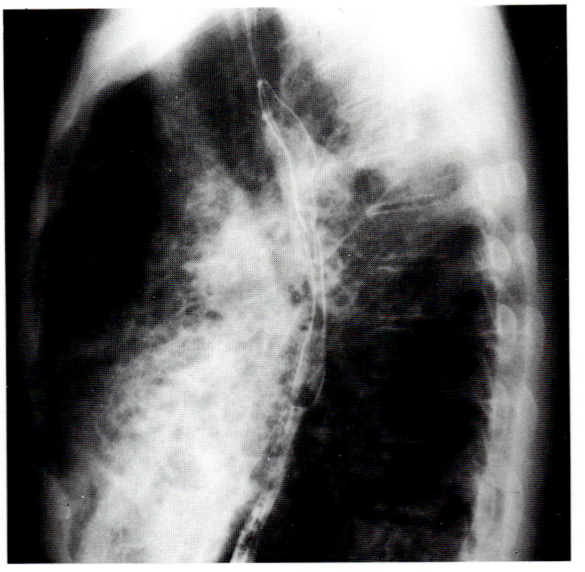

106.2 Lateral chest radiograph showing a similar pattern.

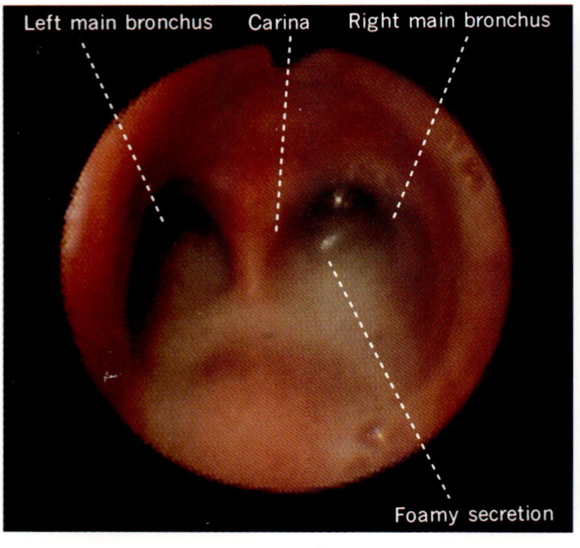

106.3 During fibreoptic bronchoscopy under oxygen inhalation, the patient suddenly became dyspnoeic and masses of frothy sputum flooded out of the bilateral main bronchi. The mucosa appeared cyanotic.

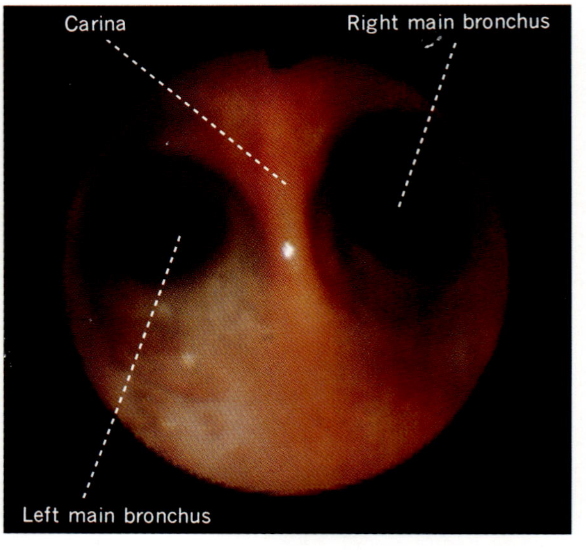

106.4 In spite of suction, the frothy sputum was so great in volume that examination was curtailed. It was considered that acute heart failure had been induced by fibreoptic bronchoscopy.

14 Mucoepidermoid carcinoma

Case 107: Mucoepidermoid carcinoma in a 22-year-old female.

The patient presented with a small haemoptysis without any other symptoms, in the summer of 1979. However, a medical examination, including chest radiograph and erythrocyte sedimentation rate, revealed all was normal. An episode of haemoptysis recurred in October 1980 and in February 1981, when RML atelectasis was revealed on her chest radiograph. On April 1st a third episode of haemoptysis brought her to the clinic. Fibreoptic bronchoscopy was performed on April 16th.

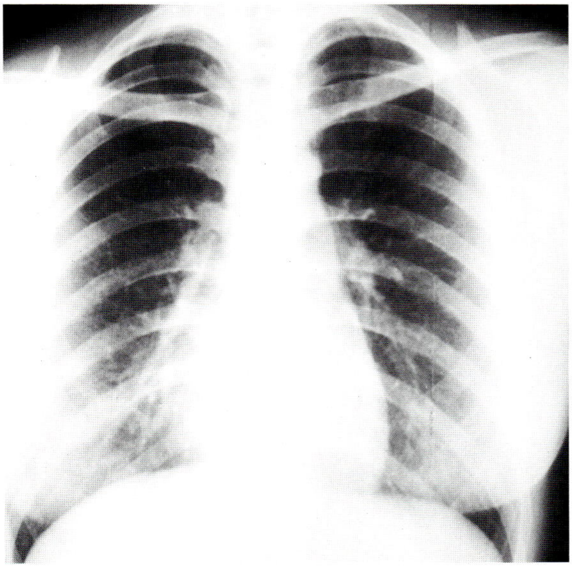

107.1 Posteroanterior chest radiograph. The right heart border is obliterated, suggesting RML atelectasis.

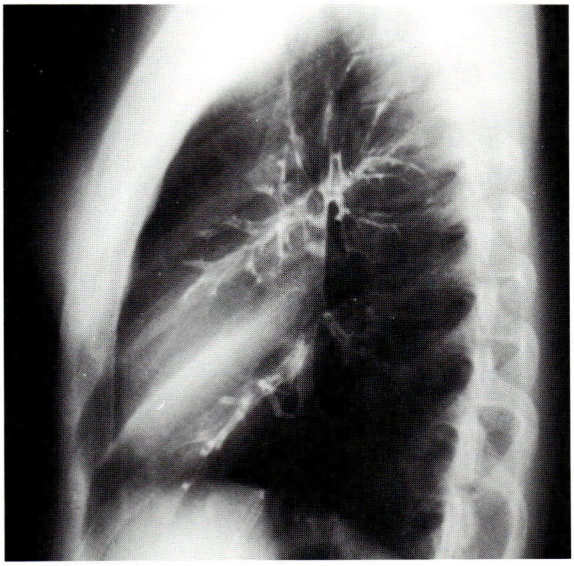

107.2 Lateral bronchogram. The RML bronchus is completely occluded at the orifice.

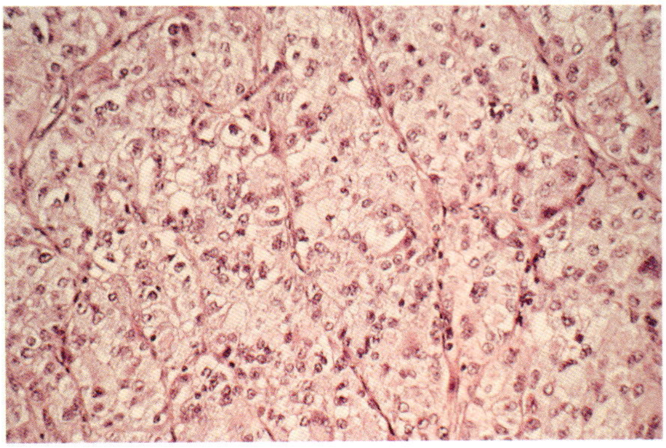

107.3 Histopathological findings of the biopsy. The tumour cells with round nuclei and eosinophilic, granular cytoplasm proliferate in sheet-like fashion, forming nests divided by the thin layers of connective tissue.

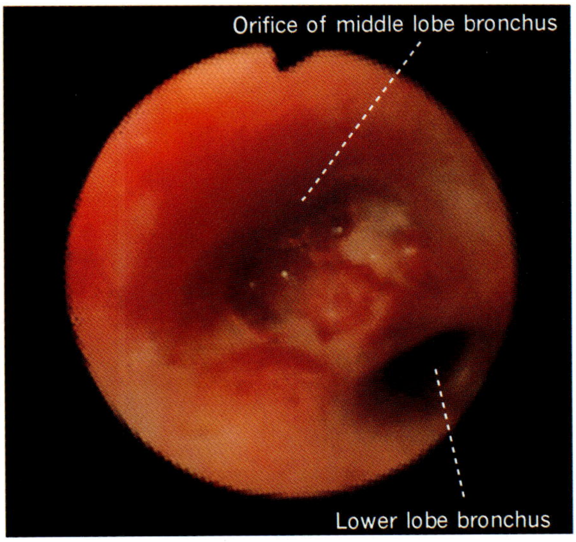

107.4 Bronchoscopic findings in the RML and RLL bronchi. The orifice of the RML bronchus is completely occluded by the tumour which is red, resembling red caviar, partly covered with a white coating. The surrounding mucosa is deeply reddened.

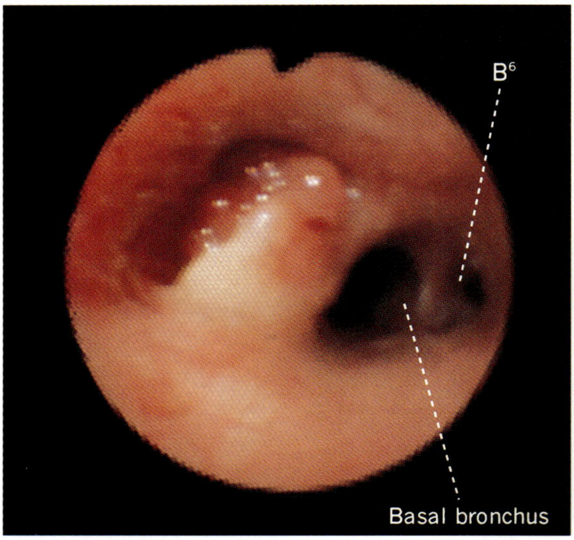

107.5 Close-up of the tumour. Its surface looks like red caviar. The surrounding mucosa shows dilated vessels.

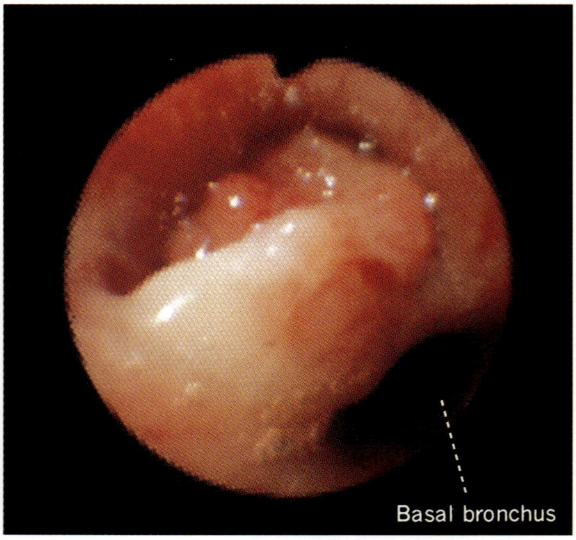

107.6 Further close-up of the tumour. The red caviar-like surfaced tumour is partly covered with a white coating, biopsy of which confirmed histological diagnosis.

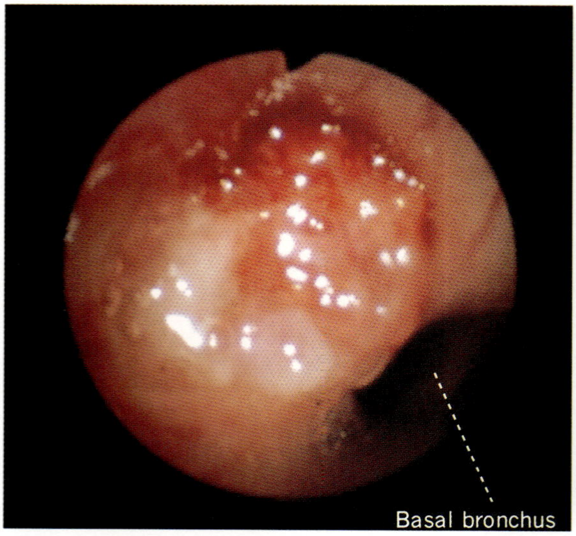

107.7 Bronchoscopic findings 2 months later. The tumour shows the same findings.

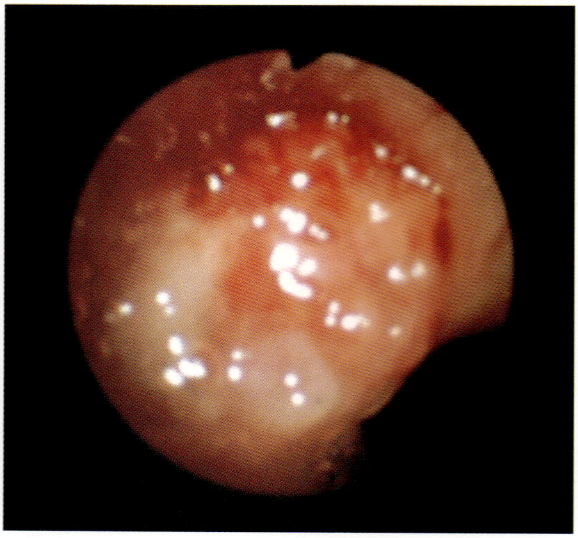

107.8 Further close-up of the tumour. It has abundant mucosal vessels and bleeds easily.

Case 108: Mucoepidermoid carcinoma in a 60-year-old female.

The patient complained of a cough and occasional haemoptysis.

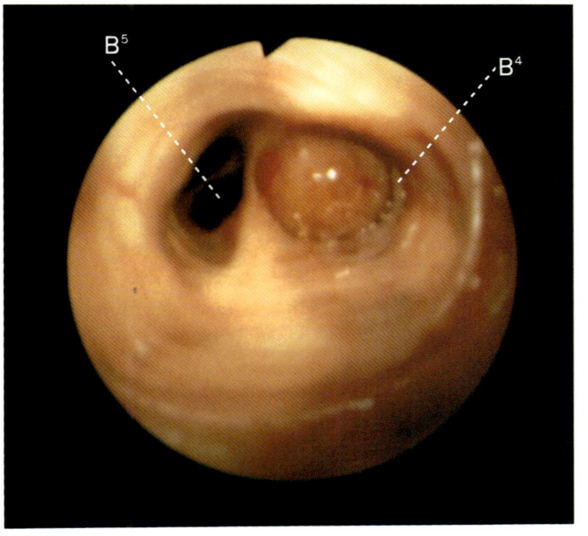

108.1 Bronchoscopic findings in the RML bronchus. B^4 is totally obstructed by the spherical tumour with a smooth surface, although B^5 remains patent.

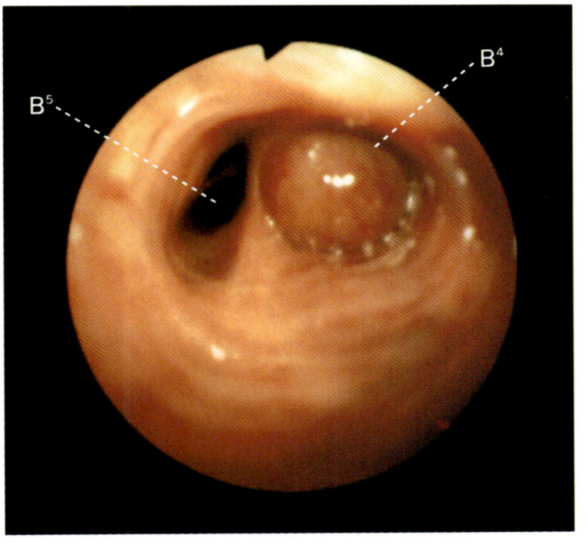

108.2 Close-up of **108.1**. The surface of the tumour is smooth, and slightly dark and the mucosal vessels are visible on it. The surrounding mucosa is reddened and oedematous.

Case 109: Acute bronchopneumonia in a 51-year-old male.

The patient, a non-smoker, presented with a productive cough with left chest pain and fever in April 1981. Laboratory tests revealed a white blood-cell count of 9,000 cell/mm^3 with leftward shift of the differential count to a mild degree. The erythrocyte sedimentation rate was 45 mm/h and C-reactive protein negative. The cold agglutinin titre was increased four-fold. He underwent fibreoptic bronchoscopy at the end of May.

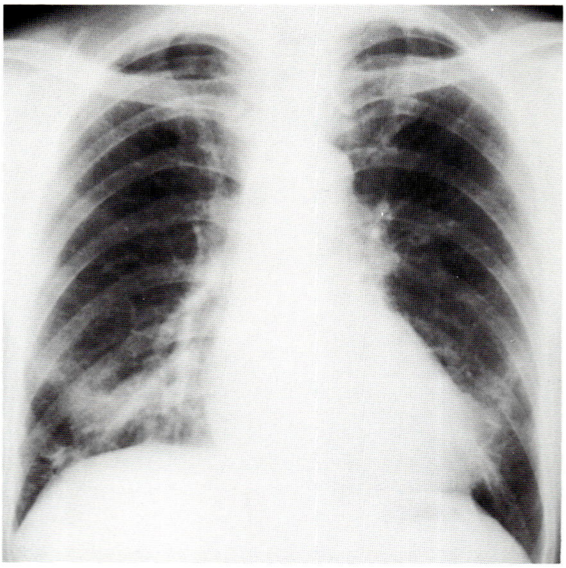

109.1 Posteroanterior chest radiograph. An infiltrate is present in the right lower zone and the lower half of the left heart border is obliterated.

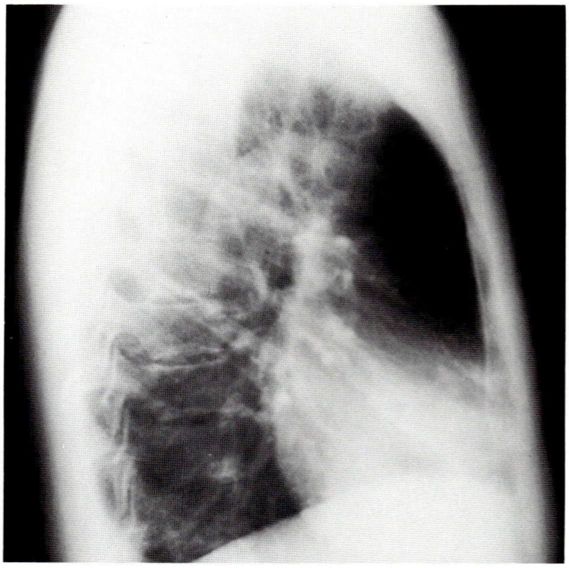

109.2 Lateral chest radiograph. Infiltrates in the RML and lower lung zone are visible.

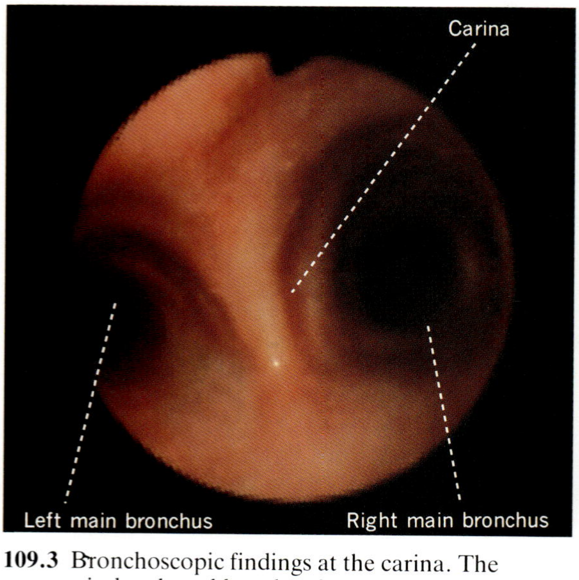

109.3 Bronchoscopic findings at the carina. The mucosa is deeply reddened and swollen.

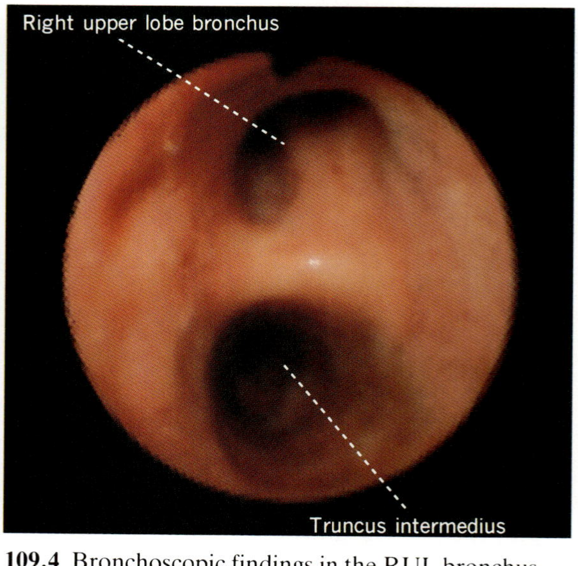

109.4 Bronchoscopic findings in the RUL bronchus. The mucosa shows similar findings to those of **109.3**. The bifurcation is widened and the longitudinal corrugations have disappeared.

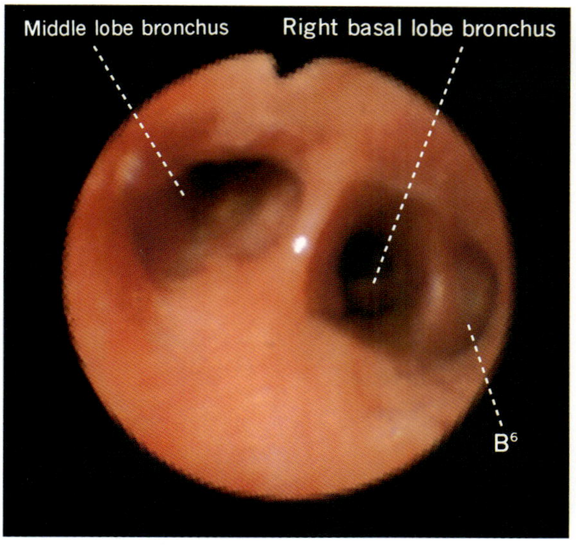

109.5 Bronchoscopic findings in RML and RLL bronchi. The mucosa is reddened and swollen; note the widened bifurcation.

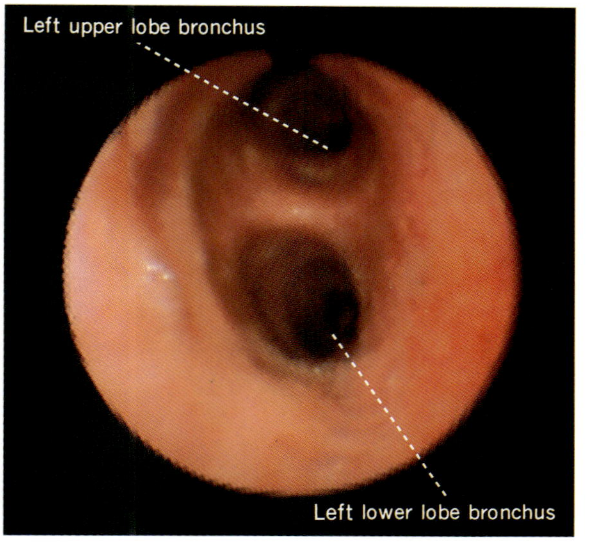

109.6 Bronchoscopic findings in the LUL and LLL bronchi. The mucosa is prominently reddened and bifurcation is widened.

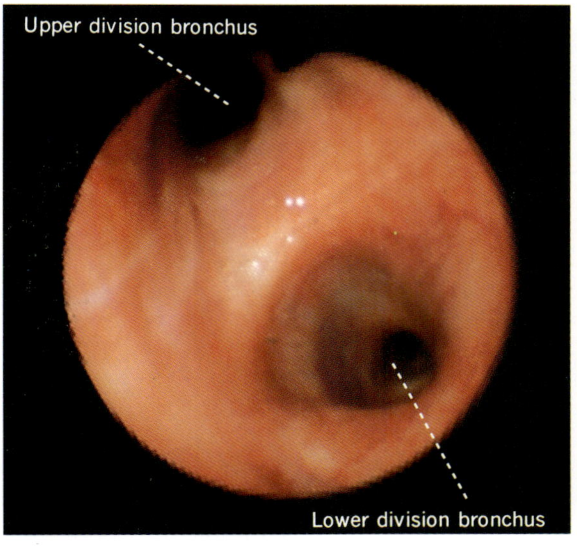

109.7 Bronchoscopic findings in the LUL bronchus. The mucosa is markedly reddened, with engorged vessels. The bifurcation is slightly swollen as well as widened.

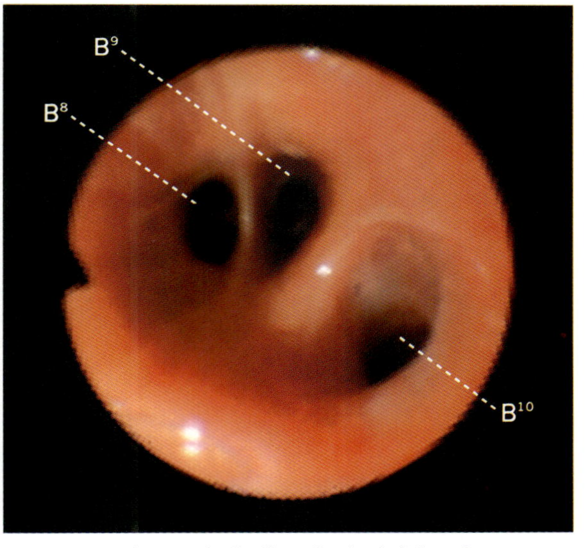

109.8 Bronchoscopic findings in the left basal bronchus. The mucosa is deeply reddened and swollen. The bifurcations between each segmental bronchi are oedematous and widened.

Case 110: Eosinophilic granuloma in a 22-year-old female.

This patient, with a history of smoking 7,000 cigarettes per year since 15 years of age, had complained of frequent coughs and flu-like sympoms. Upper-respiratory-tract infections with 38.5°C of fever brought her to the clinic where abnormalities were revealed on her chest radiograph. She was referred to us for further examination in November and underwent fibreoptic bronchoscopy in December.

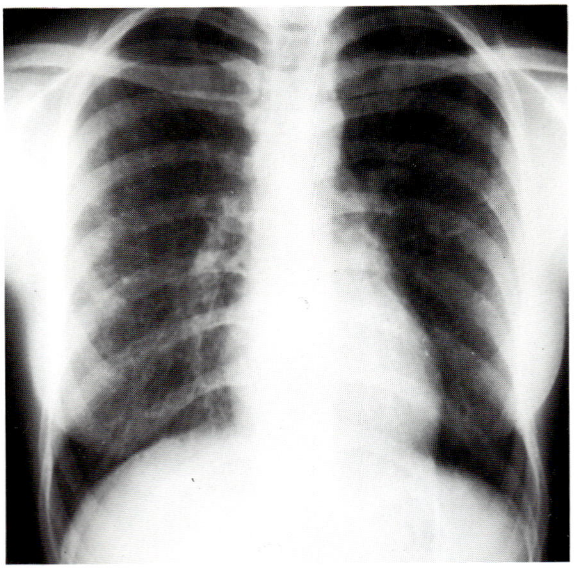

110.1 Posteroanterior chest radiograph. A diffuse reticular pattern is seen throughout the lungs. Kerley B lines are also seen in both costophrenic angles.

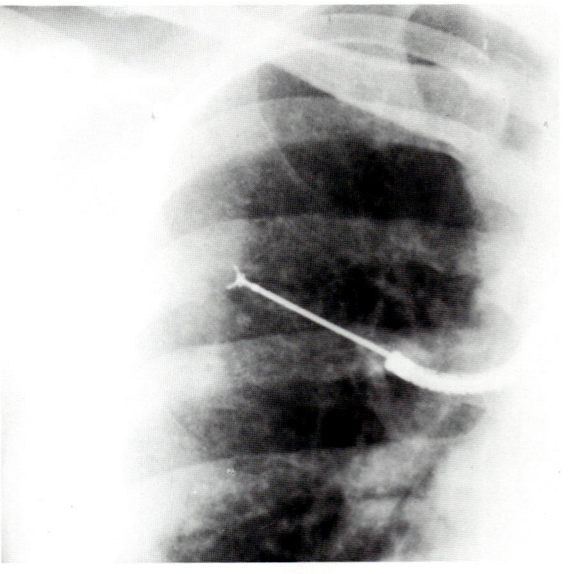

110.2 Transbronchial lung biopsy being performed under fluoroscopy. Biopsy material from right B^3ai (shown by the forceps) revealed eosinophilic granuloma.

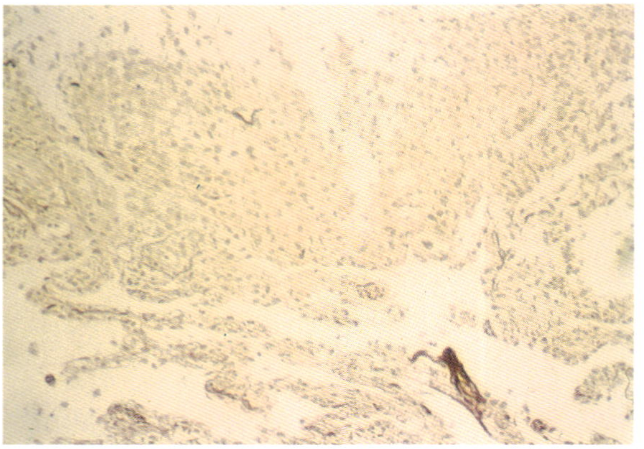

110.3 Pathological findings. Granulomas composed of histiocytes and a small number of eosinophils are scattered around the blood vessels as well as in the alveoli in part; alveolitis is present to a mild degree.

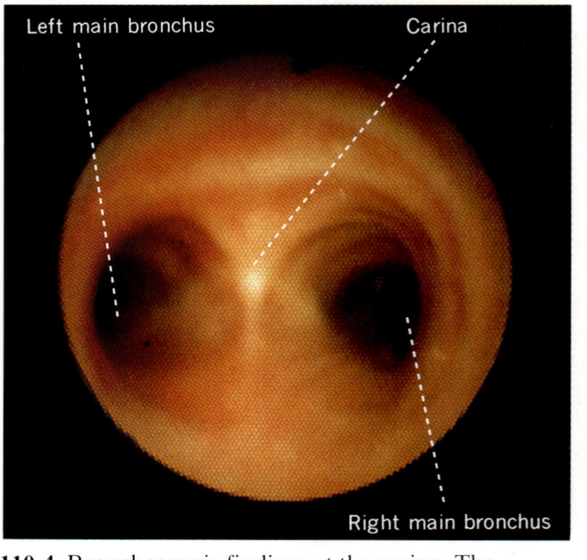

110.4 Bronchoscopic findings at the carina. The mucosa is deeply reddened.

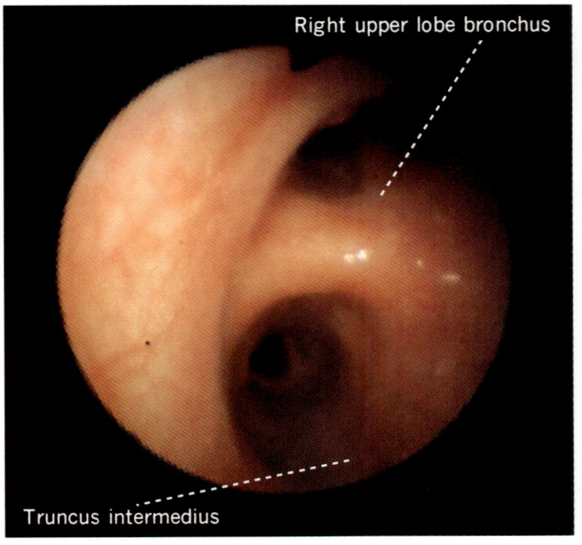

110.5 Bronchoscopic findings in the RUL bronchus and truncus intermedius. The mucosa is markedly reddened and swollen, in addition to the vascular dilatation. The bifurcation is oedematous and widened.

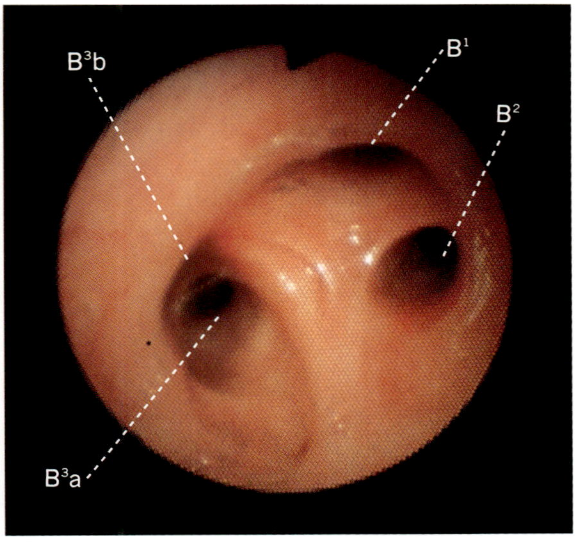

110.6 Bronchoscopic findings in the RUL bronchus. The mucosa is prominently reddened and swollen.

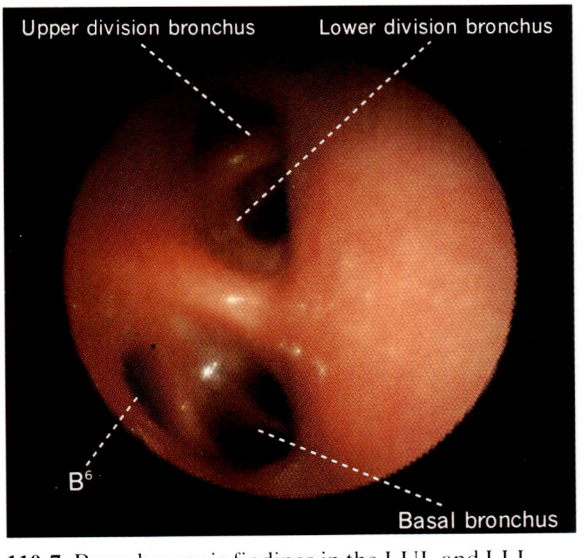

110.7 Bronchoscopic findings in the LUL and LLL bronchi. The mucosa is generally reddened and swollen. Vascular engorgement and widening of the bifurcations into segmental and subsegmental bronchi are clearly visible.

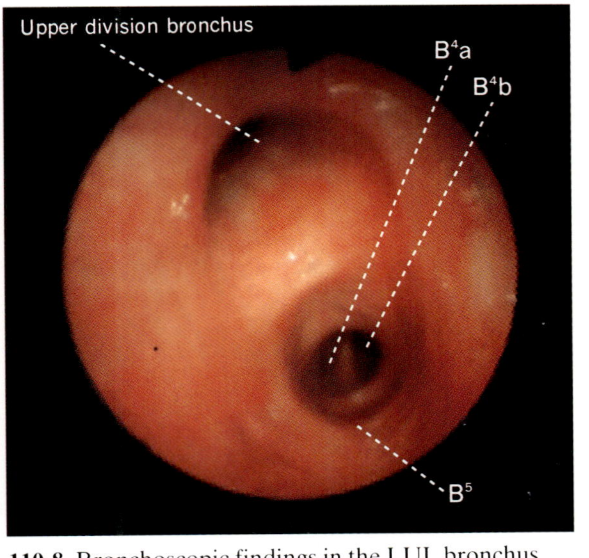

110.8 Bronchoscopic findings in the LUL bronchus. The mucosa is reddened as well as swollen, with dilated vessels.

Case 111: Diffuse panbronchiolitis in a 57-year-old male.

The patient, who had undergone surgery for paranasal sinusitis, complained of a cough with purulent sputum in 1977. He visited our clinic in January 1981.

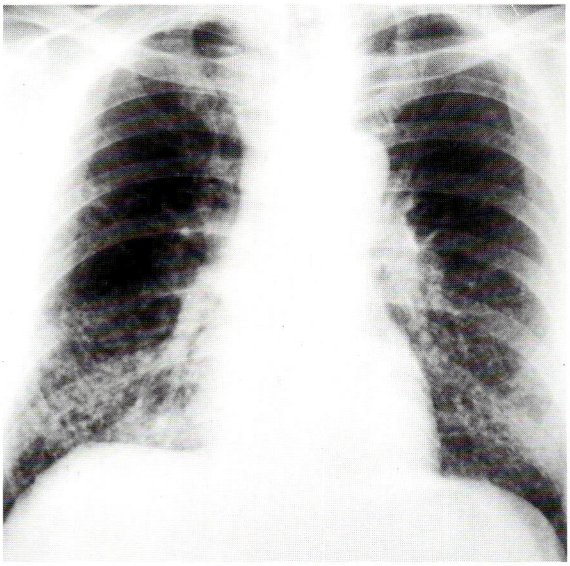

111.1 Posteroanterior chest radiograph. Diffuse micronodular shadows, 2-3 mm in size, are visible throughout the lungs, particularly in the lower lung zone.

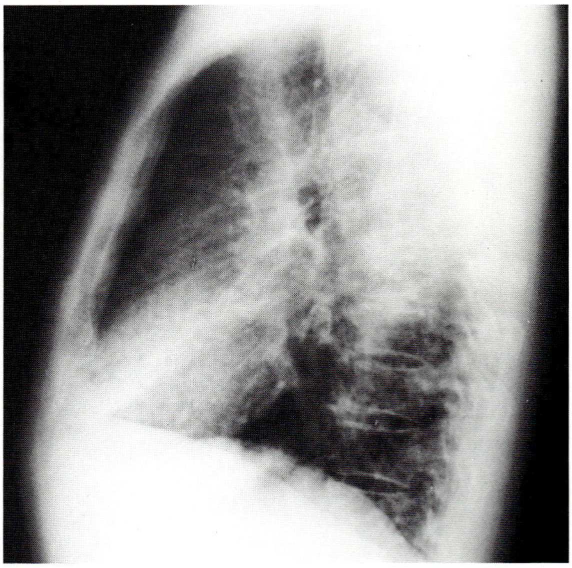

111.2 Lateral chest radiograph. Diffuse micronodular densities are visible.

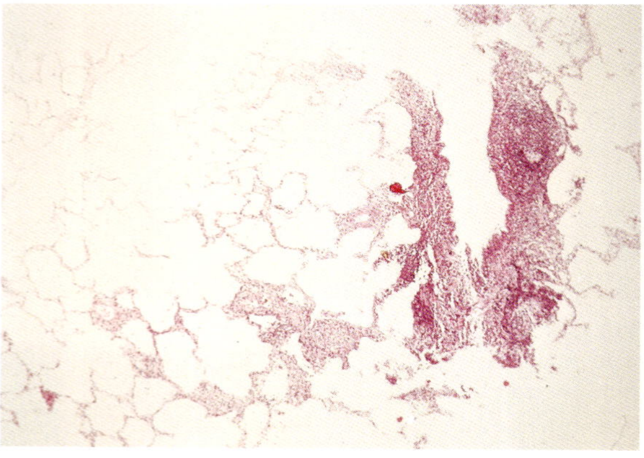

111.3 Histology of the biopsy material taken from right S^3 using transbronchial lung biopsy. A cellular infiltrate of lymphocytes or histocytes around the bronchi is observed, forming granulomas.

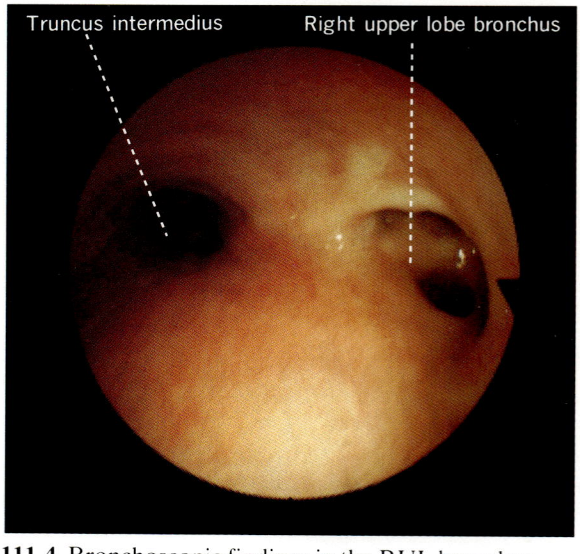

111.4 Bronchoscopic findings in the RUL bronchus and truncus intermedius. The bifurcation is widened and purulent secretion lies on it.

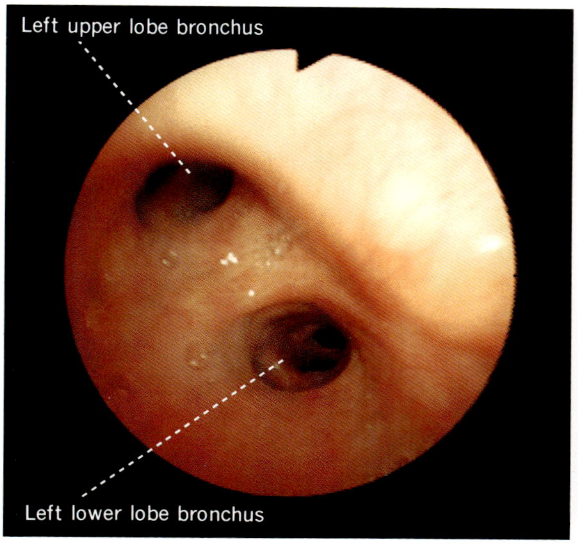

111.5 Bronchoscopic findings in the LUL and LLL bronchi. The bifurcation is widened and dilated vessels are seen on the mucosa, in addition to purulent secretion.

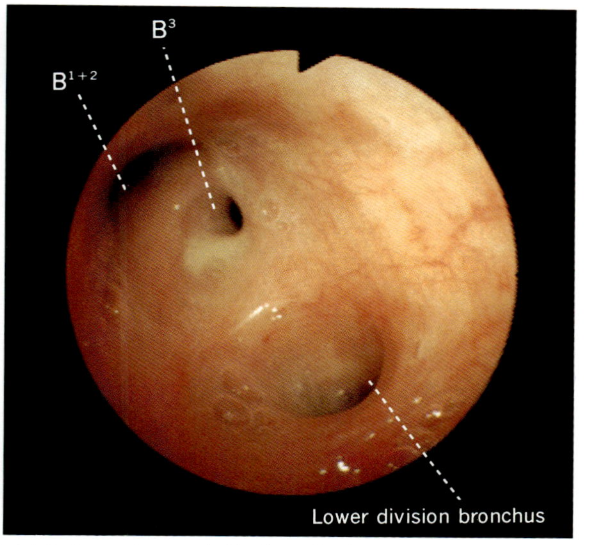

111.6 Bronchoscopic findings in the LUL bronchus. Each bifurcation is oedematous and widened and dilated vessels are seen on the mucosa, in addition to purulent secretion.

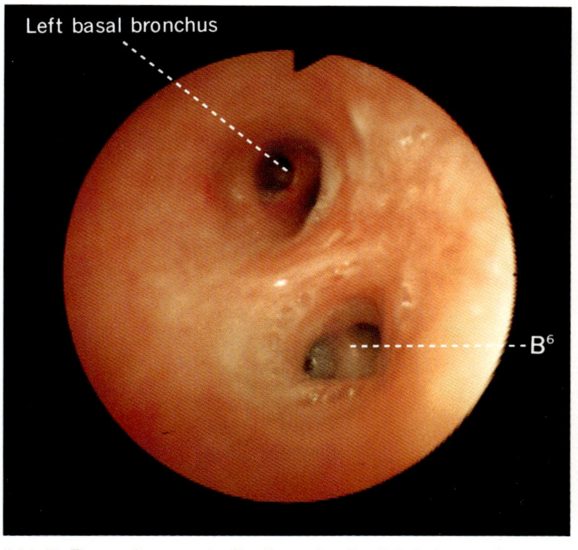

111.7 Bronchoscopic findings in the LLL bronchus. The mucosa is reddened and bifurcations into segmental and subsegmental bronchi of B^6 are widened.

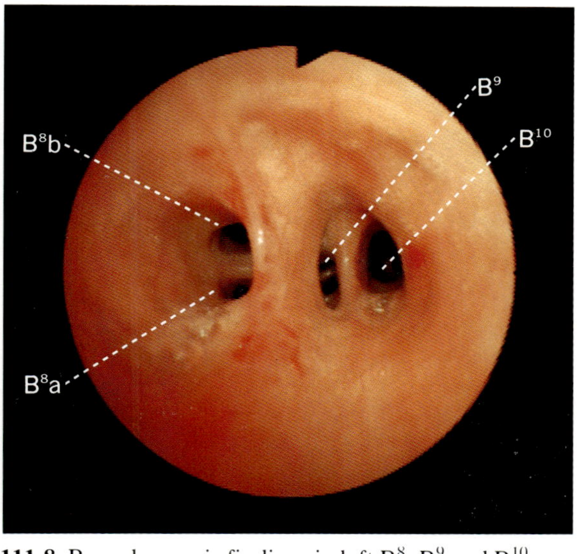

111.8 Bronchoscopic findings in left B^8, B^9 and B^{10}. The mucosa around B^8 is deeply reddened and swollen, with purulent secretion. The bifurcation between B^9 and B^{10} is widened.

Case 112: Diffuse panbronchiolitis in a 56-year-old female.

The patient presented with a productive cough with occasional fever from the time she was 20 years of age. She visited hospital for further evaluation in August 1978. Cold aggulutinin titre was elevated to 1:8192.

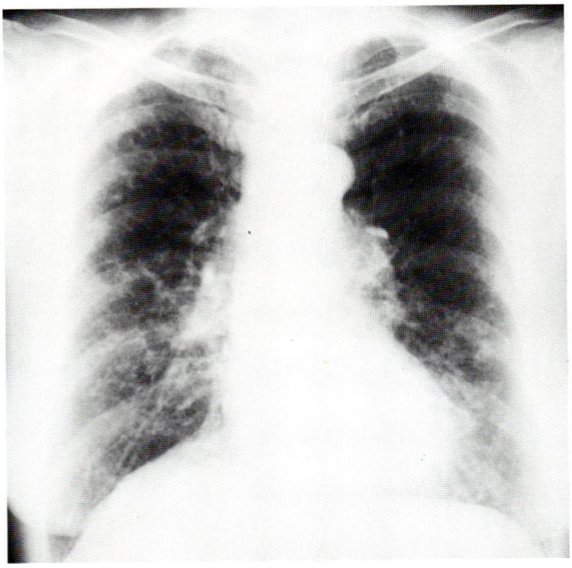

112.1 Posteroanterior chest radiograph. Micronodular shadows are diffusely seen throughout the lungs and the lower half of the heart border is obliterated.

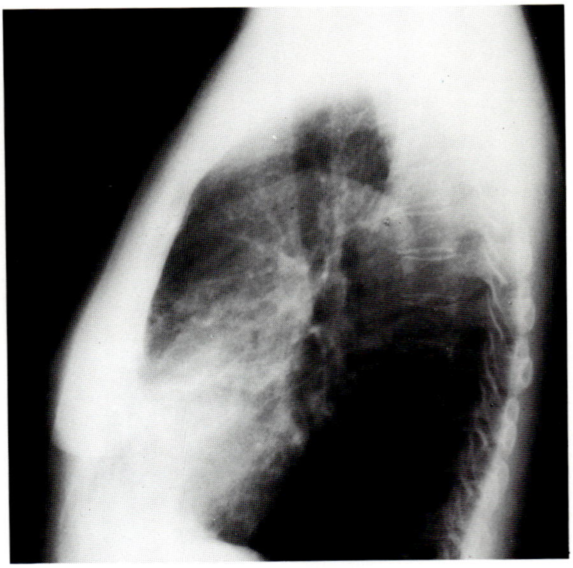

112.2 Lateral chest radiograph. Micronodular shadows are more prominent in S^4, S^5 and $S^{10}c$.

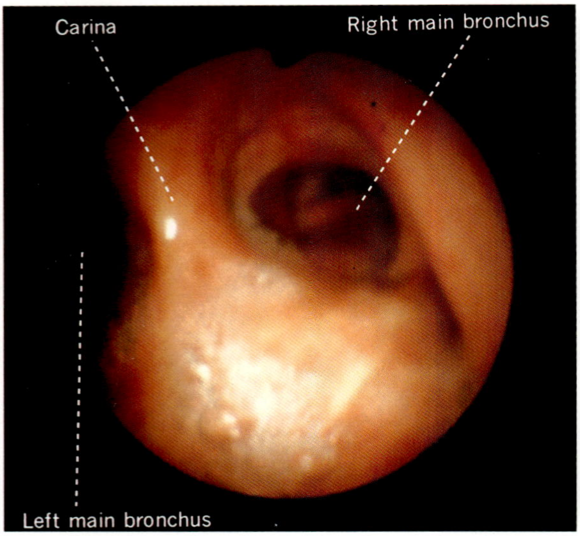

112.3 Bronchoscopic findings at the carina. The mucosa is reddened and swollen, with copious secretion. The bifurcation is oedematous and widened.

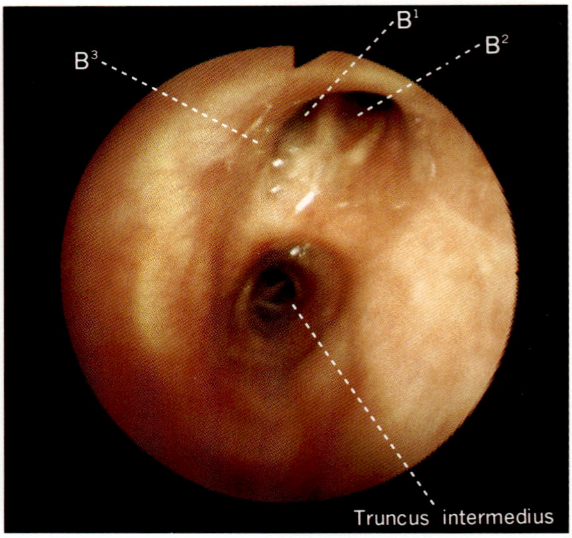

112.4 Bronchoscopic findings in the RUL bronchus and truncus intermedius. The bifurcation is widened and covered with secretion.

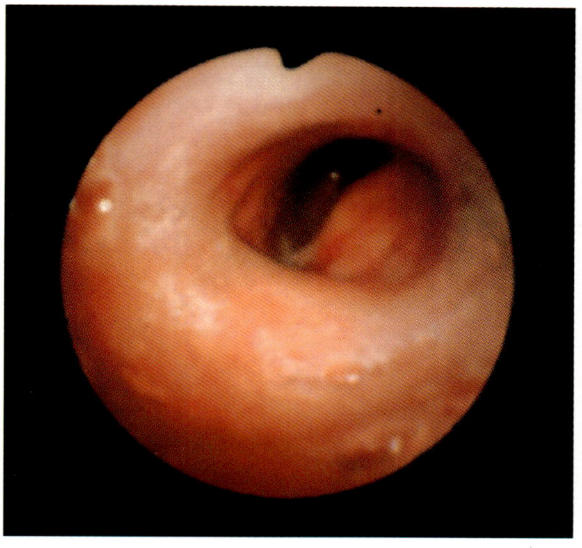

112.5 Bronchoscopic findings in the truncus intermedius. Copious secretion is present and the mucosa is markedly reddened and swollen, narrowing the bronchial lumen.

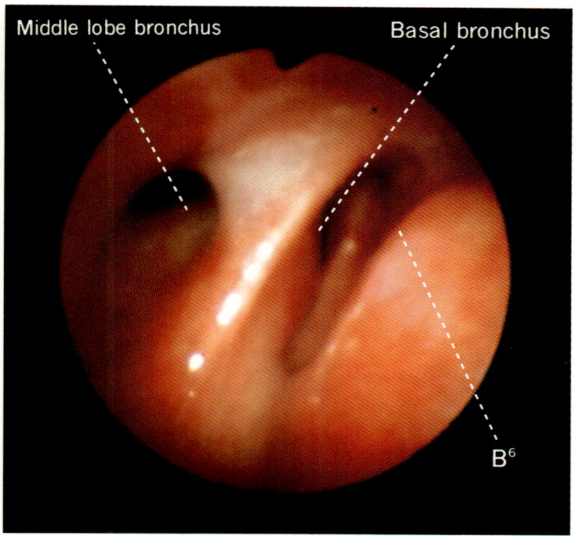

112.6 Bronchoscopic findings in the RML and RLL bronchi. The mucosa is prominently reddened and swollen and the bifurcation is widened, narrowing particularly the orifice of the RLL bronchus.

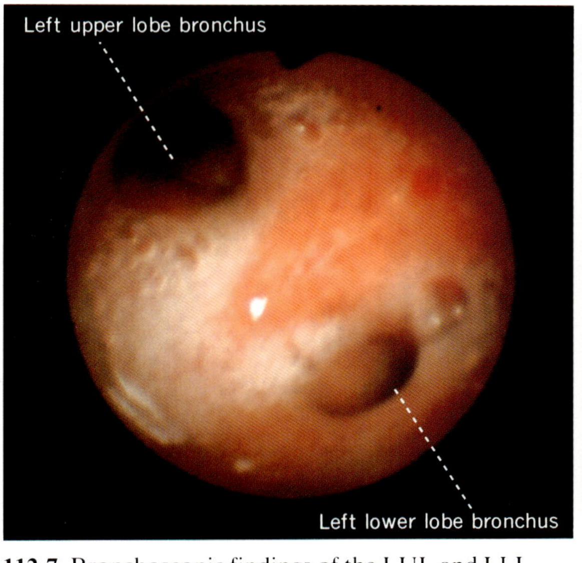

112.7 Bronchoscopic findings of the LUL and LLL bronchus. The mucosa is markedly reddened and swollen, and there is copious purulent secretion.

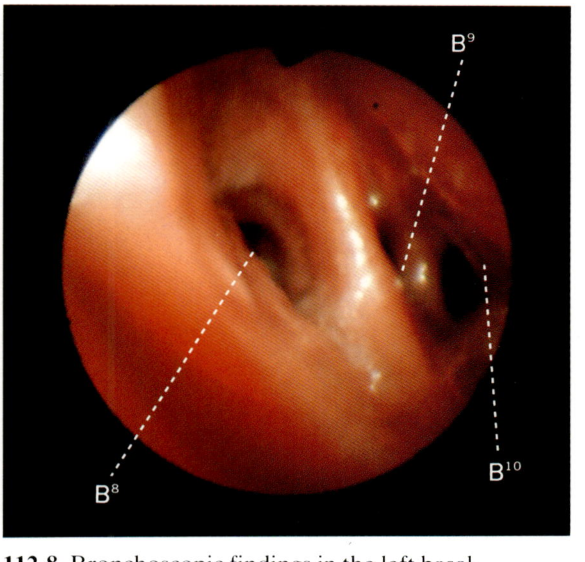

112.8 Bronchoscopic findings in the left basal bronchus. The mucosa is reddened and swollen. Each bifurcation is so widened as to narrow the orifice of each segmental bronchus.

Case 113: ND-Yag laser treatment of epidermoid carcinoma of the lung in a 69-year-old male.

This patient had an epidermoid carcinoma of the lung, and had already been treated with chemotherapy which impaired renal function. He underwent fibreoptic bronchoscopy because of increasing dyspnoea. Because there was a possibility that the RLL bronchus might have been occluded by the tumour, laser treatment was performed.

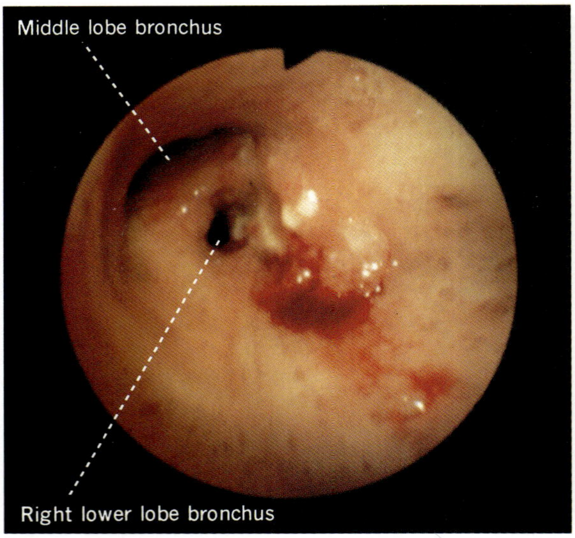

113.1 Bronchoscopic findings in the RML and RLL bronchi before laser treatment. The tumour involves the lower half of the truncus intermedius, the orifice of the RLL bronchus and the bifurcation into the RML bronchus, which is so wide that it narrows the RLL bronchus.

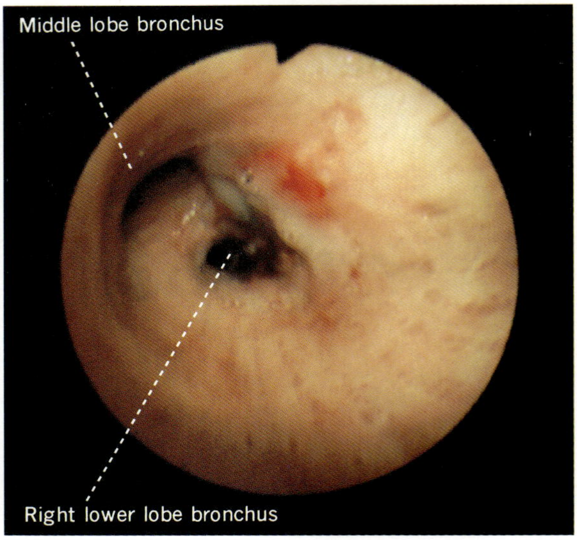

113.2 Bronchoscopic findings in the same portion after laser treatment. The tumour of the truncus intermedius is reduced in size to increase the narrow RLL orifice.

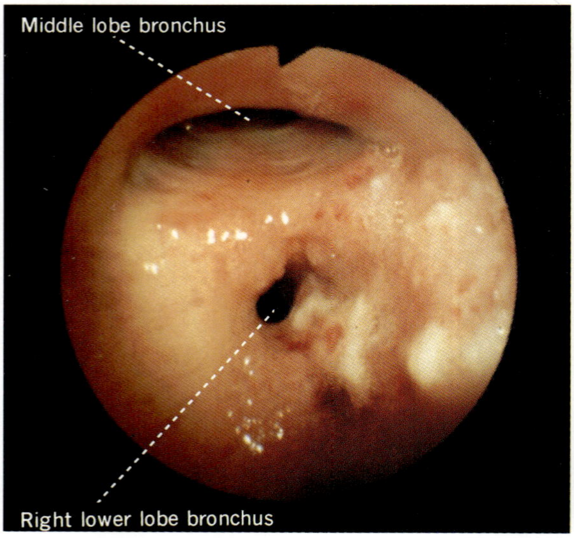

113.3 Bronchoscopic findings in the RLL bronchus before therapy. At the orifice of the RLL bronchus there is a nodular tumour which narrows the lumen.

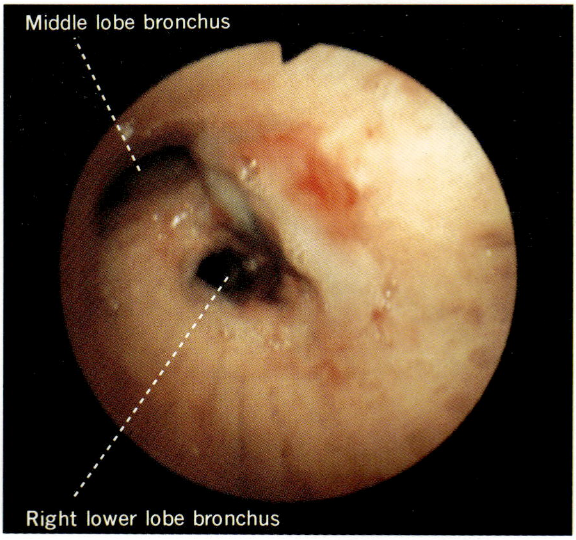

113.4 Bronchoscopic findings in the same portion as that of **133.3** after therapy. The nodular tumour has almost disappeared and the orifice of the RLL bronchus is patent.

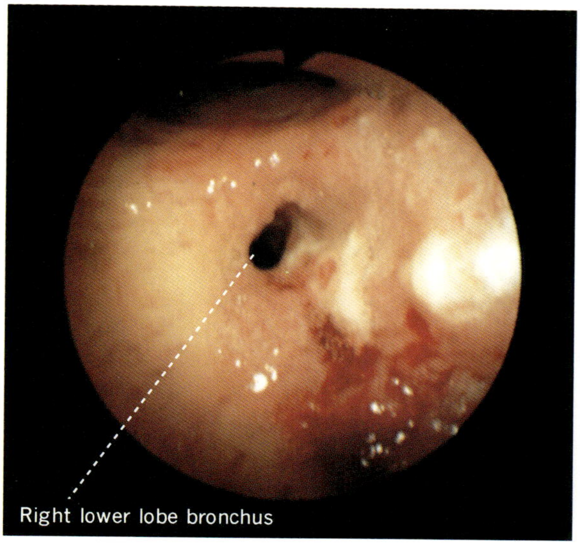

113.5 Another view of the RLL bronchus before laser treatment. The truncus intermedius is invaded by a white tumour. The orifice of the RLL bronchus is markedly stenotic.

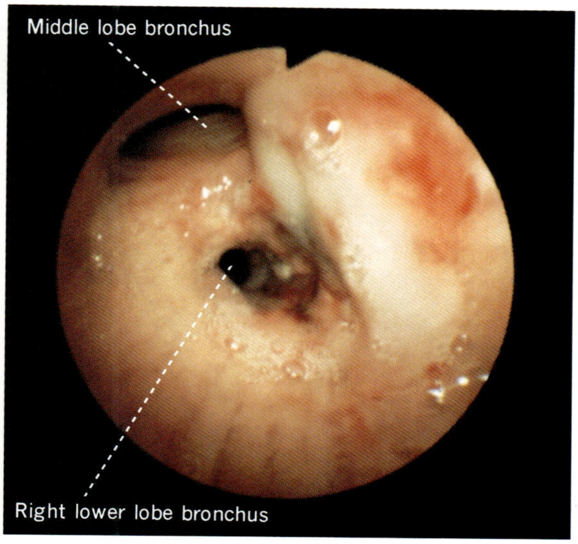

113.6 Bronchoscopic findings of the same region as that of **113.5** after treatment. The stenotic orifice of the RLL bronchus is now patent. The previously irregular wall of the truncus intermedius has flattened and is covered with white necrotic tissue.

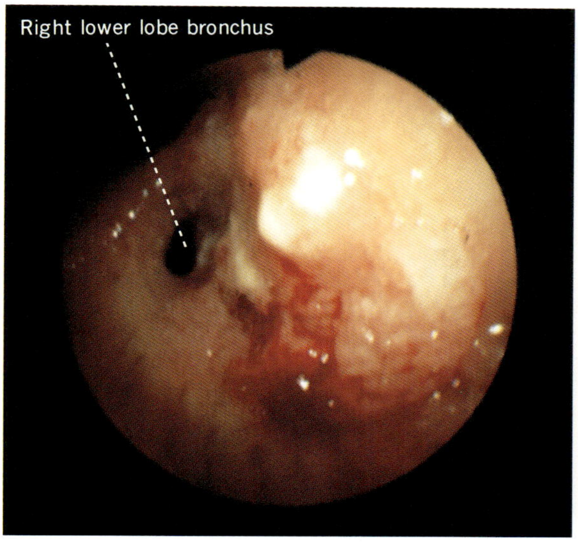

113.7 Bronchoscopic findings of the tumour of the truncus intermedius before therapy. A white nodular tumour is clearly visible.

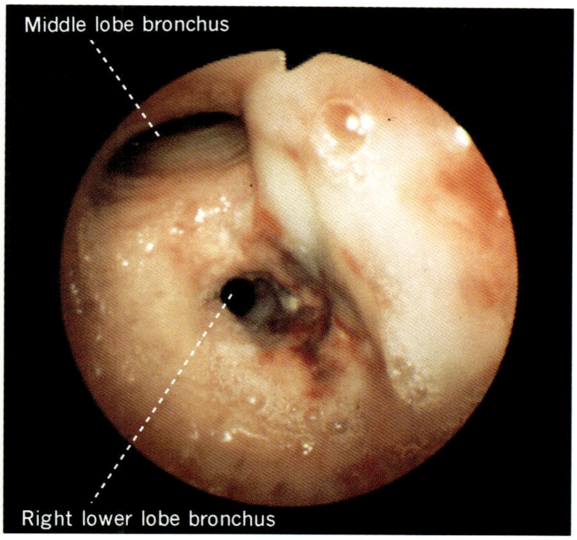

113.8 Bronchoscopic findings of the same region as that of **113.7**. The tumour has almost disappeared and the wall of the truncus intermedius is flattened. The previously stenotic orifice of the RLL bronchus is now patent.

Index